How to Use This Saunders Nursing Survival Guide

This book presents need-to-know information on fluids and electrolytes in a complete, easy-to-learn format to help you master one of the most difficult subjects in nursing.

These headings walk you through each chapter:

What You WILL LEARN An introductory list of checkpoints to outline what is covered in each chapter.

What It IS A "short and sweet" section devoted to the definition and description of the topic.

What You NEED TO KNOW The essential information and skills to be mastered, with a discussion of why they are important.

What You DO Nursing interventions that apply everything you learned in the What You NEED TO KNOW section.

Do You UNDERSTAND? Various activities and exercises (with answers) so you can review and make sure you understand each topic.

Technical terms (and common hospital terms) are given easy-to-understand explanations, and if you're likely to hear something referred to in a certain way in the hospital setting, we've highlighted the term in color.

These icons punctuate the text:

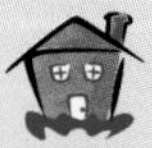
Highlights the most important points to study or use in the clinical atmosphere.

Alerts you to urgent information about dangerous conditions and how to avoid them.

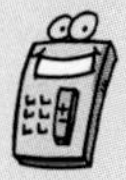
Guides you through formulas and problem-solving (with examples).

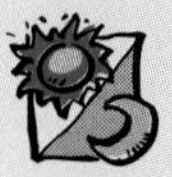
Points out age-related variations in signs and symptoms, nursing interventions, and patient teaching.

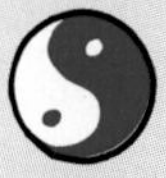
Clues you in to possible variations related to a patient's cultural background.

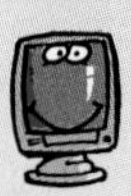
Instructs you to head to the Internet for additional resources.

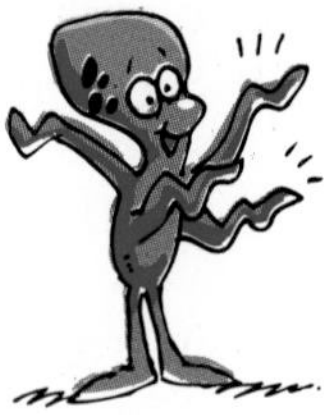

Tell Us What YOU Think

The *Saunders Nursing Survival Guide Series* has been created with the help of student feedback to serve your nursing review needs. In order to continue this tradition we invite you to voice your opinion. A website has been created to allow you the opportunity to Tell Us What YOU Think. Please, go to the website SNSGSurvey.elsevier.com, and help us continue to provide you with student focused and friendly review activities. Your ideas will be used to create new and fun ways for students like you to learn and review the difficult topics they face throughout their nursing education.

Go to: SNSGSurvey.elsevier.com and Tell Us What YOU Think.
YOU Think.

Saunders Nursing Survival Guide

Fluids & Electrolytes

Second Edition

Cynthia Chernecky, PhD, RN, CNS, AOCN
Professor, Department of Physiological and Technological Nursing
Medical College of Georgia, School of Nursing
Augusta, Georgia

Denise Macklin, BSN, RN, BC
President
Professional Learning Systems, Inc.
Marietta, Georgia

Kathleen Murphy-Ende, PhD, RN, AOCNP
Nurse Practitioner, Associate Researcher, and Clinical Assistant Professor
University of Wisconsin Hospital and Clinics
University of Wisconsin
School of Nursing
Madison, Wisconsin

SAUNDERS
ELSEVIER

SAUNDERS
ELSEVIER

11830 Westline Industrial Drive
St. Louis, Missouri 63146

SAUNDERS NURSING SURVIVAL GUIDE:
FLUIDS & ELECTROLYTES

ISBN-13: 978-1-4160-2879-6
ISBN-10: 1-4160-2879-X

Previous edition copyrighted 2002

ISBN-13: 978-1-4160-2879-6
ISBN-10: 1-4160-2879-X

Acquisitions Editor: Catherine Jackson
Developmental Editor: Amanda Sunderman Politte
Publishing Services Manager: Jeff Patterson
Designer: Jyotika Shroff

Printed in the United States of America

Last digit is the print number: 9 8 7 6 5 4 3 2 1

About the Authors

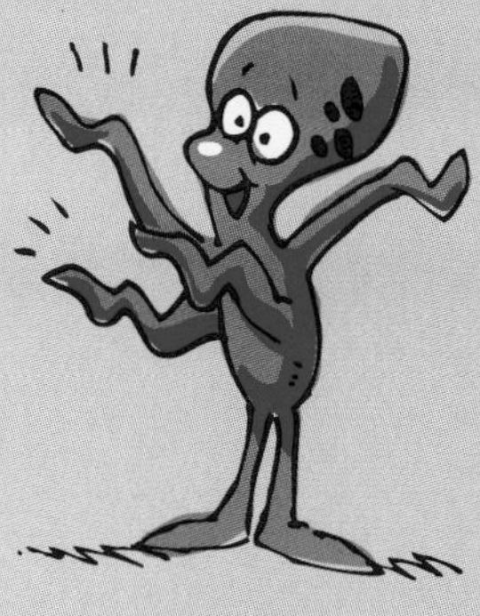

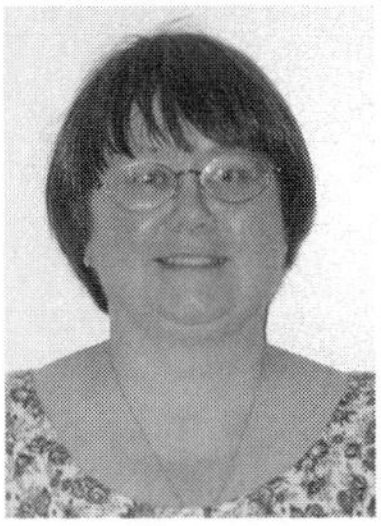

Dr. Cynthia Chernecky earned her degrees at the University of Connecticut (BSN), the University of Pittsburgh (MN), and Case Western Reserve University (PhD). She also earned an NCI fellowship at Yale University and a postdoctorate visiting scholarship at UCLA. She is the coordinator of the Acute & Critical Care Clinical Nurse Specialist track and an Advanced Oncology Certified Nurse (AOCN) with over 25 years of clinical practice experience. Her clinical area of expertise is critical care oncology, with over 22 book publications including *Laboratory Tests and Diagnostic Procedures* (fourth edition) and Advanced *and Critical Care Oncology Nursing: Managing Primary Complications.* She is a national and international speaker, researcher, and published scholar in cancer nursing as well as the recipient of numerous awards. She is also active in the Orthodox Church and enjoys life with family, friends, colleagues, and a West Highland white terrier.

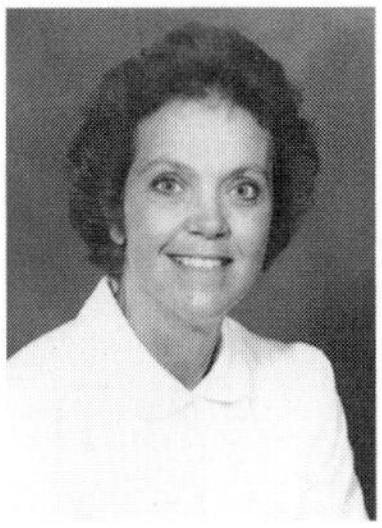

Denise Macklin is President and founder of Professional Learning Systems (PLS), Inc., and the creator and editor-in-chief of ceuzone.com, a continuing education Internet site. She is certified in adult/staff education. She has over 25 years of nursing experience (17 years in the specialty of IV therapy). She was included in *Who's Who in Media and Communications 1998* and is a member of the Council of Healthcare Advisors. She is a past chairperson of the National Research Committees for Intravenous Nursing Society and the current chairperson of research for the National Association of Vascular Access Networks. She has lectured around the United States on a wide variety of topics related to IV therapy and has published articles in various publications, including the *American Journal of Nursing, Journal of Intravenous Nursing, Journal of Vascular Access Devices,* and *Nursing Management and Dimensions of*

Critical Care. Her work includes extensive experience in the production of training videos for vascular access and interactive programs for medical manufacturers and the Centers for Disease Control and Prevention. PLS's videos, CD-I programs, and web CE offerings are being used to educate nurses not only in the United States but also in Canada, England, mainland Europe, Turkey, and several countries on the Pacific rim.

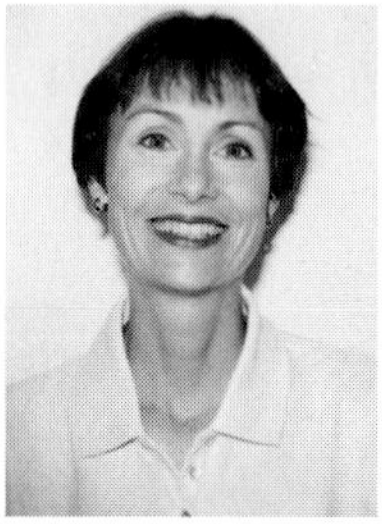

Kathleen Murphy-Ende has been in nursing for over 25 years and has been a practicing Certified Nurse Practitioner for the past 20. She currently specializes in adult and pediatric palliative care and oncology at the University of Wisconsin Hospital and Clinics in Madison, Wisconsin, and holds the position of Associate Researcher and Clinical Associate Professor in the School of Nursing. She received an Associate degree from Cardinal Stritch College, Bachelor of Nursing Science degree from the Medical College of Wisconsin in Milwaukee, Masters in Community Health Nursing & Family Nurse Practitioner Program at Rush University in Chicago, and PhD from the University of Wisconsin. She worked as a staff nurse on the medical and oncology units at St. Joseph's Hospital in Milwaukee, as a nurse practitioner in a family practice clinic in Chicago, and in oncology and palliative care in Madison. Her interest in patient education, program development, and professional clinical education compelled her to obtain a doctorate with a focus on the psychoeducational needs of those with life-limiting illness. Currently her role is dedicated to providing care and education to patients, families, and staff and publishing and speaking on symptom management. She is certified as an Advanced Oncology Certified Nurse and as a Family Nurse Practitioner. She lives in the forest with David and Jamie Rae.

Contributors to the First Edition

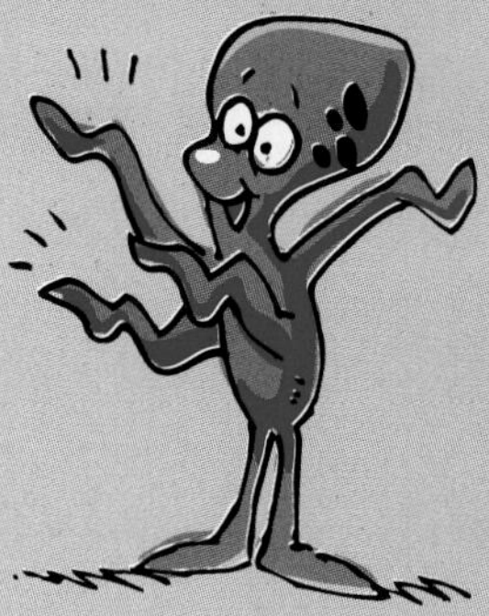

Jeanette Adams, PhD, RN, MS, CRNI, CS
Consultant
Mercer Island, Washington

Jane Brazy, MD
Neonatologist and Professor of Pediatrics
University of Wisconsin Medical School
Madison, Wisconsin

Diane Cope, PhD, RN, AOCN
Nurse Practitioner
Private Practice in Oncology
Fort Meyers, Florida

Christine Marie Fong, MD
Neonatologist
Meriter Hospital
Madison, Wisconsin

Michelle Frey, RN, MS, AOCN
Administrative Director of Children's Services
Consulting Associate at the Duke University School of Nursing
Duke University Medical Center
Durham, North Carolina

Mary Ann Ihlenfeld, RN, BSN
Staff Nurse, Oncology
Meriter Hospital
Madison, Wisconsin

Barbara S. Kiernan, PhD, RN, CS, PNP
Assistant Professor of Nursing,
Parent-Child Nursing
Medical College of Georgia
School of Nursing
Augusta, Georgia

Collette L. McKinney, MSN, RN
OIC, Urgent Care Center
Bassett Army Community Hospital
Fort Wainwright, Alaska

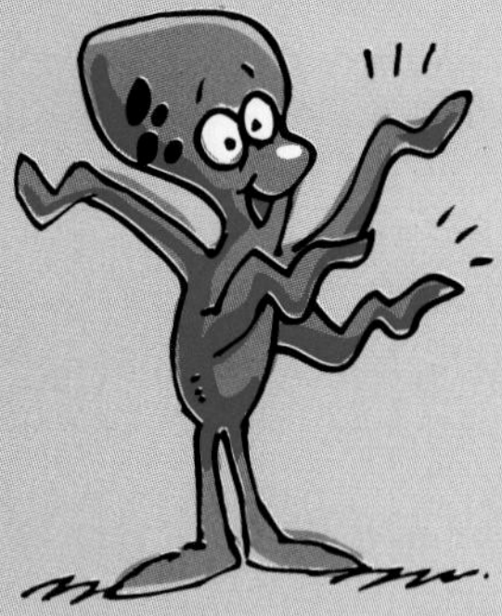

Faculty and Student Reviewers of the First Edition

FACULTY

Luvencia Connor, RN
Pediatric Nurse, Memorial Hospital West
Pembroke Pines, Florida

Eileen Marie Griffiths, MSN, RN
Miami-Dade Community College
Miami, Florida

Shirley A. Hemminger, MSN, RN, CCRN
Instructor, Kent State College of Nursing
Kent, Ohio;
Staff Nurse, University Hospitals of Cleveland
Cleveland, Ohio

Joyce LeFever Kee, MS, RN
Associate Professor Emerita
College of Health and Nursing Sciences
University of Delaware
Newark, Delaware

Dorothy B. Liddel, MSN, RN, ONC
Retired Associate Professor of Nursing
Bethesda, Maryland

Mary Ellen Mitchell-Rosen, BSN
Instructor
Deck Department
RTM Simulation Training and Research Center
Dania Beach, Florida

Michelle A. Mongillo, RN, BSN, CRRN
Independent Nurse Consultant
Coral Springs, Florida

Michael Tomak, RN, BSN
Assistant Professor
Miami-Dade Community College
Miami, Florida

STUDENTS

Kimberly Ann Bloom
Bloomsburg University
Bloomsburg, Pennsylvania

Lori Burton
Medical College of Georgia, School of Nursing
Athens, Georgia

Lorrie Kirby, CNA
Austin Community College
Austin, Texas

Melissa Schondelmayer
Medical College of Georgia
School of Nursing
Athens, Georgia

Series Reviewers

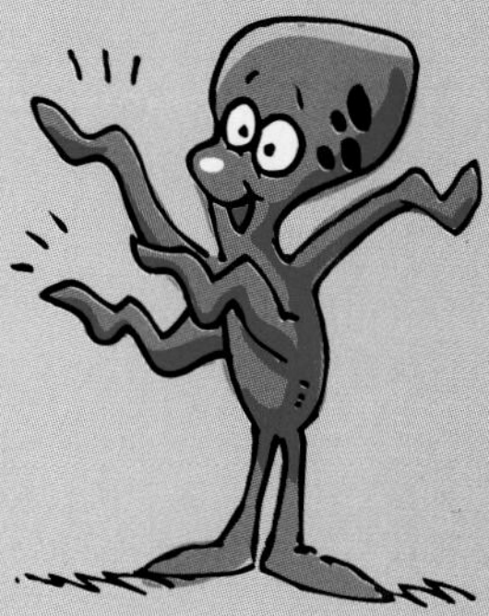

FACULTY

Edwina A. McConnell, PhD, RN, FRCNA
Professor
School of Nursing
Texas Technical University Health Sciences Center
Lubbock, Texas;
Consultant
Gorham, Maine

Judith L, Myers, MSN, RN
Health Sciences Center
St. Louis University School of Nursing
St. Louis, Missouri

STUDENTS

Joy Kutlenios Amos, RN, BSN
Piedmont Medical Center
Rock Hill, South Carolina;
Former Student
Wheeling Jesuit University
Wheeling, West Virginia

Angela M. Boyd, AS
University of Tennessee at Martin
Martin, Tennessee

Shayne Michael Gray, RN, BSN
University of Arkansas
Little Rock, Arkansas

Jill Hall, RN
Miller Children's Hospital
Long Beach, California

Jennifer Hamilton
University of Virginia
Charlottesville, Virginia

Elizabeth J. Hoogmoed, RN, BSN
Valley Hospital
Ridgewood, New Jersey

Katie Scarlett McRae, BA, BSN
Oregon Health Sciences University
Portland, Oregon

Preface

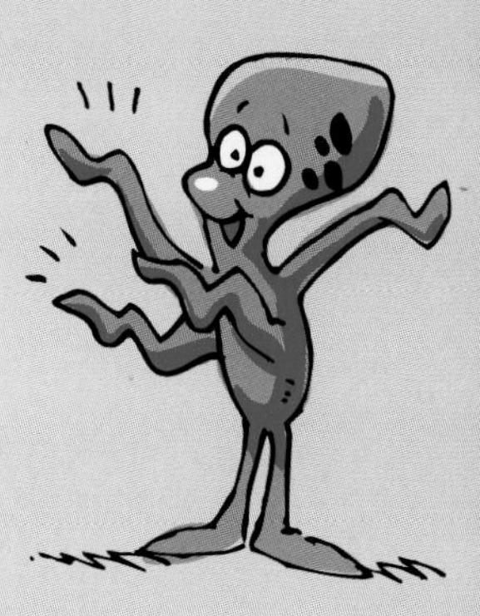

The *Saunders Nursing Survival Guide* series was created with your input. Nursing students told us about the topics they found more difficult to master, such as fluids and electrolytes, drug calculations, ECGs, pathophysiology, and pharmacology. Focus groups were held at the National Student Nurses Association meeting, and we asked you what the best way would be to learn this difficult material. Your responses were certainly interesting! You said we should keep the text to a minimum; use an engaging, fun approach; provide ample space to write on the pages; include a variety of activities to appeal to students with different learning styles; make the content visually appealing; and provide NCLEX review questions so you could check your understanding of key topics and perform any necessary review. The *Saunders Nursing Survival Guide* series is the result of your ideas.

Fluids & Electrolytes simplifies and clearly explains the complex concepts and processes of fluids and electrolytes in the human body. Each chapter begins with a discussion of the basics and advances to cover complex issues. The early chapters of the book address electrolyte dysfunctions. The later chapters describe common age-related conditions and diagnoses associated with fluid and electrolyte imbalances, covering lifespan issues through groups. For each age group we have included the most common and most complex dysfunctions to enhance learning and represent real clinical problems. We recognize that fluids and electrolytes involves concepts that are difficult to understand, so we have taken a step-by-step learning approach based on adult learning principles and the nursing process. The material has been reviewed extensively by nursing students across the nation to ensure that it is presented clearly, concisely, and in an appropriate manner.

We include many features in the margins to help you focus on the vital information you'll need to succeed in the classroom and in the clinical setting:

- **TAKE HOME POINTS** are composed of both study tips for classroom tests and "pearls of wisdom" to assist you in caring for patients. Both are drawn from our many years of combined academic and clinical experiences.
- Content marked with a **CAUTION** icon is vital and usually involves nursing actions that may have life-threatening consequences or significantly affect patient outcomes.
- The **LIFESPAN** icon and the **CULTURE** icon highlight variations in treatment that may be necessary for specific age or ethnic groups.
- A **CALCULATOR** icon will draw your eye to important equations and examples that will help you calculate proper medication dosages.
- A **WEB LINKS** icon will direct you to sites on the Internet that give more detailed information on a given topic.

Each of these icons specifically helps you focus on real-world patient care, the nursing process, and positive patient outcomes.

We also use consistent headings that emphasize specific nursing actions:

- **What You WILL LEARN** provides a list of the concepts to be learned in that chapter.
- **What It IS** provides a definition of a topic.
- **What You NEED TO KNOW** provides the explanation of the topic.
- **What You DO** explains what you do as a practicing nurse.
- **Do You UNDERSTAND** provides questions and exercises that are both appropriate and useful to reinforce the topic's concepts.

This five-step approach provides you with information and helps you learn how to apply it to the clinical setting.

We have used our own clinical experiences, our memories of being nursing students, and the expert experiences of nursing faculty, clinicians, and current nursing students to bring you a text that will help you understand fluids and electrolytes and therefore implement better patient care. We believe that understanding is the key to critical thinking and that critical thinking is the key to the art and science of nursing. We believe that this book and this series will result in excellent nursing care. The race to acquire knowledge is never-ending; just take one step at a time!

Cynthia Chernecky, PhD, RN, CNS, AOCN
Denise Macklin, BSN, RN, BC
Kathleen Murphy-Ende, PhD, RN, AOCNP

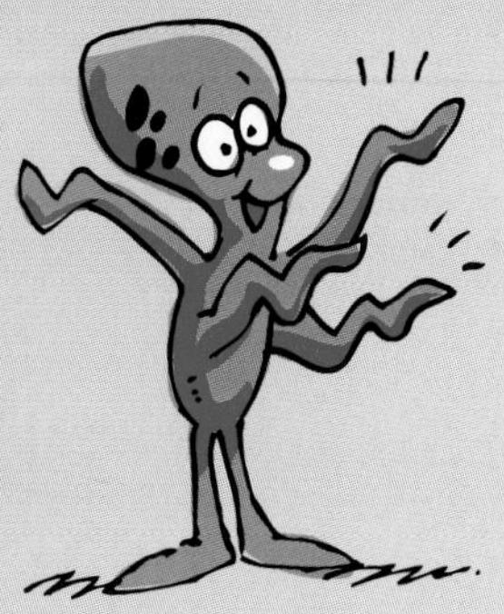

Acknowledgments

I would like to thank those colleagues who have professionally supported me and been my mentors: Dr. Ann Marie Kolanowski of Pennsylvania State University, Dr. Linda Sarna and Dr. Leda Danao of the University of California at Los Angeles, Dr. Jean E. Brown of The State University of New York at Buffalo, Dr. Mary Cooley of Dana Farber Cancer Institute, Harvard University, Dr. Marlene Rosenkoetter of Medical College of Georgia, and Dr. Geri Padilla of The University of California at San Francisco. Your faith, integrity, and time have made all the difference. I also owe a great deal of thanks to my colleagues who have worked, and some who still work, at the Medical College of Georgia. Your support and encouragement have been a tribute to your character. A special degree of thanks to nursing students who are the essence of what is good and who always make my clinical days a joy and a challenge!

To my parents, my mother Olga and late father Edward; to Mother Thecla, Mother Helena, and Mother Seraphima at Saints Mary and Martha Orthodox Monastery in South Carolina; and to my Godparents Helen Prohorik and the late Andrew Chernecky, nieces Ellie and Annie, nephew Michael, cousins Tyler and Benjamin Sztuka, Godchildren Priscilla, Vincent, and Jonathon, and Orthodox Catholic Christians everywhere, you add so much to my life that I dare say I am a lucky and blessed person.

I would also like to thank the professional personnel at Elsevier for their support and commitment to excellence, for without them, learning would be a chore.

Finally, to my coeditors Denise and Kathleen, who worked endlessly burning the midnight oil, I can truly say we have completed a necessary text that carries with it real world experiences that future nurses need to know. Thank you for your commitment, professionalism, colleagueship, and friendship.

Dr. Cynthia (Cinda) Chernecky

I would like to thank my sister and partner Judith Carnahan for her never-ending support and assistance. I would also like to thank my husband, Dana, who has believed in me and understood the long hours, missed meals, and trips that were required to complete this book. Last but not least, I would like to thank Cynthia Chernecky, who has been my mentor throughout this and many other professional activities. Her generosity of spirit and enthusiasm for life mean so much to me.

Denise Macklin

Many professionals have made this work possible; their dedication to the mission of teaching nurses is endless. The staff at Elsevier helped us stay on schedule and provided numerous resources and feedback from students, and staff nurses helped shape this book into a practical tool for students and clinicians. A special dedication and message of appreciation to Dave and Jamie for their endless patience and excitement over the writing and editing of this book!

Kathleen Murphy-Ende

Contents

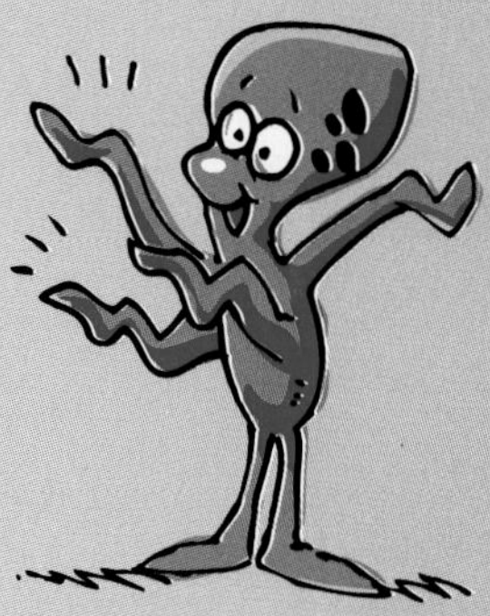

Dynamics of Fluids and Electrolytes

Chapter 1

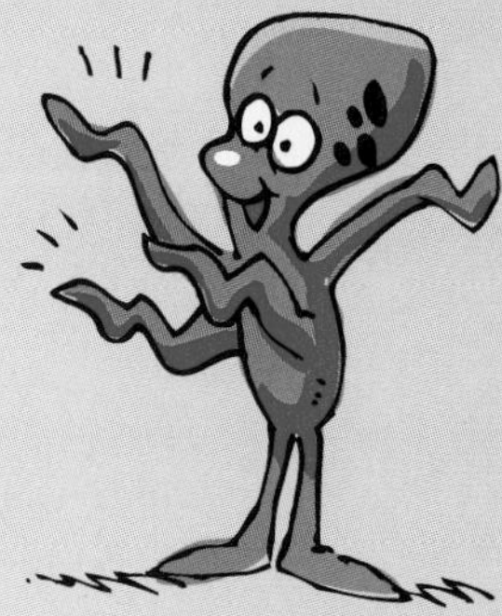

What You WILL LEARN

After reading this chapter, you will know how to do the following:

- ✔ Describe the effect of fluid and electrolytes on the body's environment.
- ✔ Differentiate intracellular from extracellular movement.
- ✔ Define fluid and state its relationship to body requirements.
- ✔ Define what an electrolyte is and one role it plays in homeostasis.

The human body is made up of approximately 100 trillion cells, each cell performing a specific function and each relying on all other cells to maintain a complex environment in which they can function. The maintenance of this environment is the responsibility of fluids, electrolytes, and acid-base balance in the body. Fluids travel throughout the body and are composed of water, electrolytes, minerals, and cells. Electrolytes are components that, when in water, are capable of carrying electric current.

Electrolytes are measured in milliequivalents per liter (mEq/L), a measure of chemical activity that occurs when the electrolyte reacts with hydrogen. Electrolytes are particularly vital to neuromuscular function and acid-base balance (the concentration of hydrogen ions in body fluid, expressed as a pH value). Fluids and electrolytes are also referred to as F & Es.

What IS the Effect of F & Es on the Body's Environment?

There are three major factors that influence the body's environment: body water, capillary permeability, and lymphatic drainage.

Body water ranges from 45% to 80% of total body weight, depending on age, sex, and body fat. Fat tissue contains no water; thus, obese people have lower amounts of body water than thin people.

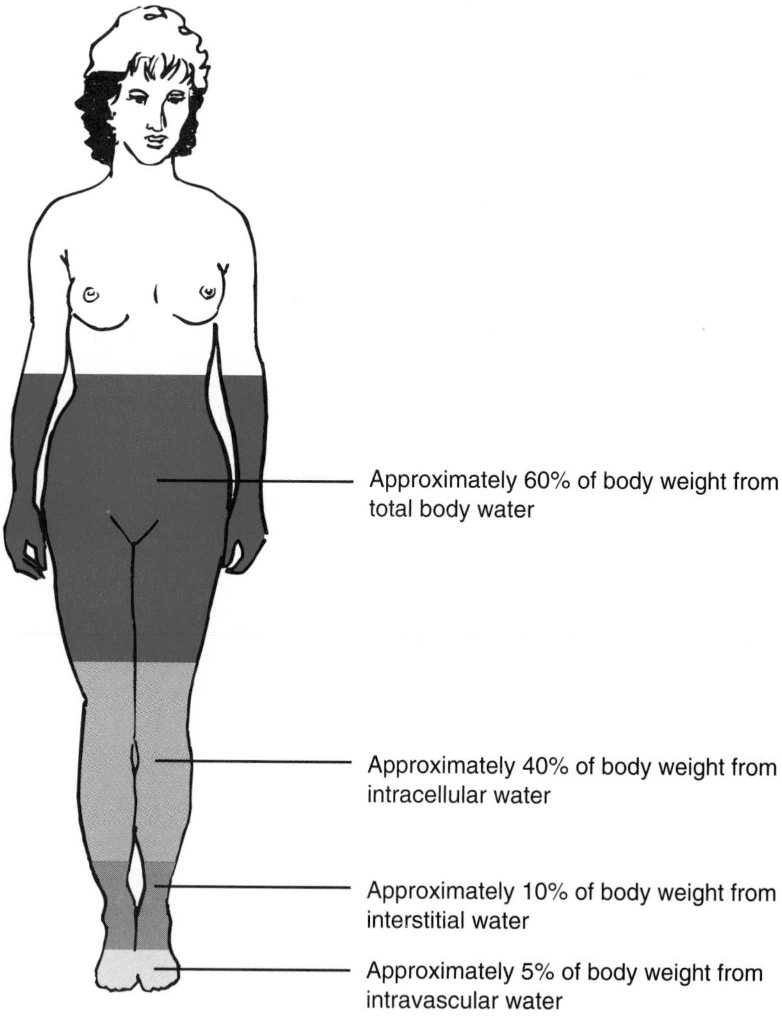

Redrawn from Monahan FD, Neighbors M: *Medical-surgical nursing: foundations for clinical practice,* ed 2, Philadelphia, 1998 M, Saunders.

Capillary permeability is the movement of fluid components (e.g., electrolytes, glucose, minerals) between organs and between cells. This movement depends on the ability of the cell membrane to allow the passage of fluid components within the vascular system. This movement, known as *capillary permeability,* occurs because of one of four transport mechanisms: diffusion, osmosis, filtration, or active transport. These transport mechanisms allow the body to pass along metabolic requirements to where they are needed, such as transporting oxygen to the brain and waste to the kidneys. Therefore any disease that interrupts capillary permeability interrupts major work of the body and brain (e.g., breathing for oxygen, thinking, walking).

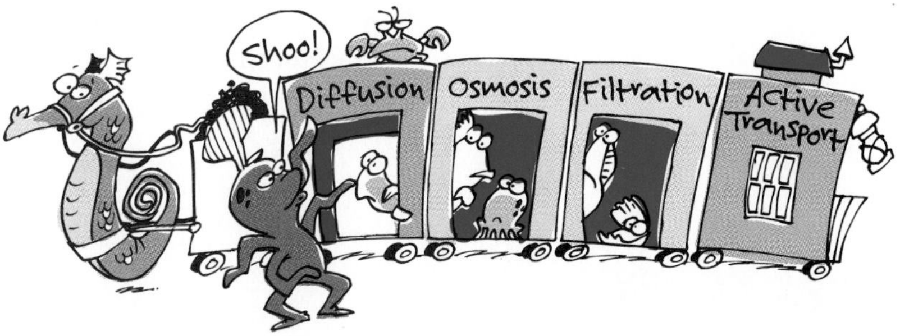

Capillary permeability occurs because of one of four transport mechanisms: diffusion, osmosis, filtration, or active transport.

Lymphatic drainage is a road system that begins at the tissues, travels toward the heart, and then travels into the bloodstream, carrying with it food materials known as *lymph.* This drainage system also contains a filter that traps bacteria, cancer cells, and other invading cells that are harmful to the body. These trapped cells are then consumed by the body's immune system and excreted as waste through the bowel or urinary systems. Any disease or condition that affects the lymphatic systems, such as lymphoma or mastectomy, affects vital organs receiving food, as well as the ability to remove waste and to be healthy through the maintenance of a good immune system.

Water Loss: Physical Assessment

1. Tachycardia > 100 beats per minute
2. Decreased blood pressure
3. Cool, dry skin
4. Weakness
5. Confusion

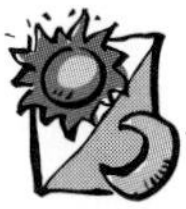

LIFE SPAN

Percentage of water to total body weight:
- 60% male adults
- 50% female adults
- 45% older adults
- 8% infants

TAKE HOME POINTS

Thirst is a late sign of a water deficit.

LIFE SPAN

- Loss of water is more crucial in infants, because more of the body is composed of water in proportion to body size, and in older adults, because water amounts are low for actual body size.
- Older individuals are prime candidates for fluid volume deficit (hypovolemia) and shock because of a reduced ability to sense thirst, kidneys with a decreased ability to hold water, and a reduction in total body size.

TAKE HOME POINTS

- Respiratory rate of 24 breaths per minute for 24 hours or more indicates that the patient is dehydrated (loss of body fluid) by 3 liters.
- When extremities are warm and nail beds blanche, good perfusion is occurring.

What You NEED TO KNOW

Water intake is controlled by thirst. Water is saved by the kidneys through the pituitary gland's secretion of antidiuretic hormone (ADH). Water reabsorption is also regulated by aldosterone, produced by the adrenal cortex, which increases sodium (Na^+) and water (H_2O) reabsorption in the body and decreases sodium and water excretion in the urine.

Water is excreted through the skin (e.g., sweating, surgery) and through feces, urine, and respiration.

Water loss results in tachycardia, lowering of blood pressure, cool and dry skin, weakness, confusion, decreased cardiac output, falsely decreased electrolyte laboratory values in general, and hemoconcentrated red blood cells that cause falsely increased hematocrit and hemoglobin laboratory values.

What You DO

- Assess for a history of conditions causing excess water loss: hemorrhage, burns, diarrhea, diabetes insipidus, vomiting, sweating, and diuretic or laxative medication abuse.
- Assess for history of conditions of excess water gain: heart failure, renal failure, high salt intake, pancreatitis.
- Assess for adequate body water requirements: serum osmolarity or concentration per liter of water (increased in dehydration), specific gravity of urine (increased when urine is concentrated as in dehydration), skin turgor (decreased in dehydration), dryness of lips or oral cavity, daily intake of fluids.
- Assess for good capillary permeability of 3 seconds or less in nail blanching; blood pressure for an adult of systolic between 110 and 140 mm Hg and diastolic between 60 and 84 mm Hg; and serum blood urea nitrogen (BUN) level between 5 and 20 mg/dL for all ages, or serum creatinine level between 8 and 21 mg/dL for an adult and 5 and 18 mg/dL for an infant or child.
- Assess for adequate lymphatic drainage: lymph nodes not enlarged, no extremity enlargement (postmastectomy, elephantiasis).

Do You UNDERSTAND?

DIRECTIONS: Provide the correct answer.

1. What age group is most prone to dehydration because their body's weight is mostly water?

____

DIRECTIONS: Place a check next to the correct answer.

2. The movement of fluid between cells depends mostly on:
   a. _____ Body weight
   b. _____ Oxygenation
   c. _____ Capillary permeability
   d. _____ Lymphatic drainage

DIRECTIONS: Fill in the correct answers on the lines provided.

3. Mr. Swanson is 89 years old and is 16 hours post-surgery for a permanent colostomy. His colostomy is functioning with 100 mL of soft liquid output. List three reasons why Mr. Swanson is at risk for fluid and electrolyte problems.

____

____

____

Answers: 1. **infant;** 2. **c;** 3. **age, surgical or postoperative status, fecal liquid output in colostomy.**

DIRECTIONS: Circle the correct pictures of organ or organs.

4. Water gain is evident in which of the following organ failures?

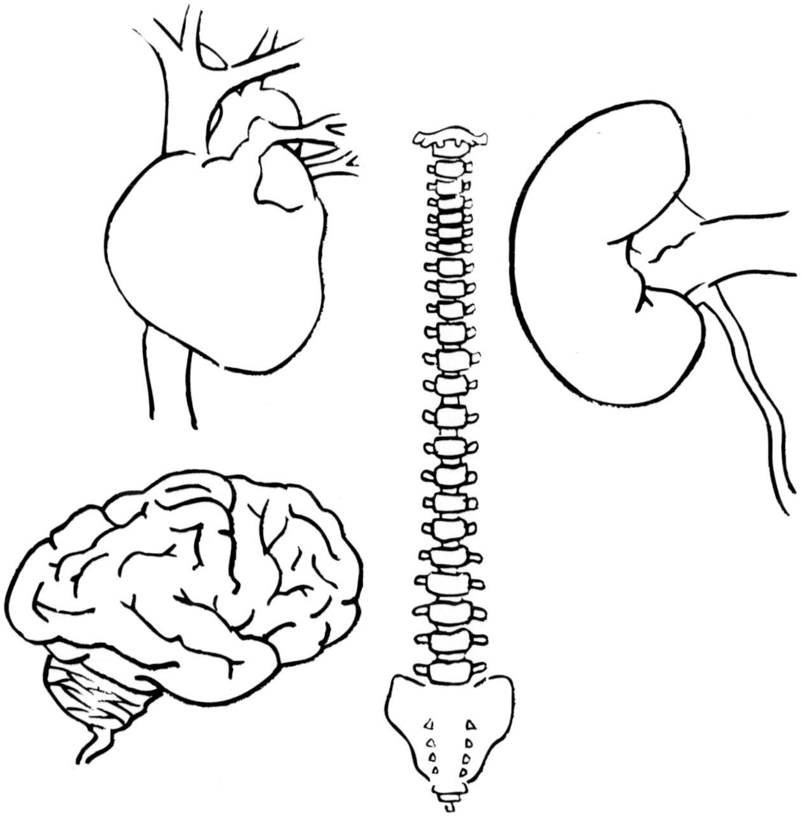

DIRECTIONS: Place an arrow indicating increased (↑) or decreased (↓) next to the following words as they relate to dehydration:

5. _____ Serum osmolarity
6. _____ Specific gravity of urine
7. _____ Skin turgor
8. _____ Dryness of oral lips

Answers: **4. heart and kidney; 5. increased; 6. increased; 7. decreased; 8. increased.**

What You NEED TO KNOW

Total body water is found within cells **(intracellular)** and outside cells **(extracellular)**. Approximately 40% of total body water is intracellular (25 L), with approximately 35% of this amount found within muscle cells. Large amounts of electrolytes (e.g., sodium) are also normally found in the extracellular fluid (ECF). ECF makes up 20% of total body water or approximately 15 L of fluid. Therefore approximately 60% of the body is water, making it an important substance.

Gender Differences in Total Body Water

Female:	**Male:**
more fat	less fat
less muscle	more muscle
less water	more water

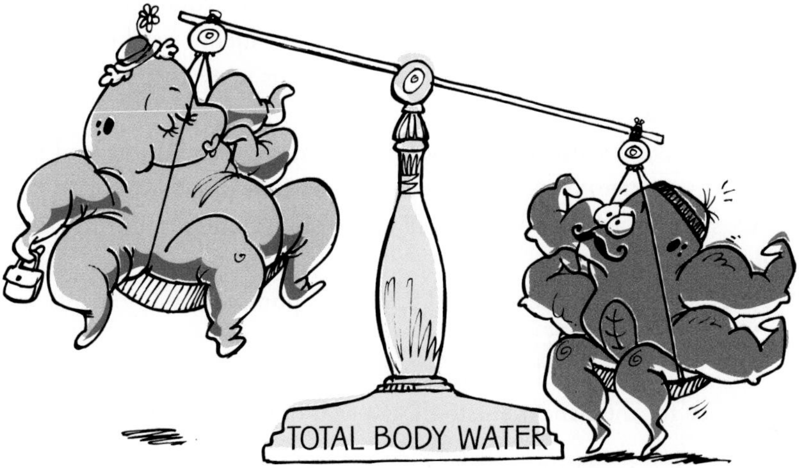

Because women have more fat than men, and fat contains no water, and because men have more muscle mass than women, men have more total body water than women.

ECF is further subdivided into three types: interstitial, intravascular, and transcellular. Interstitial fluid constitutes 80% of the ECF that surrounds the cell. Intravascular fluid, or plasma, is the only ECF that is influenced by changes in the body's fluid balance. Transcellular fluid is found in the spaces of the gastrointestinal (GI) tract, the cerebrospinal fluid, and the intraocular spaces of the eyes.

TAKE HOME POINTS

Because women have more fat than men, and fat contains no water, and because men have more muscle mass than women, men have more total body water than women.

- The average adult intake is 1000 mL of water a day.
- The body produces 250 mL of water a day as a result of oxidation of food.
- The lungs excrete, in vapor form, 500 mL of water a day.
- The skin evaporates, through sweating, 500 mL of water a day.
- The kidneys excrete excess body fluids as urine.

What You DO

- Monitor intake and output every hour in the intensive care hospital environment and every 8 hours in the general medical-surgical hospital or home-care environments.
- Assess urine-specific gravity; 1.012 to 1.025 is normal. The specific gravity is increased when the urine is concentrated and the patient is dehydrated.
- Assess skin turgor using the sites over the sternum, inner aspect of the thigh, or forehead.
- Measure daily weights. Remember, every pound is worth approximately 450 mL of water.
- Assess for edema of the lower extremities and dependent edema of the trunk. Bilateral leg edema usually indicates heart failure.
- Note thirst, decreased tears, decreased saliva production, or change in saliva consistency as being more "sticky."
- Assess blood pressure, which decreases during dehydration.
- Assess vein distension in the neck with the patient's head of the bed elevated 45 degrees. Positive distension occurs in overhydration, heart failure, and edema.
- Assess mental status for changes. Disorientation, confusion, and personality changes may indicate dehydration (low plasma volume).
- Assess pulse, which will be rapid and weak in intensity during dehydration.
- Assess hydrostatic pressure and the heart's pumping ability by placing the patient's hand in a dependent position, and determine whether the veins in the hand fill within 3 to 5 seconds (normal). Longer than 5 seconds for the hand veins to fill is a sign of dehydration.

TAKE HOME POINTS

For diabetes insipidus, the specific gravity of urine decreases as the urine is more dilute.

LIFE SPAN

- Older adults normally have a decreased specific gravity of urine because their kidneys have a reduced ability to concentrate.
- Older adults are at increased risk for dehydration caused by a decreased ability to sense thirst, decreased ability of the kidneys to concentrate urine, decreased intake of total body water, decreased intake of food, and increased confusion and cognitive impairment.

Do You UNDERSTAND?

DIRECTIONS: **Fill in the blanks with the appropriate word, either *intracellular* or *extracellular*.**

1. Water found within muscle cells is called __________ fluid.
2. Large amounts of electrolytes are found in the __________ fluid.

Answers: 1. intracellular; 2. extracellular.

3. Most body water is found in the ______________ fluid.
4. Interstitial fluid is a type of ______________ fluid.

DIRECTIONS: Color in the correct picture.

5. Transcellular fluid is found in the:

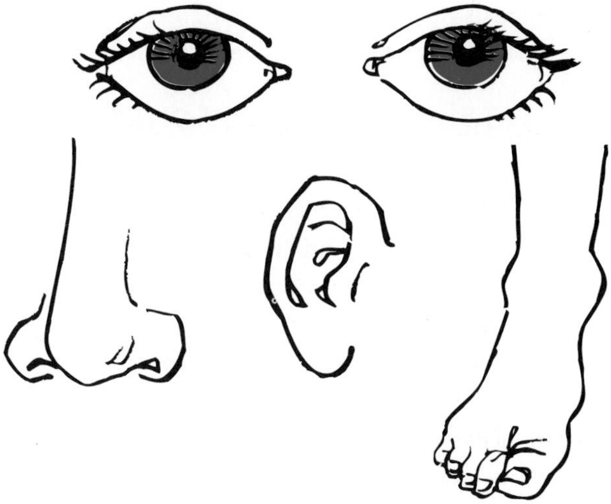

DIRECTIONS: Place a check to indicate the specific gravity of urine in the following diseases or conditions.

6. Diabetes insipidus (_____ decreased, _____ increased)
7. Heart failure (_____ decreased, _____ increased)
8. Kidney failure (_____ decreased, _____ increased)
9. Overhydration (_____ decreased, _____ increased)

DIRECTIONS: Place an arrow indicating increased (↑) or decreased (↓) next to the following words as they relate to dehydration.

10. _____ Pulse
11. _____ Blood pressure
12. _____ Neck veins distended
13. _____ Saliva production

DIRECTIONS: Provide the correct answer.

14. A method of quickly assessing a patient's hydrostatic pressure and the heart's pumping ability is to place his or her hand in a dependent

Answers: 3. intracellular; 4. extracellular; 5. eyes; 6. decreased; 7. increased; 8. increased; 9. decreased; 10. increased; 11. decreased; 12. decreased; 13. decreased; 14. dehydration.

position (below the level of the heart) and determine whether the veins in the hand fill within 3 to 5 seconds (normal). If a patient's hand veins take 10 seconds to fill, would this be a sign of overhydration or dehydration?

TAKE HOME POINTS

- Diffusion does not require energy and is not pressure dependent.
- Diffusion is responsible for maintaining nutrition in body tissues.

TAKE HOME POINTS

- The infusion of an isotonic intravenous (IV) solution will have no effect on the volume of fluid within cells because water neither leaves nor enters the cell.
- D5W (saline solution) is isotonic in the bag but hypotonic once it enters into the body.

What IS Intracellular and Extracellular Movement?

Intracellular fluid (ICF) and ECF contain water, electrolytes (charged particles such as sodium, potassium [K^+], and chloride [Cl^-]), minerals (e.g., iron, zinc, metals), compounds (e.g., hormones, urea), and cells (e.g., red blood cells, white blood cells, platelets). All of these contents within fluid need to circulate to give the body the food it needs to do its work. For example, the brain needs glucose so that an individual can think; the heart needs potassium so it can pump; the nervous system needs sodium so the person can move; and the muscle system needs calcium so that the legs can walk. For the body parts (organs and cells) to get their required food from the foods and liquids you consume, several processes must occur. These processes are diffusion, osmosis, filtration, and active transport.

Diffusion

Diffusion is the process during which a solid, such as sugar, in a fluid moves across an area, such as a cell membrane, from an area of higher concentration to an area of lower concentration. The result is that the solid is evenly distributed in the fluid. For example, iced tea with added sugar tastes the same whether you drink the tea from the top of the glass or from the bottom through a straw. No energy is used in this process of diffusion. Diffusion occurs between fluids and cells in the body when solids permeate the cell membrane. If the solids are small enough, they dissolve the solids by attaching themselves onto lipids in the cell walls. If the solids attach themselves to hormones, then they will carry them across the cell membrane, such as when glucose attaches to insulin and is transported across the cell membrane. The process of diffusion is clinically important to glucose transportation and use.

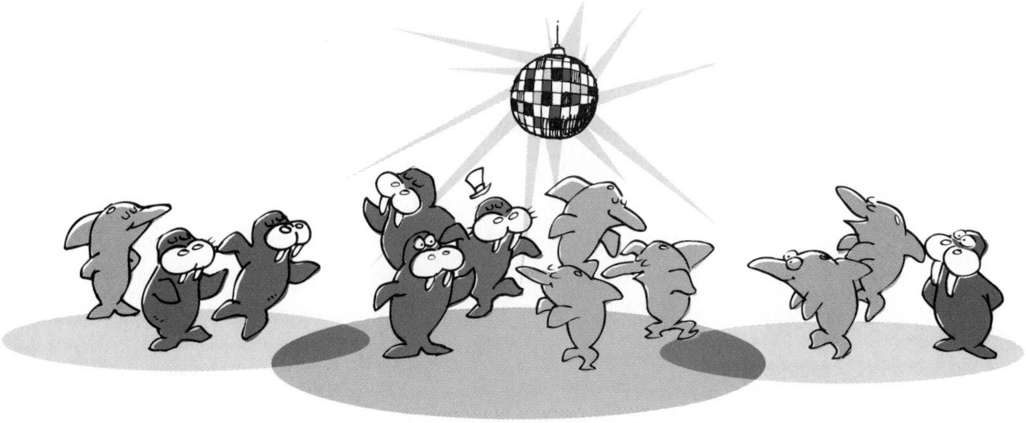

Active diffusion is the process during which a solid in a fluid moves across an area from an area of higher concentration to an area of lower concentration.

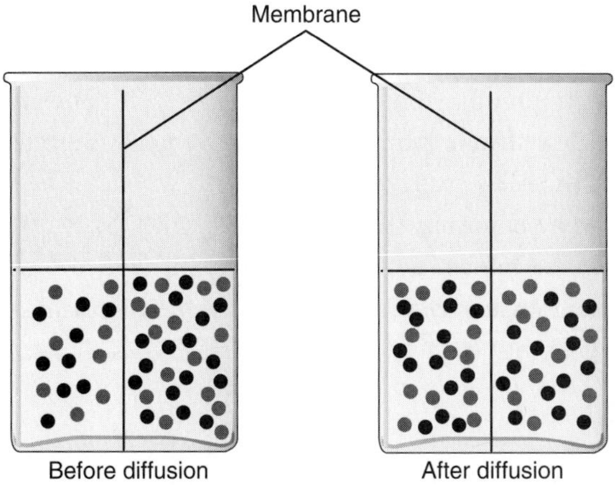

Diffusion.

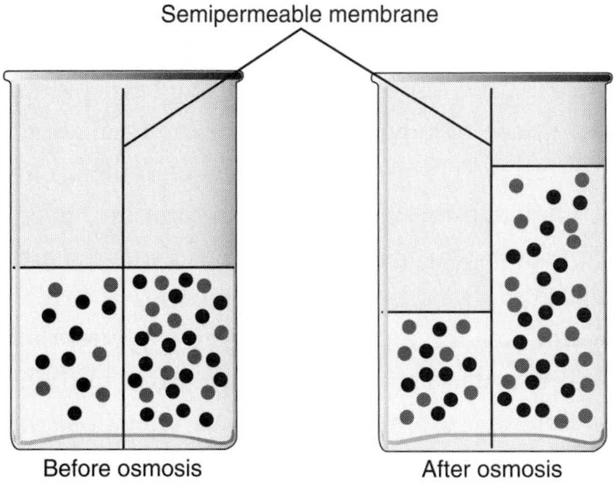

Osmosis.

Hypotonic IV promotes movements of water into cells, causing cell to swell.

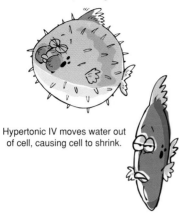

Hypertonic IV moves water out of cell, causing cell to shrink.

Osmosis

Osmosis is the movement of water from an area of lesser concentration to an area of more concentration; thus, both sides can be equal in number of particles per quantity of water. The pressure exerted by water to equalize both sides is called osmotic pressure or osmolality. Osmolality is influenced, to a large extent, by sodium, the principal extracellular (outside the cell) cation (electrically positive-charged electrolyte). The clinical importance of osmosis can be demonstrated by the mechanism of thirst. When a person loses water (e.g., by sweating, when exercising, through diuretic abuse) the ECF volume is decreased, and a message is sent to the hypothalamus in the brain. This message creates thirst, and the person drinks fluids. When enough fluid is consumed, and the ECF volume has been replaced, the message is no longer sent to the brain, and the person stops drinking fluid.

Hypotonic IV solutions (i.e., 0.20% normal saline [NS], D_5W, 0.45% NaCl, or 0.50% NS), also known as hypoosmolality or hyposodium-containing solutions, have a lesser concentration than plasma. These solutions help promote movement of water into cells, which makes the cells swell.

Hypertonic IV solutions (e.g., D_5NS, D_{5+} 1/2NS, $D_{10}W$, $D_{20}W$, 3% NS, 5% NS), also known as hyperosmolality or hypersodium-containing solution, have a greater concentration than that of plasma. These solutions move water out of cells, which makes the cells shrink.

TAKE HOME POINTS

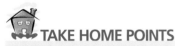

- Osmosis does not require energy and involves the movement of water only.
- Osmosis depends on hydrostatic and osmotic pressure.
- **Isotonic** = cells remain same; water does not move.
- **Hypotonic** = cells swell; water moves in.
- **Hypertonic** = cells shrink; water moves out.
- Hydrostatic pressure resulting in the heart pumping blood is known as blood pressure. Therefore a measure of blood pressure is actually a measure of hydrostatic cellular pressure.
- When intravascular fluid leaks into the interstitial spaces, the resulting state is known as hypovolemia, which can lead to shock or tissue edema.
- Filtration does not require energy and usually occurs in the capillaries. Filtration depends on differences in hydrostatic pressures.

Filtration

Filtration is the movement of fluid through a cell membrane as a result of liquid pressure (e.g., hydrostatic pressure, blood pressure) differences on both sides of the cell membrane.

The process of filtration is active in capillaries and is often referred to as capillary pressure because it is a result of the heart pumping blood to the capillaries. As the blood and fluid enter the capillaries, the pressure moves fluid, electrolytes, and waste out of the capillaries into the interstitial spaces. However, there is an opposing pressure called plasma colloid osmotic pressure that moves the fluid, electrolytes, and waste back into the capillaries. The plasma pressure, composed of plasma proteins (known as albumin, globulin, and fibrinogen) is greater than the hydrostatic pressure, thereby preventing leakage back into the interstitial spaces. If for some reason proteins leak into interstitial fluid, then the lymph system quickly returns the proteins to the plasma.

Active Transport

Active transport is the process by which some energy is spent to move a large molecule or substance across an area of high pressure. This "uphill" movement is also known as pumping, such as in the body's sodium and potassium pumps. For example, when the body's oxygen intake has been decreased as a result of a chest injury, there is insufficient oxygen to produce adenosine triphosphate (ATP). Without ATP, the sodium and potassium pumps fail to work efficiently, which leads to cellular swelling. Eventually the cells burst **(lysis)**, causing cellular death.

What You NEED TO KNOW

Diffusion

There are two major reasons why solids or particles may not be distributed evenly by diffusion: there is a difference in electrical pull (potential positive and negative charges of ions) existing on one side of the cell membrane, or there is an increase in pressure on one side of the cell membrane, such as in chronic heart failure.

Osmosis

A solution that has the same osmolality as plasma is isotonic (i.e., 0.9% NaCl, 0.9% NS; or lactated Ringer's), which prevents shifting of fluids and electrolytes from intracellular (inside the cell) to extracellular compartments.

Filtration

Clinically, filtration is important in the exchange of water, nutrients, and waste products when blood reaches the capillaries. If the pressure from the heart changes, such as in right-sided heart failure, then tissue swelling **(edema)** results. This condition occurs because capillary pressure exceeds hydrostatic pressure in the interstitial fluid, causing fluid to travel from the capillaries into the interstitial spaces.

TAKE HOME POINTS

Active transport is the medium whereby substances are absorbed into cells to carry out metabolic activities.

Active Transport

Sodium and potassium are transported into the ICF by active transport. However, the active transport of sodium and potassium occurs in opposite directions. The energy needed for active transport comes from breaking off a phosphate group from an ATP molecule.

Clinically, if active transport does not work, then cellular death occurs.

What You DO

Because of intracellular and extracellular movement, the health care provider will do the following:

- Assess whether the patient has sufficient fat **(lipids)** for cellular diffusion to occur.
- Assess the patient's insulin status for diffusion and active transport to occur.
- Assess blood pressure to maintain adequate hydrostatic pressure.
- Assess serum osmolality as part of fluid equilibrium **(homeostasis)**.
- Assess for thirst and other signs of dehydration.
- Assess for edema and other signs of overhydration.
- Monitor electrolytes, especially serum potassium and sodium levels.
- Assess the pumping ability of the heart by apical pulse (i.e., rate, rhythm, intensity) or by Swans-Ganz catheter by obtaining the pulmonary capillary wedge pressure (PCWP) or central venous pressure (CVP). See *Saunders Nursing Survival Guide: Hemodynamic Monitoring* for more information.
- Evaluate peripheral circulation by assessing dorsalis pedis, popliteal, and brachial pulses.
- Monitor oxygen saturation using a pulse oximeter, because oxygen is required for active transport.

Do You UNDERSTAND?

DIRECTIONS: **Fill in the blanks.**

Why do men have more water content, in general, than women?

1. ________________ mass is greater in men than in women, and ________________ contains water.
2. Fat content is ________________ in women than in men, and fat contains ________________ water.

Answers: **1. Muscle, muscle; 2. greater, no.**

DIRECTIONS: **Older adults are at increased risk for dehydration. Next to each picture that follows, state a reason for this increased risk.**

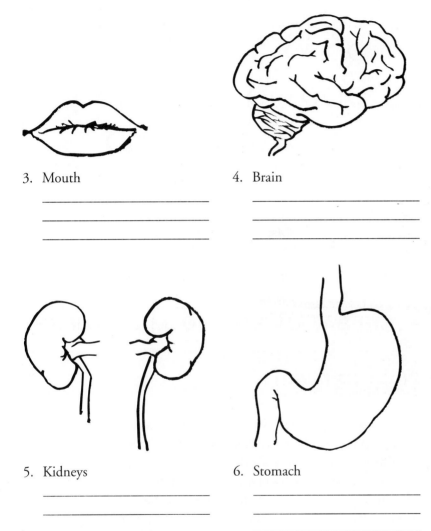

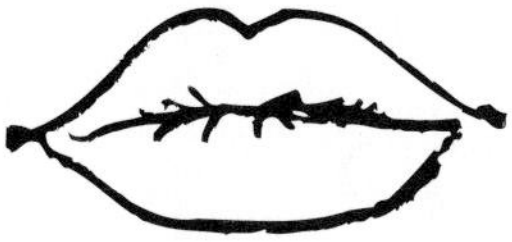

3. Mouth

____

____

____

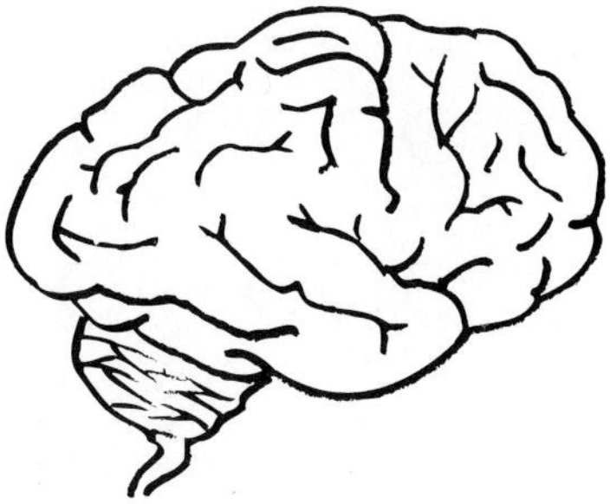

4. Brain

____

____

____

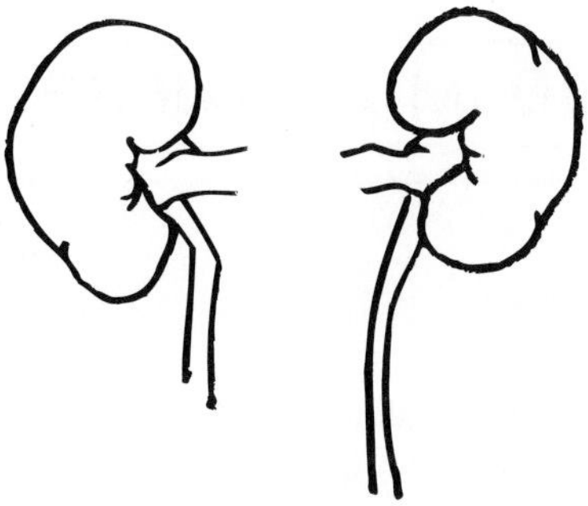

5. Kidneys

____

____

____

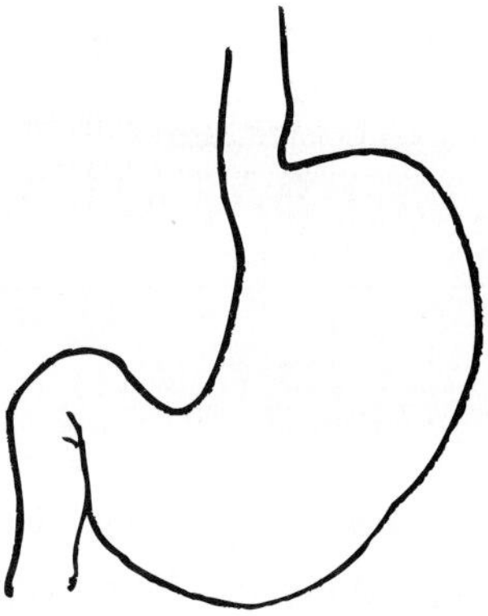

6. Stomach

____

____

____

Answers: 3. mouth is where thirst occurs and where intake of food and liquid occurs; 4. older adults are at risk for increased confusion or cognitive impairment, and the hypothalamus is in the brain where thirst occurs; 5. decreased ability of kidneys to concentrate urine; 6. stomach and GI tract are for decreased total food intake.

DIRECTIONS: The following pictures depict the processes of diffusion, osmosis, filtration, or active transport. Write the word next to the picture of the process it best represents.

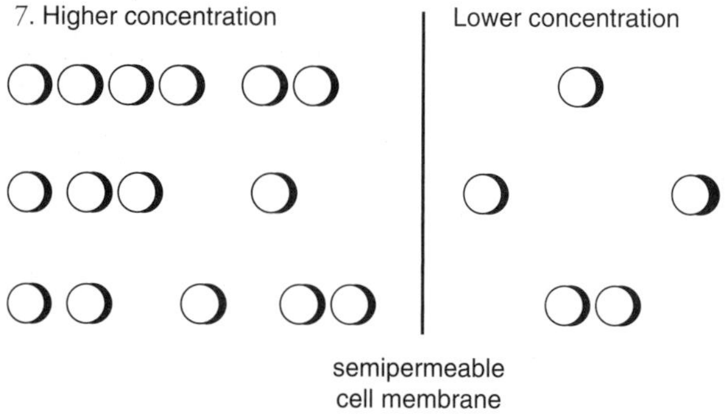

8. Intracellular	Extracellular
Na+ Na+	Na+ Na+ Na+
ATP →	Na+ Na+ Na+ Na+
Na+ ATP →	Na+ Na+ Na+ Na+

FLUID BALANCES AND IMBALANCES

What IS Fluid?

Fluid is essential to all bodily functions. Even small imbalances can cause multiple problems, from hypovolemic shock to hypervolemic heart failure. Careful assessment and monitoring by the health care provider is necessary, including a history, physical examination, interpretation of laboratory data, and clinical observation. Causes of fluid imbalance include suctioning, fistulas, medication usage of prednisone or diuretics, heart failure, kidney dysfunction, diarrhea, vomiting, excessive exercise, peritonitis, burns, diabetes insipidus, and syndrome of inappropriate antidiuretic hormone (SIADH). SIADH is a syndrome, usually associated with disorders of the central nervous system, tumors, or drugs, during which there is an increase in ADH activity, despite a reduced plasma osmolarity. SIADH initially includes the symptom of hyponatremia.

Answers: 7. diffusion; 8. active transport.

What You NEED TO KNOW

Signs of fluid depletion (e.g., hypovolemia, hyperosmolar imbalance) include the following:

- **Early signs:** dry tongue, thirst, cool hands or feet, decreased capillary nail refill, decreased pulse pressure (the difference between the systolic and diastolic blood pressures)
- **Late signs:** decreased blood pressure, increased pulse, rapid and weak respiration

Signs of fluid overload (i.e., hypervolemia, hypoosmolar imbalance) include the following:

- **Early signs:** wheezy dry cough, bilateral leg or ankle edema, upper eyelid (periorbital) edema when getting out of bed in the morning
- **Late signs:** increased blood pressure, breathlessness, pulmonary edema, rapid respirations, moist cough, frothy sputum, increased intracranial pressure

Serum osmolality is the number of particles of sodium, urea, proteins, and glucose in solution.

The formula for serum osmolality is as follows:

$$2 \times Na^{+} + \frac{BUN}{3} + \frac{glucose}{18}$$

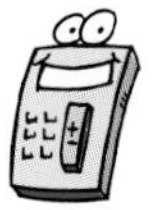

During dehydration, the serum osmolality increases; during overhydration (fluid overload) the serum osmolality decreases.

Hematocrit (HCT) is the volume of red blood cells in plasma, represented as a percentage. During dehydration, the HCT is increased (**hemoconcentrated**), such as with burn patients. During fluid overload, the HCT is decreased, such as with overhydrated patients.

Serum urea and albumin increase during hypovolemia and decrease during hypervolemia (fluid volume excess). Water excess can be caused by excessive secretion of ADH, such as in SIADH, which occurs in individuals with cancer. In addition, cancer can cause cerebral edema to occur, which can lead to coma and death.

When there is a loss of extracellular fluids, and the fluid gets trapped in a body space (third space syndrome or third spacing), a severe fluid volume deficit occurs. This condition is found in patients with small bowel obstruction, peritonitis, burns, and portal hypertension.

TAKE HOME POINTS

- The body responds to increased blood osmolality or water deficit by the posterior pituitary gland releasing ADH, which promotes water reabsorption from the distal tubules of the kidneys; thus the production of urine is decreased.
- For every increase of 1 kg of weight, there is an increase of 1000 mL of water, or approximately 450 mL of water for every 1 pound increase.

What You DO

- Measure the CVP and the PCWP as indicators of intravascular fluid volume, when possible.
- Assess serum osmolality (285 to 295 mOsm/kg is normal in an adult).
- Assess HCT (40% to 52% in adult men; 37% to 48% in adult women).
- Assess serum urea (normal is 5 to 21 mg/dL in an adult) and serum albumin (normal is 3.5 to 5.0 g/dL in an adult).

Do You UNDERSTAND?

DIRECTIONS: **Circle all medications that apply.**

1. Medications or classifications of medications that are known to cause fluid imbalances include:

   Antibiotics   Diuretics
   Prednisone   Vitamins

DIRECTIONS: **Write the sign or symptom that represents hypovolemia for the following:**

2. Tongue:
3. Fingernails:
4. Feet:
5. Pulse pressure:
6. What is the name of the gland that releases ADH in response to a body water deficit?

DIRECTIONS: **Place an arrow indicating increased (↑) or decreased (↓) next to the following laboratory tests as they relate to dehydration.**

7. _____ HCT
8. _____ Serum albumin
9. _____ Serum osmolality

Answers: 1. prednisone, diuretics; 2. dry; 3. decreased capillary refill; 4. cool; 5. decreased; 6. pituitary; 7. increased; 8. increased; 9. increased.

DIRECTIONS: **Place a check next to the correct answer.**

10. CVP and PCWP pressures are indicators of what type of fluid volume?
    a. _____ Extracellular
    b. _____ Interstitial
    c. _____ Intravascular
    d. _____ Fat concentration

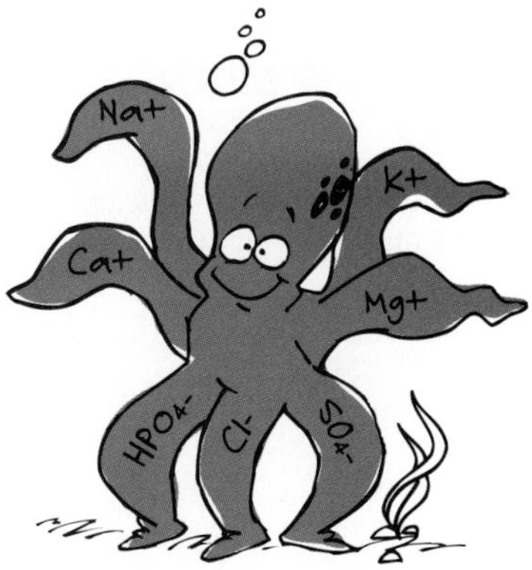

Electrolytes are positive (+) or negative (–) charged ions

ELECTROLYTE BALANCE AND IMBALANCE

What IS an Electrolyte?

Electrolytes are chemical substances that, when placed in a solution, break apart into electrically charged particles **(ions)** with positive (+) or negative (–) charges. The positive ions **(cations)** are sodium (Na^+), calcium (Ca^+), potassium (K^+), or magnesium (Mg^+); the negative ions **(anions)** are chloride (Cl^-), phosphate (HPO_4^-), and sulfate (SO_4^-). Most electrolytes differ in their concentrations in ICF and ECF.

TAKE HOME POINTS

It is important to maintain equilibrium **(homeostasis)** of electrolytes so that the body can function normally. The maintenance of electrolyte homeostasis is controlled by dietary intake and kidney output.

What You NEED TO KNOW

Sodium is the major cation in ECF and is responsible for muscle contraction, for heart contraction, for transmission of nerve impulses, and for maintaining kidney urine concentration.

Low amounts of sodium in the blood stream, which draws water back into the cells, is called hyponatremia; excess serum sodium, which draws water out of the cells, is called hypernatremia.

Potassium is the major cation in ICF and is important for protein synthesis, use and storage of glucose, and maintenance of excitability of cellular membranes in the heart and nervous system. A low level of serum potassium is known as *hypokalemia;* excess serum potassium is called

TAKE HOME POINTS

- Common causes of hyponatremia include vomiting, diarrhea, and GI suctioning. A common cause of hypernatremia is an excessive ingestion of Na^+ (salt) orally or via IV (NaCl). Common food sources of Na^+ are table salt, cheese, milk, bread, ketchup, and soy sauce.
- Common sources of K^+ are fish, bananas, cantaloupe, raisins, avocados, carrots, potatoes, spinach, orange juice, and other fruit juices.

Answer: **10.** c.

LIFE SPAN

Newborns can quickly develop hypochloremia from diarrhea.

hyperkalemia. Causes of hypokalemia include diuretic use, diarrhea, vomiting, Cushing's syndrome, and excessive sweating. Causes of hyperkalemia include renal failure, burns, large amounts of IV or oral intake of potassium, acidosis, and adrenal insufficiency.

Chloride is the major anion of ECF, which works with sodium to maintain osmotic pressure. A low serum amount of serum chloride is known as *hypochloremia*; a high amount is known as *hyperchloremia.* Chloride is important in the formation of hydrochloric acid in the stomach, which aids in the digestion of food and in the maintenance of the respiratory system, blood pressure, and the metabolism of hydrogen within the body (acid-based balance). Causes of hypochloremia are fistula drainage, excessive nasogastric (NG) drainage, vomiting, and diarrhea. Causes of hyperchloremia include metabolic acidosis, decreased ventilation, shock, starvation, and diabetic ketoacidosis.

What You DO

- Assess serum laboratory values and compare with normative values. Normal values in adults are as follows:
  Sodium: 136 to 145 mEq/L or mmol/L
  Potassium: 3.5 to 5.3 mEq/L or mmol/L
  Chloride: 98 to 107 mEq/L or mmol/L
- Monitor intake and output, and evaluate specific gravity of urine, which will be increased as a result of increased urine concentration.
- Assess for hyponatremia: poor skin turgor, sunken eyes, dry tongue.
- Assess for hypernatremia: thirst, confusion, hallucinations.
- Assess for medications that influence electrolytes: diuretics, steroids, laxatives, chemotherapy, IV fluids, total parenteral nutrition (TPN), hyperalimentation (HPA).

TAKE HOME POINTS

Output needs to include fluid loss from wounds or dressings (pad count), drains (Penrose, Hemovac, vacuum wound care system), GI tubes, chest tubes, urinary catheters, and kidney **(nephrostomy)** tubes.

Do You UNDERSTAND?

DIRECTIONS: Match column A with column B.

Column A	Column B
1. _____ NG suctioning	a. Hypokalemia
2. _____ Overhydration with IV 1000 mL NS	b. Hyperkalemia
3. _____ Use of diuretics, such as furosemide	c. Hypernatremia
4. _____ Renal failure	d. Hyponatremia

DIRECTIONS: Place the foods *(salt, fish, bananas, raisins, cheese, potatoes, soy sauce, ketchup)* in the correct category of whether they are sources of potassium or sodium.

5. Sources of potassium:	6. Sources of sodium:
____________________	____________________
____________________	____________________
____________________	____________________
____________________	____________________

DIRECTIONS: Circle the correct italicized word.

7. A person is brought into the emergency department with a gun shot wound, shallow breathing, and in shock. Would his serum electrolyte results indicate that he is *hyperchloremic* or *hypochloremic?*

DIRECTIONS: Place a check in the space(s) provided in front of the correct answer(s).

8. Which of the following tubes represents fluid loss caused by drainage from a kidney tube?
   a. _____ Nephrostomy
   b. _____ Nasogastric
   c. _____ Chest
   d. _____ Otic

Answers: 1. d; 2. c; 3. a; 4. b; 5. fish, bananas, raisins, potatoes; 6. salt, cheese, soy sauce, ketchup; 7. hyperchloremic from decreased ventilation and shock; 8. a.

DIRECTIONS: Provide the correct answer in the space provided.

9. Your patient is experiencing 100 mL output per hour from her NG tube, and she has received 80 mg of the diuretic furosemide (Lasix). What two electrolyte laboratory values would you expect under these circumstances?

10. Your patient is admitted with a diagnosis of renal failure. What major cation would you assess for in his/her laboratory results and why?

References

Guazzi M: Alveolar-capillary membrane dysfunction in heart failure: evidence of a pathophysiologic role, *Chest* 124(3):1090, 2003.

Kramer GC: Hypertonic resuscitation: physiologic mechanisms and recommendations for trauma care, *J Trauma Injury Infect Crit Care* 54(5S):Suppl:S89, 2003.

Smith AE, Helenius A: How viruses enter cells, *Science* 304(5668):237, 2004.

Answers: **9. hyponatremia from GI suctioning, hypokalemia from diuresis; 10. potassium for hyperkalemia.**

NCLEX® Review

1. Mrs. Rodriquez is 77 years old, somewhat confused, and tachycardic. Her blood pressure is 88/64, and she has cool but dry skin. Her daughter, who lives in the same town, states that in the past few days her mother has gotten weaker. What would be your first probable diagnosis?
   1 Acute myocardial infarction
   2 Hypertensive crisis
   3 Hypovolemia
   4 Shock

2. Skin turgor is among the assessment criteria for hydration status. Where is the most reliable area to assess for skin turgor in the adult?
   1 Hands
   2 Forehead
   3 Under the axilla
   4 Webs of the toes

3. Which one of the following conditions would lead to some solids or particles not being distributed evenly by diffusion?
   1 Tumor mass
   2 Overhydration
   3 Infusion of isotonic saline intravenously
   4 Tachycardia, in an adult, of 92 beats per minute

4. When plasma pressure is lower than hydrostatic pressure, the result is leaking of fluid into the interstitial spaces. What laboratory value would reflect a decrease in plasma pressure?
   1 Decreased sodium
   2 Increased potassium
   3 Increased fibrinogen
   4 Decreased albumin

5. Mrs. Maria Frank has come into the emergency department with severe volume deficit caused by hypovolemia and burns. What would you expect her hematocrit and serum albumin levels to be?
   1 Increased hematocrit and increased albumin
   2 Increased hematocrit and decreased albumin
   3 Decreased hematocrit and decreased albumin
   4 Decreased hematocrit and increased albumin

6. Which of the following are the four transport mechanisms associated with capillary permeability?
   1 Osmosis, diffusion, interstitial passive transport, extracellular autolysis
   2 Filtration, osmosis, active transport, transcellular electrophoresis
   3 Active transport, electrical current, diuretic transport
   4 Diffusion, osmosis, filtration, active transport

7. Older adults have a decreased ability to hold water caused by the decreased capability of what body organ(s)?
   1 Heart
   2 Lungs
   3 Kidneys
   4 Gallbladder

8. You place your patient's hand below the level of the heart and note that it takes 15 seconds for the hand veins to fill. This is a classic sign of which fluid volume problem?
   1 Dehydration
   2 Overhydration
   3 Cerebrovascular stroke
   4 Sepsis

9. What part of the brain is responsible for receiving messages when extracellular fluid volume is decreased, thereby creating thirst in an individual?
   1 Midbrain
   2 Hypothalamus
   3 Brain stem
   4 Subcortical adrenal hypophysis

10. You have determined that you should assess for perfusion q1h in Mrs. Walters' left leg because she is

2-hour status post vein stripping and ligation. For which signs and symptoms should you assess?

11. True or False: Bradycardia is a sign of water loss.

12. True or False: Laxative abuse can be a cause of excess water loss.

13. What occurs to the specific gravity of urine in a person with diabetes insipidus?

14. Infusion of _______ tonic intravenous solutions promotes movement of water into cells, thus making the cells swell.

15. Failure of filtration, such as in right-sided heart failure, causes fluid to travel from the capillaries into the interstitial spaces, causing swelling or _______.

NCLEX® Review Answers

1. 3 Dry, cool skin, confusion, and tachycardia are the signs of hypovolemia, and older adults are prone to dehydration. There are no signs of myocardial infarction. Mrs. Rodriguez's blood pressure is low, and there are no usual signs of shock, including decreased pulmonary capillary wedge pressure, decreased oxygen saturation, increased respirations, and restlessness.

2. 2 The forehead, inner aspect of the thigh, and sternum are good sites for assessing skin turgor because they are not sites that lose elasticity. The hands often lose elasticity from frequent use, as well as increased and constant environmental exposure. The axilla is moist from nonexposure. There is not enough tissue to assess in the webs of the toes.

3. 1 Tumors create increased pressure on one side of the cell membrane. In overhydration, the particles would be distributed evenly, but there is more fluid. Isotonic fluids do not affect diffusion. This heart rate is not tachycardia and will not affect membrane diffusion.

4. 4 Albumin is a plasma protein that helps maintain plasma pressure. Sodium and potassium are not plasma proteins. Increased fibrinogen will increase plasma pressure, thereby allowing no fluid into the interstitial space.

5. 1 Hematocrit and albumin are increased with hypovolemia and dehydration. Decreased albumin reflects hypervolemia. Decreased hematocrit and albumin reflect hypervolemia. Decreased hematocrit reflects hypervolemia.

6. 4 Diffusion, osmosis, filtration, and active transport are the four transport mechanisms associated with capillary permeability. Interstitial passive transport, extracellular autolysis, and transcellular electrophoresis are not valid terms. Electrical current and diuretic transport are not associated with capillary permeability.

7. 3 The kidneys are responsible for holding water. The heart circulates blood. The lungs are responsible for exchanging oxygen and carbon dioxide. The gallbladder aids in digestion.

8. 1 Failure of the veins in the hand to fill within 5 seconds indicates dehydration. An outward characteristic of overhydration would be edema. Cerebrovascular stroke is characterized by a weakness in muscles on one side of the body—perhaps resulting in a sagging profile. Sepsis outwardly appears as fever with positive blood gases.

9. 2 The hypothalamus in the brain is responsible for receiving messages of fluid volume depletion and creating thirst in a person, which leads them to drink fluids. The midbrain is responsible for eye and head reflexes. The brainstem controls automatic functions, such as respiration. The subcortical adrenal hypophysis is not a physiologic entry.

10. To see whether the extremities are warm and the nail beds blanche.

11. False. Tachycardia is a compensatory mechanism to increase blood circulation.

12. True.

13. Specific gravity decreases because the urine is more dilute.

14. "Hypo" as in "hypotonic."

15. Edema.

Dynamics of Acid-Base Balance

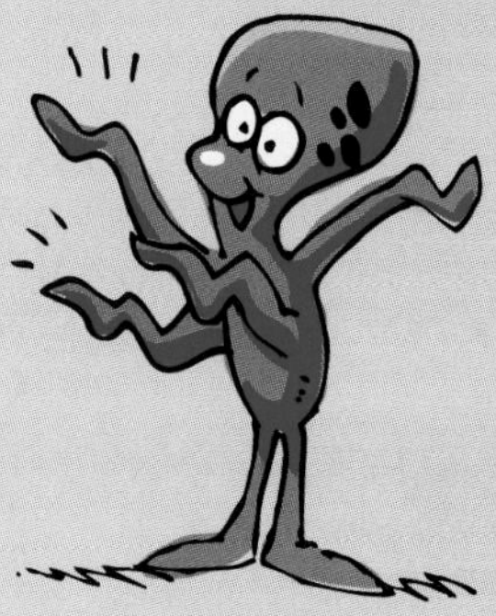

Chapter 2

What You WILL LEARN

After reading this chapter, you will know how to do the following:

- ✔ Define acid-base balance.
- ✔ Differentiate between regulation by buffers, respirations, and the renal system.
- ✔ Define acidosis.
- ✔ Differentiate acidosis from metabolic acidosis.
- ✔ Define alkalosis.

What IS Acid-Base Balance?

Body fluid is measured in units of hydrogen (H^+) ion concentration or pH units. Acids (substances that release hydrogen when dissolved in water) and bases (substances that bind hydrogen ions when in water) affect hydrogen ion production and elimination, thus affecting pH. Any substance that acts as either an acid or a base is called a *buffer*. Even small changes in the pH of body fluids can create major problems in the body. The normal pH of arterial blood is 7.35 to 7.45; normal pH of venous blood is 7.32 to 7.42.

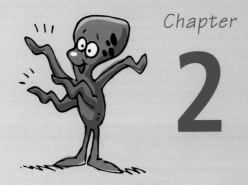

Fatal blood pH levels are less than 6.9 or greater than 7.8.

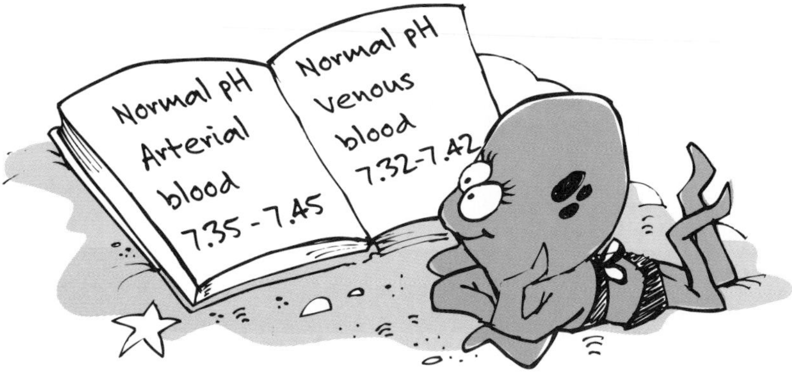

TAKE HOME POINTS

An acid gives up a hydrogen ion, and a base takes on a hydrogen ion when dissolved in water. As the concentration of hydrogen ions increases, the pH decreases.

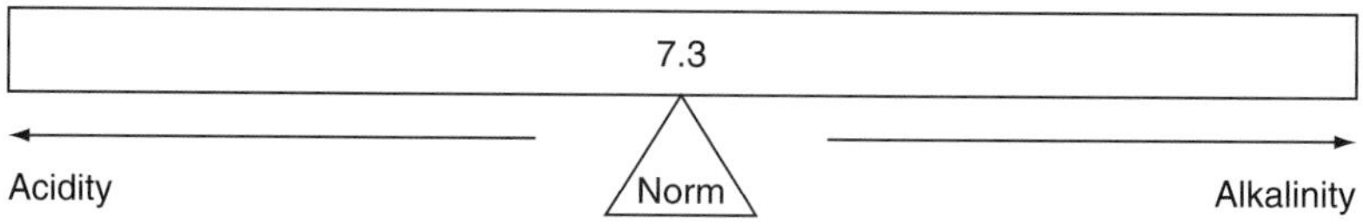

pH scale

What You NEED TO KNOW

Small changes in pH interfere with many physiologic functions: hormones, electrolytes, electrical impulses of the heart, gastrointestinal (GI) tract, nerves and muscles, and medication activity and distribution.

Disturbances that cause increased pH **(increased alkalinity** or decrease of hydrogen ion concentration) include pneumonia, dehydration, infection, and renal diseases. Disturbances that cause decreased pH **(increased acidity** or increase of hydrogen ion concentration) include overhydration, heart failure, and the use of medications such as thiazide loop diuretics, digitalis, insulin, antibiotics, and chemotherapy.

Acid-base balance is regulated by chemical, renal, and respiratory mechanisms. Sources of acids are the by-products of normal metabolism:

- Carbon dioxide (CO_2) is produced from the breakdown of glucose and the release of carbon dioxide exhaled by the lungs.
- Metabolism of fats produces fatty acids and keto acids.
- Metabolism of proteins produces sulfuric acid.
- Anaerobic metabolism of glucose produces lactic acid.
- Cell destruction causes the release of intracellular acids into the extracellular fluid (ECF).

LIFE SPAN

The pulse oximetry probe is attached to the toe for infants and the finger for adults.

The pulse oximetry probe should be placed on the cartilage on the bridge of the nose of extremely obese persons for a more accurate reading.

Sources of bases are substances that accept hydrogen ions:

- Sodium hydroxide (NaOH)
- Ammonia (NH_3)
- Aluminum hydroxide ($AlOH_3$)
- Bicarbonate (HCO_{3-})

What You DO

- Assess arterial pH on blood gases, as well as bicarbonate (base) and carbon dioxide production (acid).
- Assess serum electrolytes to ensure they are within normal limits (WNL).
- Assess serum hormone levels to ensure they are WNL.
- Assess pulse oximetry to ensure proper oxygenation for normal glucose and body metabolism to occur and to ensure that carbon dioxide does not build up in the body.
- Assess the electrocardiogram (ECG), gastrointestinal tract motility, nerve conduction, and muscle movement of the patient. Any abnormality can be a result of acid-base imbalance.
- Assess respirations for any changes in rate, rhythm, or intensity, which are early signs of most acid-base imbalances (except metabolic alkalosis).
- Assess for chronic conditions and diseases or treatments that can produce cellular destruction, such as chemotherapy, radiation therapy, cancer, systemic lupus erythematosus, and myocardial infarction.
- Monitor renal function through serum creatinine levels, and maintain the value that is WNL.
- Monitor nutritional intake, which can affect metabolism.

CULTURE

Persons with dark skin have a slightly lower (1%) pulse oximetry reading.

LIFE SPAN

Normal ranges of serum creatinine laboratory values are as follows:

- Adult woman = 0.5 to 1.1 mg/dL
- Adult man = 0.6 to 1.2 mg/dL
- Older adult = 0.4 to 1.0 mg/dL
- Child = 0.6 to 1.2 mg/dL
- Infant = 0.7 to 1.7 mg/dL
- Newborn = 0.8 to 1.4 mg/dL

Do You UNDERSTAND?

DIRECTIONS: Unscramble the word jumble.

1. The pH of body fluid is measured in units of ____________ ions. *(eyogdhrn)*

Answer: 1. **hydrogen.**

DIRECTIONS: **Fill in the blanks.**

2. The normal pH of *arterial* blood is 7._5 to 7._5.
3. The normal pH of *venous* blood is 7._2 to 7._2.
4. The substance X is placed in water and becomes substance Z. Is substance X an acid or a base?

Substance X

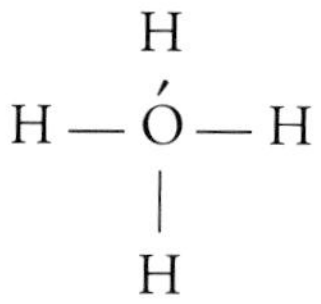

Substance Z

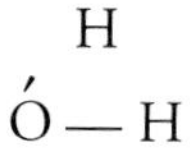

DIRECTIONS: **Match the following sources of acid with their appropriate by-product.**

Acid	By-product
5. Anaerobic metabolism of glucose	a. Keto acids
6. Metabolism of fats	b. Carbon dioxide
7. Cellular destruction	c. Sulfuric acid
8. Metabolism of proteins	d. Intracellular acids to ECF
9. Breakdown of glucose released	e. Lactic acid in lungs

What IS Regulation by Buffers, Respirations, and the Renal System?

To maintain the pH of the ECF within the narrow range of normal, there are three body-regulation mechanisms: chemical buffers, respirations, and the kidneys.

What You NEED TO KNOW

Chemical buffers are the first line of defense against a change in pH because they are always present in body fluids. Chemical buffers include bicarbonate, phosphate, and proteins.

Answers: 2. 7.35 to 7.45; 3. 7.32 to 7.42; 4. acid, because it gives up hydrogen ions; 5. e; 6. a; 7. d; 8. c; 9. b.

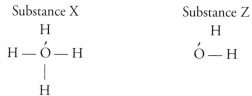

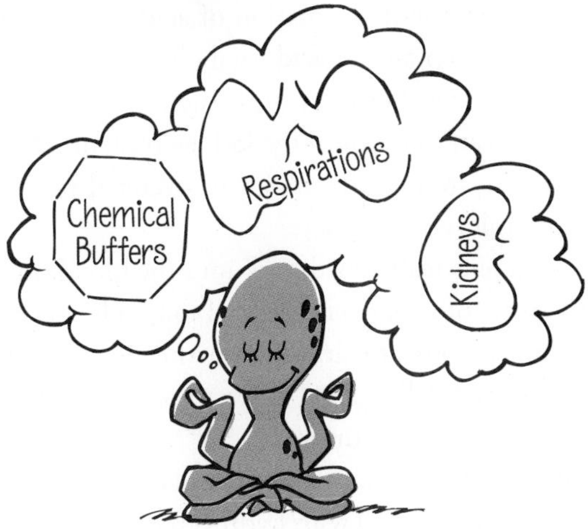

Three regulatory mechanisms for maintaining pH are chemical buffers, respirations, and the kidneys.

Bicarbonate is found in the ECF and intracellular fluid (ICF) and controls small fluctuations in pH. It responds immediately. This factor is the reason bicarbonate is often given intravenously (IV) during emergencies.

Phosphate buffers are found in the ICF as bicarbonates. They control small fluctuations in pH and respond quickly.

Proteins are found in both the ICF, as hemoglobin, and the ECF, as albumin and globulins. Proteins work rapidly.

Respiratory mechanisms, the second line of defense against changes in pH, come to the rescue when fluctuations in pH are acute and when the chemical buffers are no longer effective.

Carbon dioxide concentration ($PaCO_2$) is directly related to pH because carbon dioxide is converted to hydrogen ions by carbonic anhydrase reactions in the arterial blood. Therefore when breathing **(respiratory rate)** increases, the body rids itself of excess carbon dioxide, and when breathing decreases, carbon dioxide is retained. This mechanism is under the control of the nervous system through special receptors in the brain that are sensitive to changes in carbon dioxide. Therefore giving a patient who has chronic obstructive pulmonary disease (COPD) too much oxygen makes his or her respiratory rate decrease and makes him or her retain more carbon dioxide, which leads to acidosis.

Renal mechanisms, the third line of defense against changes in pH, are the most powerful mechanisms for regulating acid-base balance but take a longer time to begin. There are three major renal mechanisms that compensate for acid-base imbalances: tubular kidney movement of bicarbonate, kidney tubule formation of acids, and the formation of ammonium (NH_4^+) from amino acid catabolism.

Bicarbonate, made in other body areas such as the pancreas or by the kidneys themselves, can move from the kidney back into the blood when blood hydrogen ions are high, or it can be excreted in the urine when blood hydrogen ion levels are low.

When bicarbonate is reabsorbed back into the blood, the urine in the kidneys has an excess of negatively charged ion—phosphate. Because of this factor, hydrogen ions are drawn into the urine to combine with dihydrogen phosphate (H_2PO_4) and make an acid called phosphoric acid (H_3PO_4) to be excreted in the urine.

Normal amino acid catabolism produces ammonia. In the kidneys, normal amino acid is combined with hydrogen ions to form ammonium, which is excreted in the urine. The result is a loss of hydrogen ions, and, thus an increase in blood pH.

What You DO

- Assess urine pH and arterial blood pH to determine the status of renal and body pH.
- Assess urine laboratory results for an excess of ammonia and H_2PO_4 acid.
- Assess the results of serum levels for hemoglobin (ICF protein), albumin, and immunoglobulins (ECF proteins) to determine the body's clinical buffer status.
- Assess results of arterial blood gases (ABG), pulmonary function tests (PFTs), and chest radiograph (CXR) to determine the patient's respiratory status.

Do You UNDERSTAND?

DIRECTIONS: **Match the word in column A with the buffer mechanism in column B.**

Column A	Column B
1. _____ Carbon dioxide	a. Proteins
2. _____ Albumin	b. Respirations
3. _____ Ammonia	c. Kidneys

Answers: 1. b; 2. a; 3. c.

DIRECTIONS: Circle the correct answer from the italicized words.

4. Is the pH of blood *increased* or *decreased* if the kidneys excrete bicarbonate and increase absorption of hydrogen ions?
5. When you are giving a patient a bolus of IV bicarbonate, are you changing the pH of the blood to be *more acidic* or *more basic?*
6. Persons who receive chemotherapy have a potential for decreased pH. Does this reflect an *acid* or *base* disturbance?

DIRECTIONS: Fill in the correct answer.

7. When pH is excessive, the kidneys respond by making a substance. What is the name of this substance?

What IS Acidosis?

Acidosis is an excess of hydrogen ions and an arterial pH of less than 7.35. The excess of hydrogen ions can be a result of an overproduction of acids that release hydrogen ions or an underelimination of acids, causing retention of hydrogen ions. Because hydrogen ions are positively charged ions, their excess in the blood causes imbalances in other electrolytes, especially the other positive ions, such as potassium (K^+), calcium (Ca^+), and sodium (Na^+). These imbalances can lead to dysfunctions of the cardiac, central nervous, neuromuscular, and respiratory systems.

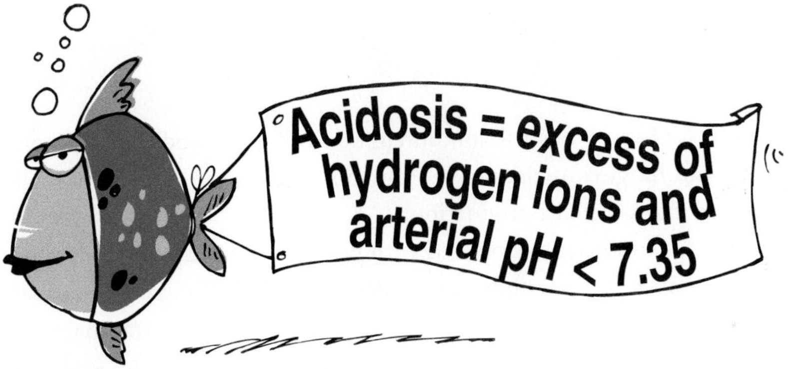
Acidosis = excess of
hydrogen ions and
arterial pH < 7.35

Answers: 4. decreased; 5. more basic; 6. acid; 7. hydrogen.

What You NEED TO KNOW

An inadequate exchange of oxygen and carbon dioxide causes retention of carbon dioxide, which causes an increase in pH. Retention of carbon dioxide creates carbonic acid that then separates into hydrogen ions and bicarbonate ions.

$$H_2O + CO_2 \rightarrow H_2CO_3 \rightarrow H^+ + HCO_{3-}$$

These free hydrogen ions in the blood create acidosis. Diseases or conditions as causes include respiratory depression, poisoning, cerebral edema, myasthenia gravis, obesity, asthma, cancer, thrombus, pneumonia, tuberculosis, adult respiratory distress syndrome (ARDS), emphysema, cystic fibrosis, and spinal cord injuries.

Airway obstruction, such as in lung cancer, leads to poor gas exchange in the capillaries, causing carbon dioxide retention and acidosis. Capillary diffusion interference decreases gas exchange between the alveoli and the capillary membranes of the lung, which causes a backup of carbon dioxide and its retention. Poor chest expansion, such as in emphysema, causes poor gas exchange and retention of carbon dioxide.

Respiratory depression resulting from either chemical or physical mechanisms causes changes in brain-stem stimulation that affects inhalation and exhalation, causing inadequate oxygen and carbon dioxide exchange.

! Persons with emphysema, ankylosing spondylitis, pleural effusion, pneumothorax, or pneumonia have decreased chest expansion and are at risk for respiratory acidosis.

What You DO

- Assess for airway obstruction: foreign body, lymph node enlargement, tight clothing, constriction of bronchioles, asthma, emphysema, lung cancer, excess mucus production.
- Assess for conditions associated with poor alveolar–capillary diffusion: aspiration of fluids, emphysema, ARDS, COPDs, lung cancer, tuberculosis, pulmonary embolism, pulmonary edema, chest trauma.
- Assess for poor chest expansion from respiratory muscle weakness, trauma, or deformities: broken ribs, flail chest, muscular dystrophy, rhabdomyosarcoma, ascites, hemothorax, severe obesity, abdominal tumors.

- Assess for chemical causes of respiratory depression: anesthetics, opioids, poisons, electrolyte imbalances of hyponatremia, hyperkalemia, hypercalcemia.

TAKE HOME POINTS

Fatal lactic acidosis is a complication of antiretroviral therapy in pediatric HIV patients.

Nursing Assessment by Systems for Acidosis

Cardiovascular	Central Nervous System
Bradycardia	Confusion
Tall T wave on ECG	Lethargy
Widened QRS complex on ECG	Stupor
Prolonged PR interval on ECG	Coma
Hypotension	
Thready peripheral pulses	
Neuromuscular	**Psychosocial**
Bilateral flaccid paralysis	Any change in behavior
Hyporeflexia	Recent uncooperative behavior
Weakness	Unable to recognize family or significant others
Respiratory	**Integumentary (Skin)**
Abnormal rate	Dry
Abnormal intensity	Flushed
Kussmaul's (deep, gasping) respirations	Pale
Cheyne-Stokes respirations	Warm
Apnea followed by deep breaths	Cyanotic (blue color)

- Assess for physical causes of respiratory depression, including head or spinal cord trauma, cerebral edema, cerebral aneurysm, cerebrovascular accident (CVA), or overhydration.
- Assess ABG: pH less than 7.35 and carbon dioxide concentration greater than 45 mm Hg.
- Monitor rate, depth, and pattern of respirations every hour.
- Monitor serum electrolytes of potassium, calcium, and sodium daily.
- Administer medications that increase alveolar capillary diffusion, such as metaproterenol sulfate (Alupent) and albuterol sulfate (Ventolin) inhalers, salmeterol xinafoate (Serevent), and pirbuterol acetate (Maxair).
- Provide patient pulmonary toilet or hygiene through physical therapy to increase diffusion and decrease airway obstruction.

- Administer oxygen therapy, chemotherapy, and/or radiation therapy as prescribed.
- Administer bronchial smooth muscle relaxant medications, such as albuterol, ephedrine, isoproterenol, terbutaline, atropine, aminophylline, and theophylline.
- Administer bronchial mucolytic medications, such as acetylcysteine sodium (Mucomyst or Mucosil), to dilute secretions.

Do You UNDERSTAND?

DIRECTIONS: **Circle the correct answer from the italicized words.**

1. Acidosis is an excess of pH. Does this make the arterial pH *increase* or *decrease?*

DIRECTIONS: **Place an increased ($\uparrow$) or decreased ($\downarrow$) sign next to each cation to reflect respiratory acidosis.**

2. The three positive cations that are affected by respiratory acidosis are listed below.
   Calcium = _____
   Potassium = _____
   Sodium = _____

DIRECTIONS: **Circle the correct answers.**

3. Which of the following are causes of respiratory acidosis as a result of airway obstruction?

Muscular dystrophy	Anxiety
Opioid use	Ascites
Asthma	Lymph node enlargement
Flail chest	Excess mucous production
Poisoning	

DIRECTIONS: **Unscramble the word jumble.**

4. Find the three causes of respiratory depression leading to respiratory acidosis in the following word jumbles:
   a. ______________________________ *(isoopn)*
   b. ______________________________ *(sciseanthet)*
   c. ______________________________ *(meypkalheria)*

Answers: 1. decreased; 2. increased calcium, increased potassium, decreased sodium; 3. lymph node enlargement, asthma, excess mucus production; 4. a. poison, b. anesthetics, c. hyperkalemia.

DIRECTIONS: Fill in the blanks.

5. Place the scientific name of the disease or condition next to the defined cause of respiratory acidosis. *Example:* Caused by tubercle bacillus: <u>tuberculosis</u>.
   a. Respiratory disease caused by inhaled allergens: ______________
   b. Chronic obstructive pulmonary disease characterized by an increase in the size of air spaces distal to the terminal bronchioles: ______________
   c. Thrombus in the lungs: ______________
   d. Rib fractures resulting in a segment of rib that is not attached on either end: ______________ chest
   e. A hereditary disease noted by marked atrophic changes in muscles: muscular ______________
   f. Fluid in the abdomen: ______________
   g. Excess serum potassium: ______________
   h. Hilar area chest neoplasm: ______________

What IS Metabolic Acidosis?

The causes of *metabolic acidosis* are related to excess acid or a deficit in base. There are four causes of metabolic acidosis: overproduction of hydrogen ions (carbon monoxide poisoning, diabetic ketoacidosis, starvation, fever, hypoxia, ethanol ingestion, salicylate toxicity, sepsis), lack of elimination of hydrogen ions (renal failure), underproduction of bicarbonate ions (renal failure, pancreatitis, liver failure, dehydration, uremia), and elimination of bicarbonate ions (diarrhea, vomiting).

What You NEED TO KNOW

Excessive breakdown of fatty acids causes increased pH, which is seen with excessive exercise, seizures, and hypermetabolic states, such as lactic acidosis caused by diabetic ketoacidosis and starvation.

TAKE HOME POINTS

- Metabolic acidosis is found in approximately 40% of children with newly diagnosed insulin dependent diabetes mellitus (IDDM).
- Metabolic acidosis usually occurs from a lack of HCO_3^- or excess acid production by the body.

Answers: **5. a. asthma, b. emphysema, c. pulmonary emboli, d. flail, e. dystrophy, f. ascites, g. hyperkalemia, h. lung cancer.**

Ingestion of excessive acid substances can also cause metabolic acidosis. These substances include ethyl alcohol, methyl alcohol poisoning, and acetylsalicylic acid (aspirin) toxicity.

Renal failure causes acidosis because the tubules cannot secrete hydrogen ions into the urine; thus retention of hydrogen ions occurs.

Because bicarbonate is made in the kidney tubules and pancreas, any diseases of the kidney or pancreas will lead to a bicarbonate deficit, thereby leaving the body's normal production of hydrogen ions in excess.

Overelimination of bicarbonate ions occurs with diarrhea and vomiting, but leaves pH levels normal, although eventually in excess proportionally to bicarbonate.

TAKE HOME POINTS

Treatment of Diabetic Ketoacidosis (DKA):

1. Fluid resuscitation with IV saline or hypotonic sodium chloride solution followed by a glucose-containing solution as plasma glucose falls
2. Soluble insulin; however, use cautiously with patients with hypokalemia or hypotension
3. IV potassium supplements
4. IV sodium bicarbonate and phosphate with selected patients

TAKE HOME POINTS

Complications of treatment of DKA include hypoglycemia, cerebral edema, and ARDS.

What You DO

- Assess skin turgor (on chest, forehead, or inner thigh) for dehydration.
- Assess for alcohol or aspirin ingestion.
- Assess serum creatinine as a sign of renal function.
- Assess for increased serum amylase as a sign of pancreatitis or pancreatic cancer
- Assess ABG: pH less than 7.35 and bicarbonate less than 24 mEq/L.
- Take a history for seizures, heavy exercise, starvation, and diarrhea.
- Assess temperature every 4 hours for fever.
- Administer IV hydration therapy.
- Administer insulin if acidosis is a result of diabetic ketoacidosis.
- Administer antidiarrheals, and rehydrate if acidosis is a result of diarrhea.
- Administer antiemetics, and rehydrate if acidosis is a result of vomiting.
- Administer IV bicarbonate if plasma venous bicarbonate level is less than 20 mmol/L (mEq/L) or arterial level is less than 21 mmol/L (mEq/L).

Do You UNDERSTAND?

DIRECTIONS: **Fill in the blanks with the words "lack of" and "excess" to complete the sentence accurately.**

1. Metabolic acidosis is caused by _____ acid or _____ base.

Answers: 1. **excess, lack of.**

DIRECTIONS: Circle the correct answer from the italicized words.

2. Persons with anorexia nervosa have metabolic starvation. Would you expect their urine pH to be *decreased* or *increased?*
3. Fill in the blank: A person with anorexia nervosa develops renal failure and has associated diarrhea from laxative abuse. The diarrhea adds to metabolic acidosis caused by the overelimination of ______________________________ ions.

DIRECTIONS: Match the patient problem associated with metabolic acidosis in column A with the health care provider intervention in column B.

Column A	Column B
4. _____ Pancreatitis	a. Assess serum creatinine
5. _____ Renal failure	b. Take patient temperature
6. _____ Fever	c. Assess skin turgor
7. _____ Dehydration	d. Assess serum amylase

What IS Alkalosis?

Alkalosis is an excess of base, especially bicarbonate, in the ECF caused by a decrease in the pH of the blood, which is evident as the arterial pH becomes greater than 7.45. Alkalosis can be caused by respiratory problems, metabolic problems, or both, similar to acidosis. Clinical signs and symptoms of alkalosis are the same whether they are metabolic or respiratory in origin.

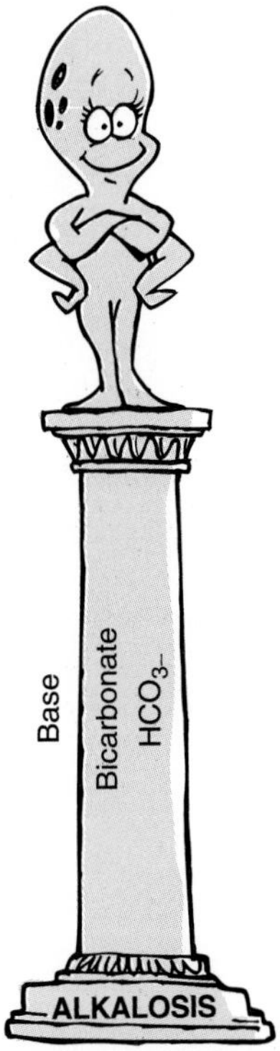

Alkalosis is an excess of base in the ECF caused by a decrease of pH in the blood.

What You NEED TO KNOW

Alkalosis can result from either an overproduction of base or a lack of elimination of base, usually bicarbonate. Treatment of alkalosis is aimed at the effective management of the underlying cause. The common systems affected by alkalosis are the nervous, cardiovascular, and muscular systems.

Answers: **2. decreased from metabolic acidosis and overproduction of hydrogen ions; 3. bicarbonate; 4. d; 5. a; 6. b; 7. c.**

TAKE HOME POINTS

- Alkalosis, as with acidosis, is a manifestation of a disease or condition, not a disease itself.
- Metabolic alkalosis is the most common acid-base disorder in acute and critically ill patients.

Many symptoms of alkalosis are related to hypocalcemia and hypokalemia.

Respiratory Alkalosis

Respiratory alkalosis is the excessive loss of carbon dioxide through rapid respirations **(hyperventilation)**, usually caused by fear, anxiety, fever, improper settings on the mechanical ventilator, central nervous system tumors or lesions, and medications, such as progesterone, aspirin, and catecholamines (e.g., isoproterenol, epinephrine).

Metabolic Alkalosis

Metabolic alkalosis is an increase in base **(base excess)** or a decrease in acid components **(acid deficit)**. The excess of base is caused by the ingestion of bicarbonates, acetates, citrate, or lactates from oral antibiotics (bicarbonate intake), blood transfusions (citrate intake), total parenteral nutrition (TPN), hyperalimentation (HPA) (lactate intake), treatment of diabetic ketoacidosis, or lactic acidosis (from administration of IV bicarbonate).

A decrease of acid components is caused by prolonged vomiting, nasogastric (NG) suctioning, Cushing's syndrome **(hypercortisolism)**, hyperaldosteronism, adrenal tumor, sepsis, postoperative status, overhydration with lactated Ringer's solution IV, hypoproteinemia, licorice ingestion, and the following medications: thiazide diuretics, steroids, high-dose carbenicillin, and penicillin.

Cardiovascular signs include tachycardia, hypovolemia, hypotension, hypokalemia, and the potential for digitalis toxicity resulting from the increased sensitivity of the myocardium to digitalis during alkalosis. Nervous system signs include agitation, confusion, lightheadedness, tingling **(paresthesias)** of mouth or toes, seizures, or hyperreflexia. Muscular signs include cramps, charley horses, continuous spasms **(tetany)**, decreased strength of the hand grip, and the inability to stand up and hold own body weight.

With metabolic and respiratory alkalosis, the serum potassium is decreased as the body tries to regain electroneutrality (see table below).

Acidosis and Alkalosis: Arterial Blood Gas Results

	pH	$PaCO_2$	HCO_3
Metabolic acidosis	< 7.35	—	< 24 mEq/L
Respiratory acidosis	< 7.35	> 45 mm Hg	—
Metabolic alkalosis	> 7.45	—	> 28 mEq/L
Respiratory alkalosis	> 7.45	< 35 mm Hg	—

What You DO

TAKE HOME POINTS

An increased bicarbonate level with a rising carbon dioxide concentration (partial pressure carbon dioxide) is the hallmark of metabolic alkalosis. A decreased bicarbonate level with a low carbon dioxide concentration is the hallmark of respiratory alkalosis or metabolic acidosis with respiratory compensation.

- Assess pH of ABG. If it is above 7.45, then metabolic or respiratory alkalosis is present.
- Assess ABG for elevated bicarbonate levels (> 29 mEq/L) in metabolic alkalosis and decreased bicarbonate levels (< 22 mEq/L) in respiratory alkalosis.
- With respiratory alkalosis, the carbon dioxide concentration of ABG is less than 35 mm Hg.
- Assess for hypocalcemia by serum value less than 8.5 mg/dL and positive Chvostek-Weiss and Trousseau's signs. The Chvostek-Weiss sign is positive if facial muscles contract when percussion is applied to the top of the facial cheek below the zygomatic bone in front of the ear, using the tip of the index or middle finger. Trousseau's sign is positive if, when the blood pressure cuff is inflated to above the patient's systolic pressure and held at that cuff pressure level for 1 to 4 minutes, the patient's hands and fingers go into spasm with palmar flexion (fingers point toward the floor).
- Assess daily for hypokalemia by serum value being less than 3.5 mEq/L.

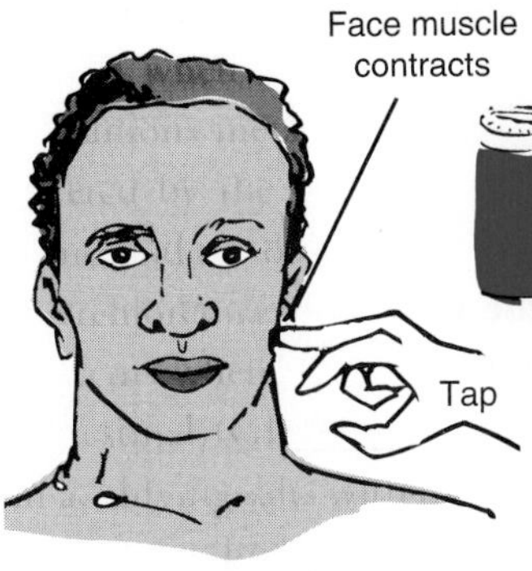

Chvostek's sign

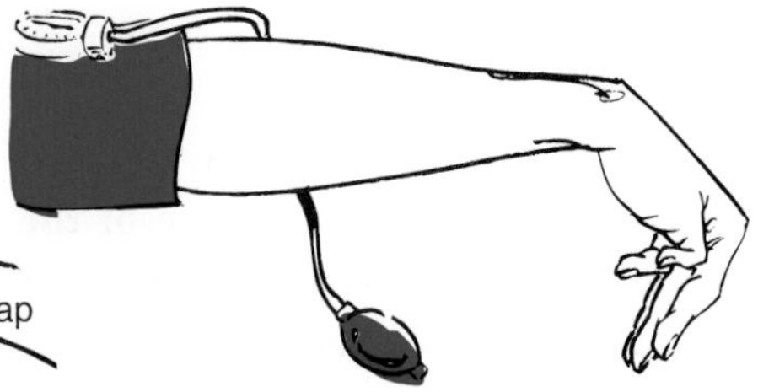
Trousseau's sign

- Assess for paresthesias using touch and for muscle weakness using push/pull and grasps.
- Assess for increased heart rate and a normal or low blood pressure as signs of alkalosis and an increased respiratory rate in respiratory alkalosis and metabolic acidosis.
- Assess serum laboratory results for digoxin toxicity. Toxicity value is greater than 2.4 ng/mL.
- Assess for hyperreflexia at the knee (patella) using a reflex hammer.

- Administer fluids and electrolytes by mouth or IV as prescribed.
- Administer antiemetics to stop nausea or vomiting as prescribed.

Basic Interpretation of Acid-Base Data

- Rule 1: Arterial pH detects acidemia or alkalemia.
- Rule 2: pCO_2 and bicarbonate levels determine if the cause of acidemia or alkalemia is metabolic or respiratory.

Do You UNDERSTAND?

DIRECTIONS: **Circle the correct answer from the italicized words.**

1. Alkalosis is an excess of base, which causes a change in pH. Does the pH *increase* or *decrease?*

DIRECTIONS: **Place an increased (↑) or decreased (↓) sign next to the phrase to make the phrase true regarding respiratory alkalosis.**

2. ______ Loss of carbon dioxide through rapid respirations
3. ______ Fever
4. ______ Aspirin toxicity
5. ______ Anxiety

DIRECTIONS: **Write in the name of the base associated with each of the three treatments listed.**

6. Oral antacids ingested: Base is ______________.
7. Blood transfusions received: Base is ______________.
8. TPN: Base is ______________.

Answers: **1. pH increases to over 7.45; 2. increase; 3. increase; 4. increase; 5. increase; 6. bicarbonate; 7. citrates; 8. lactates.**

DIRECTIONS: Circle all correct answers.

9. Which treatments decrease the acid components of the blood, causing metabolic alkalosis?
   Percutaneous endoscopic gastrostomy (PEG) tube feedings
   Thiazide diuretic administration
   NG suctioning
   Overhydration with lactated Ringer's solution IV
   Metronidazole hydrochloride (Flagyl) antibiotic ingestion
   Acetaminophen (Tylenol) ingestion

DIRECTIONS: Circle the correct answer from the italicized words.

10. Is the relationship between pH and serum calcium *directly proportional* or *inversely proportional?*

References

Banker D, Whittier FC, Rutecki G: Acid-base disturbances: 5 rules that can simplify diagnosis, *Consultant* 43(3):381-384, 2003.

Charemska D, Przbyszewski B, Klonowska B: Estimation of the severity of metabolic disorders in children with newly diagnosed insulin dependent diabetes mellitus, *Medycyna Wieku Rozwojowego* 7(2):261-270, 2003.

Chernecky C, Berger B: *Laboratory tests and diagnostic procedures,* ed 4, Philadelphia, 2004, Saunders.

McHoy A: The clinical management of diabetic ketoacidosis in adults, *J Diabetes Nurs* 7(9):332-336, 2003.

Mokhlesi B et al: Adult toxicity in critical care: Part 1: General approach to the intoxicated patient, *Chest* 123(2):577-592, 2003.

Rey C et al: Fatal lactic acidosis during antiretroviral therapy, *Pediatr Crit Care Med* 4(4):485-487, 2003.

Workman LM: Interventions for clients with acid-base balance. In Ignatavicius DD, Workman ML, Mishler MA, editors: *Medical-surgical nursing across the health care continuum,* Philadelphia, 1999, Saunders.

Answers: 9. thiazides, NG, overhydration; 10. Inversely proportional, because pH increases as the serum calcium decreases, and as pH decreases the serum calcium increases.

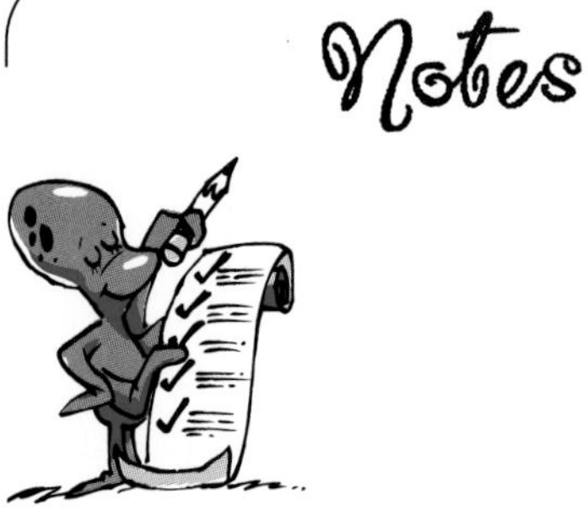
Notes

NCLEX® Review

1. The major intracellular protein buffer is:
   1 Hematocrit
   2 Hemoglobin
   3 Immunoglobulins
   4 Albumin

2. A patient comes to the emergency department from a motor vehicle accident (MVA) with a diagnosis of flail chest, hyponatremia, and illegal opioid use. What type of acid-based imbalance is most likely?
   1 Respiratory acidosis
   2 Metabolic acidosis
   3 Respiratory alkalosis
   4 Metabolic alkalosis

3. Shelly is brought to the emergency room with an attempted aspirin overdose. What type of acid-based imbalance is most likely to result from her aspirin ingestion?
   1 Respiratory alkalosis
   2 Respiratory acidosis
   3 Metabolic alkalosis
   4 Metabolic acidosis

4. A person who is anorexic, is in a starving state, and has developed subsequent renal failure would be at high risk for what acid-base imbalance?
   1 Respiratory alkalosis
   2 Respiratory acidosis
   3 Metabolic alkalosis
   4 Metabolic acidosis

5. What cardiac medication has the potential to create toxic blood levels in the person with metabolic alkalosis?
   1 Chlorpromazine (Thorazine)
   2 Hydrochlorothiazide (HydroDIURIL, Esidrix)
   3 Digoxin (Lanoxin)
   4 Furosemide (Lasix)

6. Chvostek's and Trousseau's signs are implemented to assess for:
   1 Hypokalemia
   2 Hypernatremia
   3 Hypocalcemia
   4 Hypertension

7. Your patient is hyperventilating and has the following arterial blood gas results: pH = 7.44 (high); bicarbonate = 16 mEq/L (low); pO_2 = 42 mm Hg (very low); $PaCO_2$ = 22 mm Hg (low); serum potassium = 3.2 mEq/L (low); serum calcium = 8 mg/dL (low). Based on this information alone, what is your acid-based diagnosis?
   1 Metabolic alkalosis
   2 Respiratory alkalosis
   3 Metabolic acidosis
   4 Respiratory acidosis

8. What serum laboratory value should be monitored to assess for signs of renal function?
   1 Hematocrit
   2 Amylase
   3 Creatinine
   4 Prothrombin time

9. In a patient who has metabolic acidosis, you would assess for hyperreflexia using a(n):
   1 Otoscope
   2 Blood pressure cuff
   3 Stethoscope
   4 Reflex hammer

10. Metabolic acidosis may be caused by the lack of elimination of hydrogen ions or the underproduction of bicarbonate ions. This is associated with failure of which major organ?

11. True or False: Cellular destruction, such as that seen with chemotherapy, causes an increase in acid, thus affecting the pH.

12. True or False: Carbon dioxide, produced from glucose breakdown and released by the lungs, produces an acid by-product, not a base by-product.

13. Retention of carbon dioxide causes acidosis by what mechanism?

14. Poisons, as well as opioids, are chemical causes of _____ depression.

15. Positive Chvostek's and Trousseau's signs indicate _____ calcemia.

NCLEX® Review Answers

1. 1 The intracellular protein hemoglobin carries oxygen. Hematocrit expresses a percentage of red blood cells. Immunoglobulins and albumins are found in extracellular fluid.

2. 1 Flail chest and hyponatremia decrease chest expansion and weaken respiratory muscles, and opioid use depresses respirations. Metabolic acidosis is a result of respiratory components. Respiratory and metabolic alkalosis indicates alkalosis.

3. 4 Metabolic acidosis is the overproduction of hydrogen ions caused by aspirin toxicity.

4. 4 Metabolic acidosis is caused by the overproduction of hydrogen ions by starvation, and decreased secretion of hydrogen ions is a result of renal failure.

5. 3 Digoxin (Lanoxin) is a cardiac drug with serum levels that need to be monitored for toxicity. Chlorpromazine (Thorazine) is an antipsychotic drug. Hydrochlorothiazide (HydroDIURIL, Esidrix) is an antihypertensive drug. Furosemide (Lasix) is a diuretic drug.

6. 3 Not enough calcium will cause muscles to spasm. Hypokalemia indicates potassium's effects on the heart. Sodium affects fluids. Hypertension is related to systemic blood pressure.

7. 2 The pH is high because buffering and renal compensation cannot maintain the hydrogen ion concentration. Carbon dioxide is low as a result of exhalation through hyperventilation. Bicarbonate is low in response to the increase in pH.

8. 3 Serum creatinine is the laboratory test to monitor for signs of renal function. Hematocrit monitors for blood loss. Amylase monitors for pancreatitis. Prothrombin time monitors for bleeding.

9. 4 A reflex hammer is used to assess for hyperreflexia, usually on the patella. An otoscope would be used to examine the ear. A blood pressure cuff is used to measure blood pressure. A stethoscope is used to assess heart and lung sounds.

10. Renal (kidney) failure causes metabolic acidosis from a lack of elimination of hydrogen ions and/or underproduction of bicarbonate ions.

11. True.

12. True.

13. Frees hydrogen ions in the blood from carbonic acid production.

14. Respiratory

15. "Hypo" as in "hypocalcemia."

Notes

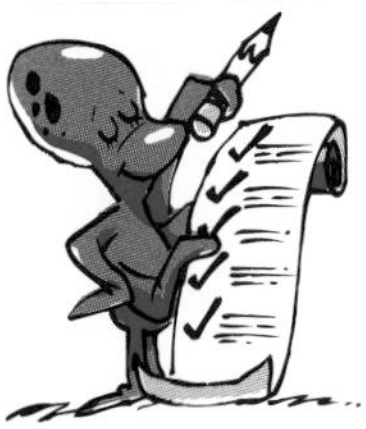

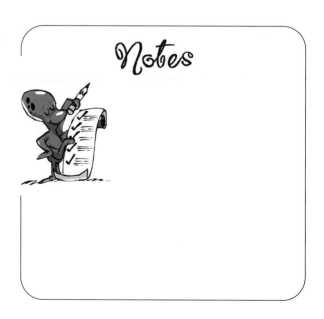

Sodium

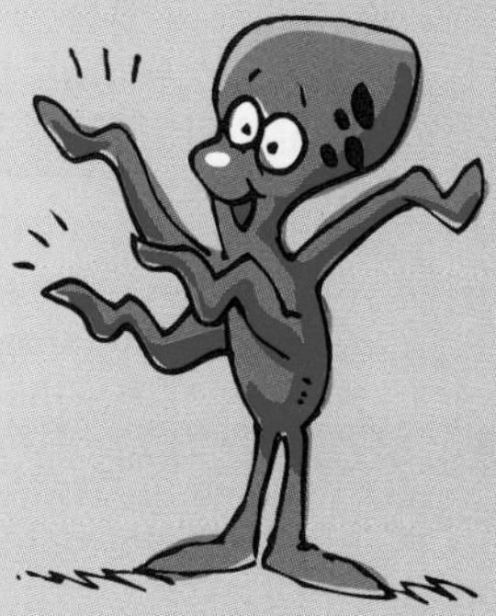

Chapter 3

What You WILL LEARN

After reading this chapter, you will know how to do the following:

- ✔ Describe sodium's role in two body functions.
- ✔ Define hypernatremia.
- ✔ Differentiate hyponatremia from hypernatremia.

Now that you understand the basic concepts of fluid and electrolyte function and the acid–base balancing act, you are ready to learn about the specific electrolytes, how they function, what problems are associated with imbalances, and the appropriate care for patients with electrolyte disturbances. Electrolytes are essential for promotion of neuromuscular impulses, maintenance of osmolality, regulation of acid–base balance, and distribution of fluids and electrolytes between compartments.

What IS Sodium?

Sodium (Na^+) is a positively charged ion **(cation)** and is the most abundant electrolyte in the extracellular fluid (ECF). Because it represents approximately 90% of all extracellular cations, it is a main factor in determining ECF volume and is important in regulating neuromuscular impulses in the nerve and muscle fibers. Only small amounts of sodium are inside the cells **(intracellular)**. The normal serum sodium in an adult is 135 to 145 milliequivalents per liter (mEq/L).

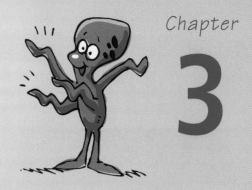

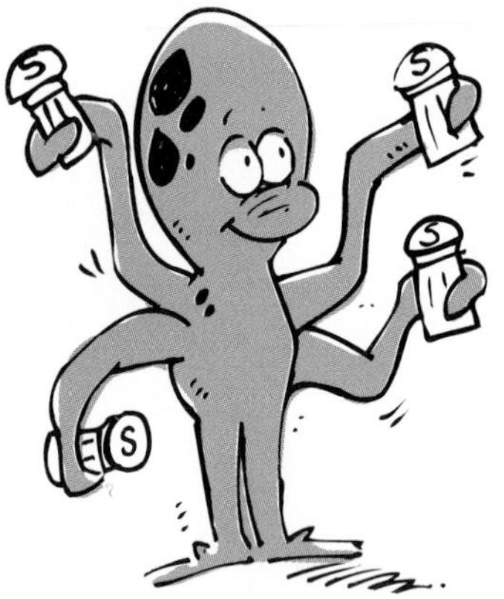

Sodium (Na^+) is a cation.

TAKE HOME POINTS

- Remember, opposites attract. Sodium is the major ECF cation, whereas chloride is the major ECF anion, which is why they are frequently observed bound to each other.
- One teaspoon of table salt contains approximately 2.3 g sodium. The average adult daily requirement is 2 g salt. Patients monitoring their sodium intake should know that in processed foods, sodium is listed in the ingredients as sodium, sodium bicarbonate, or sodium chloride.

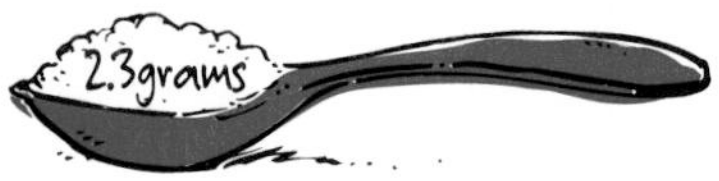

Alterations in the normal concentration of sodium can result in serious and life-threatening conditions.

Normal Sodium Values

Serum is the clear, straw-colored, liquid portion of the blood.

- Adult serum Na^+ = 135 to 145 mEq/L
- Child serum Na^+ = 138 to 145 mEq/L
- Infant serum Na^+ = 139 to 146 mEq/L
- Critical or panic level in adults is < 110 mEq/L

Normal Serum Osmolality

- Adult serum osmolality = 280 to 300 mOsm/kg water
- Child serum osmolality = 270 to 290 mOsm/kg water

Body fluids that have a high concentration of sodium include saliva, bile, and gastric, pancreatic, and intestinal secretions. Sodium is absorbed from the gastrointestinal (GI) tract and eliminated through urine, feces, and perspiration. Sodium is stored deep within the tissues and released into the ECF when levels drop. Sodium is often found attached to chloride, a negative-charged electrolyte **(anion)**, and bicarbonate to regulate the acid-base balance.

Normal Urine Sodium and Specific Gravity

- Adult urine sodium = 75 to 200 mEq/L; urine specific gravity = 1.016 to 1.022
- Child urine sodium (female) = 20 to 69 mEq/L; (male) = 41 to 115 mEq/L
- Infant urine sodium = 14 to 40 mEq/L; urine specific gravity = 1.002 to 1.006

What You NEED TO KNOW

Sources of Sodium

Sodium is primarily obtained from foods that are high in sodium content, including table salt, processed or cured meats (especially corned beef, ham, sausage, hot dogs, and pork), packaged foods, seafood (tuna), cheese and cottage cheese, pickles, and junk food, such as potato chips and salted pretzels. Most canned foods, seasonings, soy sauce, and many soft drinks have moderate-to-high sodium content. Breads, certain cereals, and fresh vegetables contain small amounts of sodium, whereas fresh fruits have minimal amounts.

Control of Sodium

Under normal physiologic conditions, sodium levels remain constant if the intake and excretion are balanced. Because most diets contain at least 2 g of sodium a day, lack of intake is usually not a problem. Fortunately, the body has a great ability to adjust the sodium and water level when there are any changes in the ratio.

Sodium balance is maintained by several physiologic mechanisms, including the thirst mechanism, antidiuretic hormone (ADH), glomerular filtration rate (GFR), renin-angiotensin-aldosterone system (RAAS), atrial natriuretic peptide (ANP), osmotic pressure, and sodium-potassium pump.

In the event that sodium levels start to rise, such as after a large salty meal or in the case of dehydration, the osmoreceptors in the hypothalamus sense increased osmolality, which triggers a nerve impulse to the brain, thereby stimulating the thirst center. In response to the sensation of thirst, the person drinks more fluid, which then increases the volume and decreases the osmolality in the ECF. The hypothalamus also sends a message to the pituitary gland to secrete antidiuretic hormone (ADH) into the bloodstream, which causes the kidneys to retain water, helping to dilute the serum sodium level, thus decreasing serum osmolality. ADH may be stimulated or suppressed, depending on the fluid-volume status. A fluid-volume deficit causes ADH to be released, and, thus, water retention.

The kidneys help maintain the proper osmolality in several ways. Remember that sodium acts as a water magnet; thus, the increase in osmolality from a high serum-sodium level leads to an increase in fluid (and, in return, blood) volume. This increased blood volume causes a greater hydrostatic pressure, pushing the fluid out of the glomerular capillaries in the renal tubules where the extra fluid is secreted into the urine **(increased GFR)**.

The RAAS plays a complex and important role in fluid balance. The kidneys directly sense the serum sodium level. When serum sodium is

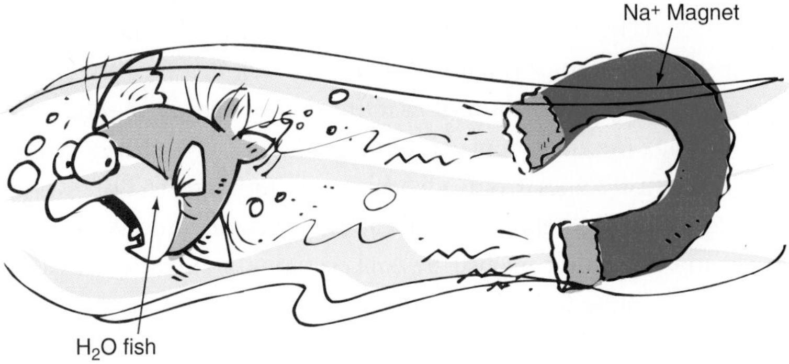

Sodium acts like a water magnet.

low, the juxtaglomerular (JG) cells in the kidney secrete renin, which stimulates the formation of angiotensin. Angiotensin acts directly on the adrenal cortex to secrete aldosterone, which causes the kidneys to retain sodium. As the serum sodium returns to physiologic levels, the JG cells secrete less renin. The RAAS is activated by decreased sodium sensed by osmoreceptors and decreased blood pressure sensed by baroreceptors.

The effects of the RAAS on sodium are opposed by the cardiac hormone atrial natriuretic peptide (ANP). Elevated serum sodium increases fluid volume, which stretches the atrial walls, causing the release of ANP into the blood. ANP suppresses the effect of aldosterone on the kidney, thereby decreasing the reabsorption of sodium in the kidney, resulting in increased urinary excretion of sodium **(natriuresis)** and decreased serum sodium.

The osmotic pressure is another way the body tries to maintain a normal extracellular sodium level. Sodium, glucose, and urea are the main solutes that affect osmolality. Because osmosis (movement of water from an area of lesser solute concentration to an area of greater concentration) takes place when the sodium level rises, water moves out of the cell into the extracellular space to help dilute the sodium concentration. Unfortunately, this mechanism can lead to cellular dehydration, especially in nerve cells, causing neurologic symptoms (see hypernatremia on page 50).

The sodium-potassium pump is another mechanism that is continually operating to maintain sodium levels. You may recall that the intracellular concentration of sodium is low and the concentration of potassium is high (see Chapter 5). Both of these ions naturally want to move from an area of higher concentration to an area of lower concentration. This characteristic means that the sodium tends to diffuse into the cell, and potassium tends to diffuse out of the cell. The sodium-potassium pump prevents this diffusion from happening by linking these ions with a carrier that accompanies the ion through the cell wall against the concentration gradient. Any time a cell tries to move a substance against a concentration gradient, energy is expended. This process of using membrane pumps is referred to as *active transport.*

The purpose of the sodium-potassium pump is to move sodium and potassium against their concentration gradients. The energy required for this activity comes from adenosine triphosphate (ATP), working with magnesium and enzymes. This active transport process of moving sodium and potassium against the concentration gradient causes a neuromuscular impulse to be transmitted.

There are many physiologic mechanisms that are continuously on guard to detect and correct any sodium imbalances. High sodium levels stimulate ADH and ANP secretion and inhibit aldosterone secretion. Low sodium inhibits ADH and ANP secretion and stimulates aldosterone secretion.

Functions of Sodium

Sodium is the most important electrolyte in regulating osmolality (sodium acts via a concentration gradient by attracting fluid), which maintains the volume of body fluids, particularly the ECFs. Think of sodium as being the king of the sea in regulating and maintaining the water volume. It is often bound to chloride, with which it works closely to maintain water distribution. Balancing water volume is important in maintaining blood pressure.

Sodium influences the permeability of cell membranes and helps to move substances across the cell membranes. Sodium works closely with potassium and calcium to maintain gradients for action potentials, which are necessary for the transmission of impulses in the nerves and muscles.

Sodium helps to regulate acid-base balance by attaching to chloride and bicarbonate and is also necessary for the initiation of cardiac contractility.

The small amount of sodium that is found inside the cell is an active participant in many intracellular chemical reactions.

TAKE HOME POINTS

- Because sodium is excreted through sweat, urine, and feces, any significant alteration in these bodily functions can result in a sodium imbalance.
- Sodium tends to cause fluid retention, which can increase blood pressure.

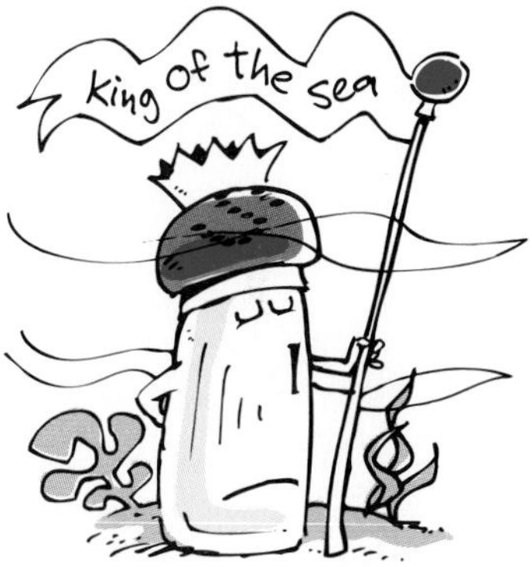

Sodium is the most important electrolyte in regulating osmolality. It is the king of the sea in water volume regulation.

Do You UNDERSTAND?

DIRECTIONS: Fill in the blanks.

1. Sodium is the most abundant electrolyte in the ____________________ ____________________ cellular fluid.
2. Sodium is often listed in nutritional ingredients as sodium ____________________ or sodium ____________________.
3. The average adult daily requirement of sodium is ____________________ ____________________ g.
4. Sodium causes fluid retention, which can ____________________ blood pressure.
5. The steroid hormone ____________________ causes the active transport of sodium from the kidney into the blood stream, increasing the serum sodium level and water volume.

Answers: 1. extra; 2. bicarbonate, chloride; 3. two; 4. increase; 5. aldosterone.

6. The ion (electrolyte) ______________________ works with sodium as a pump (active transport) to help move these ions against their concentration gradient.
7. A major function of sodium is to regulate osmolarity, which is vital in maintaining the ______________________ of body fluids.

What IS Hypernatremia?

A serum sodium level greater than 147 mEq/L is called *hypernatremia.*

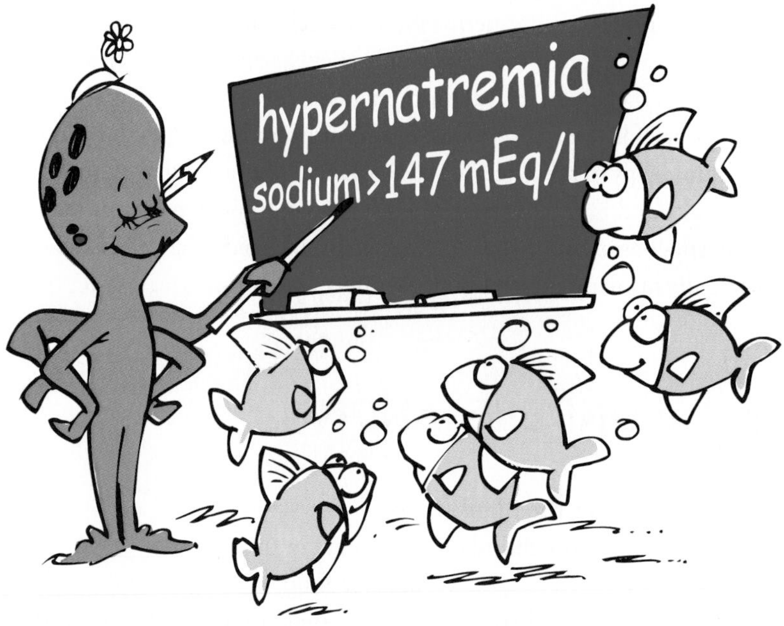

What You NEED TO KNOW

High sodium levels are not as common as low sodium levels, but this is a common electrolyte imbalance that you will encounter in your clinical practice. In general, hypernatremia is caused by an increase in sodium intake or an excess loss of water. Other causes of hypernatremia include diabetes insipidus (DI), hyperaldosteronism, and Cushing's syndrome.

Answers: **6. potassium; 7. volume.**

Hypernatremia causes the serum osmolality to become concentrated or thick **(hypertonic)**.

An excessive sodium intake is common after ingestion of a high-sodium diet for patients with renal dysfunction. Remember that sodium concentration is maintained and regulated by the kidneys with the help of the hormones aldosterone, ADH, and ANP. Therefore people with normal renal function are able to compensate for a high oral sodium load by excreting it in the urine. Another cause of excessive sodium intake may occur from intravenous (IV) fluids, such as sodium bicarbonate (which is given to treat acidosis), or hypertonic solutions, such as dextrose 5% with 0.45% ($D_5W\frac{1}{2}NS$) or 0.9% normal saline (NS), or sodium chloride solutions of 3% or 5% (hypertonic saline solutions) (see table on hypertonic intravenous solutions).

CULTURE

Inadequate intake may occur in persons who are fasting for religious practices. Many conditions can cause an excessive loss of fluids, such as vomiting, diarrhea, fever, sweating, or burns.

Hypertonic Intravenous Solutions

Solution	Osmolarity	pH	Indications and Precautions
10% dextrose in water ($D_{10}W$)	500	3.5-6.5	Water replacement; hyperglycemia May cause hyperglycemia
5% dextrose in 0.9% NS (D_5W/NS)	560	3.5-6.5	Dehydration; shock May worsen CHF
5% dextrose in 0.45% NS ($D_5W\frac{1}{2}NS$)	406	4	Diabetic ketoacidosis May cause hyperglycemia

CHF, Congestive heart failure; *NS,* normal saline.

An excessive loss or inadequate oral intake of water can result in hypernatremia with an increase in serum osmolality. Common causes of poor intake may occur with patients who are experiencing nausea, anorexia, difficulty swallowing, immobility, confusion, or malfunction of the hypothalamic thirst center from a stroke or tumor.

Other causes of excessive fluid loss may result from a physiologic process called osmotic diuresis. This process of fluid loss is caused by medications or any condition that causes the body fluids to become hypertonic. Osmotic diuretics are low–molecular-weight substances that stay in the renal tubules to increase plasma osmolality, glomerular filtration, and tubular fluid, ultimately resulting in rapid and excessive fluid loss and cellular dehydration. High-protein feedings can also cause osmotic diuresis when water is not administered concurrently, as can the administration of

TAKE HOME POINTS

An example of an osmotic diuretic is mannitol, which is given to initiate rapid diuresis, to relieve increased intracranial and intraocular pressures or spinal cord edema, or to prevent or treat acute renal failure.

iodinated contrast agents for radiographic studies. Diabetic hyperglycemic nonketotic syndrome (a hyperosmolar state) may initiate osmotic diuresis.

Diabetes insipidus, which is caused by lack of ADH production in the hypothalamus (central DI) or by the inability of the kidneys to respond to ADH (nephrogenic DI), causes excessive urination and hypernatremia. Remember that the lack of ADH (or the lack of its effect) causes large outputs of dilute urine. The urine becomes highly diluted (**hypotonic**) with a low specific gravity.

Hyperaldosteronism is the excessive secretion of aldosterone (the major mineralocorticoid), resulting in inappropriate renal reabsorption of sodium and water with an increased renal excretion of potassium. Remember that the mineralocorticoids produced in the adrenal cortex affect homeostasis of electrolytes such as sodium and potassium. This condition can be either primary or secondary. Primary aldosteronism may be caused by adrenocortical hyperfunction (Conn's syndrome) or aldosterone-producing adenoma, or it may be the result of a primary or metastatic cancer. Secondary aldosteronism is a response to renin excess as a result of decreased renal perfusion.

Cushing's syndrome, another disorder of the adrenal gland, is the excessive production of glucocorticoids from the adrenal cortex, which causes hypercortisolism. Exogenous administration of cortisol (such as prolonged use of prednisone for the treatment of inflammatory conditions) can also lead to Cushing's syndrome, which is manifested by weight gain, hypertension, muscle wasting, weakness, and skin changes. Cortisol can cause sodium retention.

Signs and Symptoms of Hypernatremia

- Serum sodium greater than 147 mEq/L
- Serum osmolality greater than 300 mOsm/kg
- Increased urine specific gravity (decreased in DI)
- Irritability, restlessness, confusion, and agitation (Remember, in acute hypernatremia the brain cells are highly sensitive to a hyperosmolar state, which causes these neurologic changes.)
- Twitching or seizures (also from neurocellular dehydration)
- Increased thirst (increased osmolality stimulates the signal to the thirst center)
- Lethargy, muscle weakness, or coma (from altered cellular metabolism)
- Low-grade fever (from dehydration)
- Flushed skin (from dehydration)
- Dry mucous membranes (from dehydration)

Signs and Symptoms of Hypernatremia—cont'd

- Decreased urinary output **(oliguria)**
- Orthostatic hypotension (from low fluid volume)
- Hypertension, bounding pulse, and dyspnea (with hypervolemia from sodium retention)

What You DO

The goal of hypernatremia management is to correct the fluid imbalance by identifying and removing the precipitating cause or providing specific treatment of the underlying disease process. Treatment measures should produce a gradual correction of hypernatremia to avoid complications.

The health care provider's assessment and documentation is important in identifying the cause and includes the following:

LIFE SPAN

Many older patients do not develop an elevated temperature with an infection. Profound dehydration may cause a lower temperature.

Monitoring Vital Signs

Vital signs can provide helpful information on the fluid and electrolyte status of the patient. The pulse may increase with fluid volume deficit. Volume overload can be observed in a patient with underlying heart failure. The blood pressure generally will decrease with fluid deficit and increase with fluid overload. Temperature may be elevated with an infection, and a high and prolonged fever can contribute to fluid loss.

Measuring Intake and Output

Monitoring intake and output (I & O) is essential for evaluating fluid and electrolyte balance, indicating whether excess fluid is being excreted or whether the body is retaining fluid. The health care provider should initiate I & O when evaluating for fluid and electrolyte imbalances. The trends over 24-, 48-, and 72-hour periods provide information regarding the hydration status and effectiveness of treatment. Measuring intake includes accounting for all oral liquids, including foods such as gelatin, ice cream, soup, and beverages, as well as tube feedings, IV fluids, blood components, and medications. Measuring output includes urine, diarrhea, vomitus, gastric suction, and wound and tube drainage. In most hospitals, the I & O are recorded in 8-hour periods, but the registered nurse should look at the trend before the 8-hour shift is over, and in some cases, the I & O may need to be monitored as frequently as every few hours.

Monitoring Daily Weight

Daily weight is an excellent way to monitor fluid retention or loss, but it needs to be measured at the same time of day, on the same scale, and with the patient wearing the same amount of clothing for the reading to be accurate. The health care provider should initiate this intervention whenever fluid balance assessment is indicated.

Inspecting for Edema

Edema is the accumulation of excessive fluid intracellularly or extracellularly. Often classified by location, edema can be caused by a variety of conditions that affect osmotic pressure, such as hypotonic fluid overload, hypoproteinemia, excessive retention of salt and water, heart failure, and inflammatory responses.

Inspect for edema in the dependent body part, which is usually the feet or sacrum. When checking for dependent edema, inspect and palpate the pretibial region by firmly depressing the skin over the tibia or medial malleolus with a finger for 5 seconds. After releasing your finger, there should be no indentation. However, a pit imprint from the finger indicates pitting edema. Swelling of the feet and ankles is known as pedal edema. Swelling without pitting is referred to as nonpitting edema. With patients who are on bed rest, check the sacral region for edema. Facial and periorbital edema should be recorded.

TAKE HOME POINTS

Pitting should be graded and recorded using the following scale as a general subjective guideline.

1 + Mild pitting: slight indentation, with no perceptible swelling of leg or foot.

2 + Moderate pitting: subsides quickly.

3 + Deep pitting: indentation remains for a brief time, and the leg or foot is swollen.

4 + Extremely deep pitting: indentation lasts longer, and the leg and foot are exceedingly swollen.

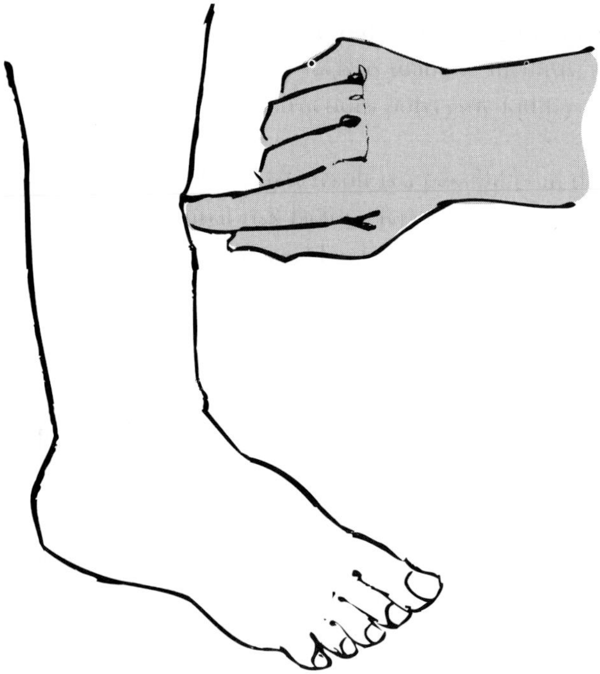

LIFE SPAN

A slight pit may be normally noted in those who are pregnant, in older adults, or in persons who have been standing for a prolonged period.

Obtaining an Initial Nutritional Assessment

Nutritional counseling regarding maintaining a low-sodium diet is important for patients who are at risk for sodium retention, such as persons with renal dysfunction or congestive heart failure (CHF). Sodium restriction is important for patients with renal compromise. Obtaining an initial nutritional assessment is necessary to identify habits, preferences, and current sources of high sodium intake that may be modified. Ask the patient what foods would be included in his or her typical breakfast, lunch, dinner, snack, and beverages. It is important to include the family member (the person who shops and prepares meals) in the teaching process.

The specific treatment depends on the exact cause of hypernatremia and will therefore vary. Some of the most common causes of hypernatremia include excessive administration of hypertonic IV fluids, dehydration, volume loss, fluid overload in treatment of central DI with vasopressin (e.g., ADH) or synthetic ADH analogs, hyperaldosteronism, and low serum cortisol, as in treatment for sudden cessation of long-term glucocorticoid therapy. Dialysis may be necessary to treat extreme cases of hypernatremia.

Isotonic Intravenous Solutions

Solution	Osmolarity	pH	Indications and Precautions
0.9% NS	308	5	Hyponatremia Hypercalcemia transfusions diabetic ketoacidosis Can cause fluid overload
D_5W	272	3.5-6.5	Hypernatremia Dehydration May cause hyperglycemia or fluid overload
Ringer's lactate	273	6.5	Dehydration Burns Hypovolemia Do not use in liver or kidney disease

D_5W, 5% dextrose in water; *NS*, normal saline.

When hypernatremia is caused by hypertonic IV fluids, switching to an isotonic solution such as D_5W or slowing the rate is useful (see table on isotonic intravenous solutions). Mild hypernatremia from dehydration is treated by oral or IV fluid replacement, given gradually over several days.

Generally, dehydration is caused by poor oral intake or increased loss. The health care provider needs to explore the cause of dehydration by assessing the patient's mental status, home situation, psychosocial situation, and physical symptoms, such as fever, nausea, vomiting, anorexia, dysphagia, diarrhea, or polyuria. In addition to reporting these findings, the health care provider should explore medication options (e.g., antipyretics, antiemetics, appetite stimulants or nutritional supplements, analgesics, antidiarrheals) for treating symptoms and consider referral for home-care assistance.

In acute or severe cases, medical management includes the slow administration of sodium-free isotonic fluids, such as D_5W, to dilute the serum sodium, which may be followed by NS (0.45%) to prevent hyponatremia.

Diuretic therapy may be initiated to restore sodium and water balance. The most commonly used diuretic is furosemide (Lasix), which may be given orally or IV. Patients who are on diuretic therapy should be monitored for blood pressure, sodium and potassium levels (I & O, noting and documenting the extent of diuresis), and daily weight (noting changes). Assess for signs and symptoms of hypokalemia (such as changes in muscle strength, tremor, muscle cramps; changes in mental status, and cardiac arrhythmias) and signs and symptoms of hyponatremia (such as confusion, thirst, and cold, clammy skin).

If hypernatremia was caused by osmotic diuresis or volume loss, then hypotonic IV fluids are indicated (see table on p. 57).

Central DI may be treated with the hormone vasopressin (e.g., ADH) in natural or synthetic form. Desmopressin acetate or lypressin are synthetic analogs of ADH and may be given by nasal spray. Side effects of these agents include circum-oral pallor, abdominal cramping, nausea, sweating, tremor, headache, and diarrhea. The rationale of fluid restriction (to avoid hypervolemic hyponatremia) should be explained to the patient and family. The type of IV fluid replacement depends on serum sodium levels.

The treatment of hyperaldosteronism depends on the cause. Adrenocorticotrophic hormone (ACTH)–secreting tumors may be treated with surgical excision or pituitary irradiation. Occasionally, a bilateral total adrenalectomy is performed, followed by lifelong hormone replacement. In mild cases, adrenal enzyme inhibitors such as ketoconazole, aminoglutethimide, or the adrenocorticolytic agent mitotane are used.

For patients taking steroids (glucocorticoids), the appropriate dose and gradual tapering of dose are important in preventing acute adrenal insufficiency **(addisonian crisis)**. Long-term, high-dose steroid therapy suppresses the hypothalamic-pituitary-adrenal (HPA) axis; therefore for patients using prescribed steroids, there is no feedback mechanism that tells the adrenal glands to produce more glucocorticoid hormones. A sudden cessation of glucocorticoid therapy will result in adrenal hypofunction, necessitating immediate treatment with IV hydrocortisone sodium succinate (Solu-Cortef). The low serum cortisol can cause a lower sodium and elevated potassium level. When discontinuing steroid treatment, decreasing the dosage over several days will allow pituitary production of ACTH and adrenal production of cortisol.

- It is much easier to prevent iatrogenically induced hypernatremia from IV therapy by administering hypertonic solutions cautiously, and to consider the type and rate of solution your patient is receiving.
- Rapid IV infusion can cause a shift of fluid into the cells, causing cellular edema (especially of the neurocells), central nervous system changes, seizures, or fluid overload, resulting in CHF and shortness of breath.
- Administration of IV furosemide should be performed slowly, not exceeding 4 mg per minute, to avoid ototoxicity.

Hypotonic Intravenous Solutions

Solution	Osmolarity	pH	Indications and Precautions
0.45% NS (½NS)	154	5	Hyponatremia Hypercalcemia—dehydration (GI fluid loss) Diabetic ketoacidosis May cause increased intracranial pressure

NS, Normal saline; *GI*, gastrointestinal.

TAKE HOME POINTS

Signs of hypokalemia include changes in muscle strength, tremor, muscle cramps, change in mental status, and cardiac arrhythmias.

Do You UNDERSTAND?

DIRECTIONS: **Unscramble the italicized letters to form the correct word and complete the statements.**

1. Hypernatremia causes serum osmolality to become ________________________. *(cnteyhproi)*
2. With the help of the hormones ADH and ANP, the ________________________ maintains sodium levels. *(inyedk)*
3. Mannitol is an example of an ________________________ diuretic. *(iosctmo)*
4. The cardinal sign of DI is excessive ________________________. *(rntoniaiu)*
5. ________________________ is a neurologic symptom of hypernatremia. *(yitririlitbi)*

Answers: **1. hypertonic; 2. kidney; 3. osmotic; 4. urination; 5. Irritability.**

6. Low fluid volume is suggested when the blood pressure reading demonstrates __________________________. *(cttotorhsai yoeson-intph)*
7. The hormone vasopressin (e.g., ADH) is given to treat central __________________________. *(iadsiteb dipinusit)*

What IS Hyponatremia?

A serum sodium level of less than 135 mEq/L is called *hyponatremia* and is the most common electrolyte imbalance, occurring in approximately 2.5% to 10% of hospitalized patients. In general, hyponatremia is caused by an inadequate sodium intake, an increase in sodium excretion, or a dilution of serum sodium (i.e., excess of water).

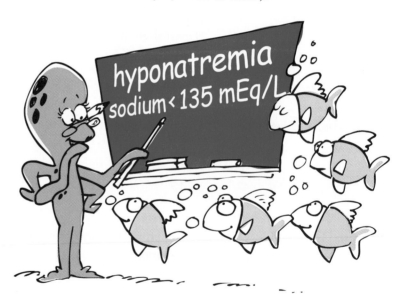

What You NEED TO KNOW

Hyponatremia is considered *true hyponatremia* when there is an actual decrease in the sodium level versus *pseudohyponatremia,* which indicates a relative decrease in sodium content.

Answers: **6. orthostatic hypotension; 7. diabetes insipidus.**

When evaluating this electrolyte imbalance, hyponatremia is classified as hypovolemic, hypervolemic, or euvolemic, depending on the amount of fluid in the patient's body.

In cases of hypovolemic hyponatremia, there is a decreased ECF volume and low sodium. With hypervolemic hyponatremia, there is an increase in ECF volume and low sodium. With euvolemic (isovolemic) hyponatremia, the ECF volume is normal and the sodium is low.

An inadequate dietary intake of sodium can be indicated in a patient who is on a strict sodium-restricted diet and is also on diuretics. This circumstance, however, is not common, because most diets contain adequate amounts of sodium.

Any condition that causes an increase in sodium excretion can deplete the serum sodium. Common causes of hyponatremia in this category include excessive sweating **(diaphoresis)**, GI wound drainage, diuretic use, decreased secretion of aldosterone, and renal disease. It is important to note that a large fluid loss from the GI tract that is treated with saline-free fluids may worsen the hyponatremia. People with cystic fibrosis have a high rate of sodium and chloride loss through the sweat glands and are at risk for electrolyte imbalance and heat prostration. Infants with cystic fibrosis are also at risk for hyponatremia because breast milk, formulas, and infant foods are low in sodium. Aggressive diuretic therapy, especially given with hypotonic IV fluids, can greatly deplete the sodium and potassium levels. Adrenal insufficiency, which causes a decrease in the production of aldosterone (the major mineralocorticoid), causes excessive renal loss of sodium and water, resulting in salt-wasting. (Remember that aldosterone helps sodium reabsorption from the renal tubules into the blood.) Renal disease may cause water retention in excess of sodium (volume excess).

Dilutional states are common causes of hyponatremia. *Pseudohyponatremia* is a term used when the sodium level is low, but the serum osmolality is normal. This condition is detected during situations in which excessive amounts of particles such as glucose, lipids, or protein reduce the amount of water in which sodium dissolves, causing the sodium level to be low relative to the other particles. Examples of these conditions are hyperglycemia, hyperlipidemia, and hyperproteinemia (seen in multiple myeloma). With hyperglycemia, the high glucose level dilutes the sodium, and the renal tubular flow rate is increased, causing further renal sodium loss in excess of water.

Other diseases that cause a dilution of serum sodium are CHF, nephrotic syndrome, cirrhosis, psychogenic polydipsia, ingestion of hypotonic fluids, and syndrome of inappropriate ADH secretion

(SIADH). Heart failure, nephrotic syndrome, and cirrhosis are diseases that have the potential to cause sodium and water retention, resulting in a hypervolemic hyponatremia.

Another cause of a hypotonic state occurs when the volume and rate of hypotonic IV fluids are excessive.

Syndrome of inappropriate ADH secretion, a common cause of hyponatremia, is caused by the continual secretion of ADH. The cause of SIADH stems from an increase in ADH levels from hypothalamic stimulation of ADH, excess production of ADH from ectopic sites, or the lack of renal responsiveness to ADH. Hypothalamic stimulation of ADH can occur with central nervous system (CNS) disorders (stroke or brain trauma), pain, excessive stress, or from narcotic medications, thiazide diuretic drugs, antineoplastic agents, oral hypoglycemic drugs, and psychoactive agents. An excess production of ADH from ectopic production can occur in paraneoplastic syndromes with malignancies, especially small cell lung cancer, and pulmonary disorders. A lack of renal responsiveness to ADH is indicated in certain types of renal disease.

In all of the previously mentioned processes, high levels of ADH result in excessive free-water retention and excessive loss of sodium in the urine, regardless of the low serum sodium levels. It is important for the health care provider to understand the basic pathophysiologic characteristics of SIADH because it is a common cause of hyponatremia. When the level of ADH rises, the renal tubules become more permeable, causing increased water retention and a rise in ECF volume (hypervolemia). This hypervolemic state causes an increased GFR, dilutional hyponatremia, decreased serum osmolality, and a decrease in aldosterone production. The hypervolemic hyponatremic status causes the fluids to shift into the intracellular space, resulting in intracellular fluid (ICF) excess, cellular edema, and water intoxication.

TAKE HOME POINTS

Patients who are NPO (nothing by mouth) without sodium replacement in the IV fluids are also at risk for hyponatremia.

When considering hyponatremia, it is important to remember that low serum sodium results in a decreased concentration gradient between the ECF and ICF. With less sodium available to move across the cell membrane, there is a delay in depolarization and excitability necessary for the transmission of neuromuscular impulse transmissions.

Another process that occurs in hyponatremia is the movement of water from the extracellular space to the intracellular space, causing the cells to swell and thus impairing normal cellular function. Knowing the basic pathophysiologic characteristics will help in understanding and identifying hyponatremia.

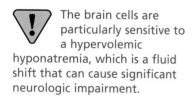

! The brain cells are particularly sensitive to a hypervolemic hyponatremia, which is a fluid shift that can cause significant neurologic impairment.

Psychogenic polydipsia, a psychiatric compulsion to drink excessive amounts of water, is a rare cause of water intoxication or ICF volume excess. During water intoxication, the excess fluid moves from the extracellular into the intracellular space, causing swelling of the cells.

Signs and Symptoms of Hyponatremia

- Serum sodium of less than 135 mEq/L
- Decreased urine-specific gravity
- Increased urinary output unless SIADH occurs
- Hallmark physical signs and symptoms: sleepiness, weakness, lethargy, nausea, vomiting, or anorexia
- Vital signs: temperature normal or below normal and possible tachypnea
- Cardiovascular signs and symptoms with hypovolemic hyponatremia: rapid pulse, hypotension, low central venous pressure, or flat neck veins
- Cardiovascular signs and symptoms with hypervolemic hyponatremia: rapid pulse, hypertension, elevated central venous pressure, or distended neck veins
- Cardiovascular signs and symptoms with euvolemic hyponatremia: rapid pulse and normal blood pressure
- Central nervous system signs and symptoms: lethargy, headache, behavioral or personality changes (depressed or excessive activity), confusion, seizures, or coma
- Muscle weakness, spasm, twitching, and diminished deep tendon reflexes
- Gastrointestinal symptoms: anorexia, nausea, vomiting, diarrhea, or hyperactive bowel sounds

What You DO

The goal of hyponatremia management is to restore the sodium level and correct the fluid imbalance by identifying and removing the precipitating cause and providing treatment aimed at the disease process. The treatment of hyponatremia should produce a gradual correction of the hyponatremia to avoid complications. Knowing which patients are at risk and the early signs and symptoms of hyponatremia is important.

The nursing assessment should include the following:

- Measurement of the patient's I & O
- Monitoring of the patient's daily weight
- Monitoring of the patient's laboratory values (e.g., serum sodium, chloride, osmolarity, glucose)

The specific treatment will depend on the cause of hyponatremia and whether it is associated with hypovolemia or hypervolemia. In general, it is safer to correct fluid retention hyponatremia by restricting fluid intake than it is to administer sodium.

Severe hyponatremia is often treated with IV fluids. Hypertonic saline solutions, which restore the sodium osmolality and fluid volume, are used to treat severe hypovolemic hyponatremia. An example of an IV hypertonic saline solution used to treat hyponatremia is 0.45% normal saline or 5% dextrose in 0.45% saline.

For hypervolemic hyponatremia, diuretics that have an osmotic diuretic effect, such as mannitol, are occasionally used. If CHF is present in patients who are hypervolemic, then loop diuretics, angiotensin-converting enzyme (ACE) inhibitors, and fluid restriction may be ordered. The registered nurse should monitor the patient for symptoms of excessive fluid loss, such as hypotension and oliguria, as well as closely follow laboratory values.

In cases of mild hyponatremia, increasing the dietary intake of sodium may be all that is necessary. Nutritional counseling may be provided for patients who need to increase their oral sodium intake. Occasionally, oral sodium supplements are ordered. Fluid restriction may or may not be indicated, depending on the cause of the hyponatremia. For example, with mild dilutional hyponatremia, fluid restriction is often the treatment of choice. Accurate measurement of I & O and daily weights are necessary. The patient and family should be taught about the importance of fluid restriction and given the specific amounts of fluid allowed per day. It is important to point out which foods are high in fluid content, such as fruits (melons) and vegetables.

When hyponatremia is caused by SIADH, the treatment is aimed at identifying and treating the causative factor. With malignancies, treatment of the primary tumor with chemotherapy or radiation is often helpful in controlling SIADH. In other situations, the discontinuation of medications that are causing SIADH alleviates the problem. Occasionally, SIADH becomes a chronic, irreversible problem and is then managed with fluid restriction of 1 liter per day and medications. Demeclocycline, a tetracycline derivative, blocks the action of ADH at the renal tubule and is often prescribed in this case. The side effects of demeclocycline include azotemia, DI, renal impairment, and liver toxicity, which are reversible when the drug is discontinued.

Other common conditions that can cause hyponatremia should be identified and treated. For example, with hyperglycemia, gaining better control of the blood sugar by managing the DI is helpful in regaining sodium balance. With thyroid deficiency, administering thyroid replacement is important. With hypoaldosteronism, mineralocorticoid replacement therapy is necessary to restore electrolyte imbalance. The health care provider plays an important role in identifying, treating, and managing patients with sodium imbalances. Through proper assessment, intervention, evaluation, and patient education, any sodium imbalance can be managed successfully.

TAKE HOME POINTS

The health care provider's assessment and documentation of signs and symptoms of hyponatremia is the first factor in identifying and treating this problem early.

- Excessive hypertonic rehydration can cause cerebral edema; therefore the health care provider needs to monitor the patient's vital signs and neurologic status.
- Severe electrolyte imbalances are life threatening, and the treatment is often managed in the intensive care unit (ICU), where rapid correction is usually restricted to raising the sodium by not more than 10 mEq/L in 24 hours.

Do You UNDERSTAND?

DIRECTIONS: **Indicate in the spaces provided whether the following statements are *true* or *false*.**

1. ______ Hypovolemic hyponatremia causes an increase in ECF volume.
2. ______ With euvolemic hyponatremia, the ECF volume is normal.
3. ______ SIADH is caused by a decrease in ADH secretion.
4. ______ Urine specific gravity will be decreased with hyponatremia.
5. ______ Venous pressure increases with hypovolemic hyponatremia.

DIRECTIONS: **Match the definitions in column A with the words in column B.**

Column A	Column B
6. ______ Osmotic injury to myelinated nerve fibers causing paralysis, which can occur from a rapid correction of hyponatremia.	a. Mineralocorticoids
7. ______ Basic treatment for mild dilutional hyponatremia.	b. Fluid restriction
8. ______ A drug that blocks the action of ADH at the renal tubule, and is used to treat hyponatremia.	c. Demeclocycline
9. ______ Agents used to restore electrolyte imbalance in patients with hypoaldosteronism.	d. Loop diuretic
10. ______ A commonly used drug given to treat CHF in patients with hypervolemic hyponatremia.	e. Osmotic demyelination syndrome

TAKE HOME POINTS

Close hemodynamic monitoring, control of the infusion rate, and assessing the patient's response are important because a correction that is too rapid may cause osmotic demyelination syndrome (central pontine myelinolysis: an osmotic injury to myelinated nerve fibers causing paralysis).

LIFE SPAN

When administering fluids, monitor the fluid balance carefully for patients with cardiovascular problems and for older adults, to prevent or detect CHF.

Answers: 1. False. In hypovolemic conditions, there is a decrease in extracellular volume; 2. True. Euvolemic, also known as isovolemic, implies normal ECF volume; 3. False. SIADH is caused by an increase in ADH, which causes excessive free water retention and excessive loss of Na^+ in the urine, resulting in hyponatremia; 4. True. The urine is more dilute with hyponatremia; 5. False. Hypovolemia implies lower fluid volume. During hypovolemic states, the central venous pressure is decreased, along with an increased pulse and hypotension; 6. e; 7. b; 8. c; 9. a; 10. d.

References

Chernecky CC, Berger BJ: Hyponatremia. In Chernecky C, Berger B, editors: *Advanced and critical care oncology nursing: managing primary complications,* Philadelphia, 1998, Saunders.

Evans MD, Evans C, Evans R: *Special tests: the procedure and meaning of common tests in hospital,* St Louis, 2003, Mosby.

Malick LB: Fluid, electrolyte, and acid-base imbalances. In Lewis SM, Heitkemper MM, Dirksen SR, editors: *Medical surgical nursing: assessment and management of clinical problems,* St Louis, 2004, Mosby.

McMullen AH, Bryson EA: Cystic fibrosis. In Allen PJ, Vessey JA, editors: *Primary care of the child with a chronic condition,* St Louis, 2004, Mosby.

Schulz K: Hypernatremia. In Chernecky C, Berger B, editors: *Advanced and critical care oncology nursing: managing primary complications,* Philadelphia, 1998, Saunders.

Skidmore-Roth L: *Mosby's 2004 nursing drug reference,* St Louis, 2004, Mosby.

NCLEX® Review

Read the following case study and answer the next five questions associated with this case study:

Mr. Joseph, an 82-year-old retired school principal, was admitted to the hospital for confusion. His medical history included hypertension, and a 50 pack-a-year smoking history. He takes furosemide (Lasix) 40 mg PO BID. The day before admission, he became disoriented and began vomiting. The admitting laboratories included a serum sodium, which was 122 mEq/L. Vital signs were temperature 37°C (98.6°F), pulse 96 and regular, blood pressure 104/58 mm Hg, and respirations 20. The Lasix was discontinued, and he was given 3 L normal saline (0.9% sodium chloride) over 12 hours and placed on a high-sodium diet. Compazine 25 mg suppository q8h PRN for nausea was ordered. The next day his sodium level was 130 mEq/L, and he was sent home on a reduced dose of Lasix 20 mg PO qd, with a follow-up appointment in 3 days with his geriatric nurse practitioner (NP). During his follow-up appointment, the NP noted that he had lost 15 pounds over the past 4 months and complained of fatigue and an occasional cough. A chest radiograph showed a 2-mm mass in the right middle lobe. Mr. Joseph was referred to a pulmonary specialist for biopsy and further work-up. The pathology report on the lung biopsy was positive for small cell lung cancer.

1. Why was Mr. Joseph's furosemide (Lasix) initially discontinued, followed by a dose reduction?
1 Nausea is a common side effect of Lasix.
2 Overdiuresis can result in hyponatremia.
3 Lasix often causes confusion in older adults.
4 Vomiting is a common side effect of Lasix.

2. What would be the danger of giving Mr. Joseph a hypertonic solution of sodium chloride and dextrose rather than the isotonic solution that was prescribed?
1 This would cause a hyperglycemic reaction.
2 This usually causes a rebound hypernatremia.
3 Too rapid a correction of the sodium level can cause cerebral edema.
4 Hypertonic solutions should only be used in the intensive care unit.

3. Mr. Joseph's pulse was slightly high, with low blood pressure. He has vomited several times and has been on diuretics. During his oral care, you note a dry mucosa. Given this history and physical findings, the health care practitioner would suspect which of the following problems:
1 Hyperglycemia
2 Alzheimer's disease
3 Hypothyroidism
4 Dehydration

4. Mr. Joseph's lung biopsy was positive for a malignancy. With this in mind, what other problems besides the dehydration may have been contributing to his hyponatremia?
1 Syndrome of inappropriate antidiuretic hormone (SIADH)
2 Hyperaldosteronism
3 Excessive use of sodium bicarbonate for nausea
4 Hyperthyroidism

5. Which type of cancer accounts for the highest incidence of SIADH in cancer patients?
1 Lung cancer
2 Breast cancer
3 Uterine cancer
4 Childhood cancers

6. The health care practitioner is caring for a 62-year-old diabetic with chronic renal failure who was admitted with dehydration, hyponatremia, and a urinary tract infection with suspected sepsis. The patient has already received several liters of intravenous (IV) fluids, and the health care practitioner has just prescribed gentamicin, an IV antibiotic. In addition to checking the serum sodium levels, the health care practitioner should check what other laboratory test before starting the IV antibiotics?

7. Which type of diet would most likely be recommended for a patient with heart failure?

1 High-fiber
2 Low-residual
3 Soft
4 Low-sodium

8. Treatment of hyponatremia includes IV sodium replacement, which needs to be done cautiously and slowly to prevent which complication?
   1 Osmotic demyelination
   2 SIADH
   3 Hypoaldosteronism
   4 Hyperglycemia

9. Your patient, who has mild hyponatremia, has been placed on a high-sodium diet. Which food groups would you encourage your patient to eat?
   1 Fresh fruits
   2 Whole grains
   3 Canned vegetables
   4 Dairy products

10. Which patient is at the highest risk for developing hyponatremia?
    1 Older male adult with chronic obstructive pulmonary disease
    2 Older female adult with congestive heart failure
    3 Young female adult with systemic lupus erythematosus
    4 Young male adult with fever, severe vomiting, and diarrhea

11. Sodium is essential for the transmission of _______________ in muscles and nerves.

12. The adrenal cortex produces the hormone _______________, which regulates sodium balance by stimulating the renal tubules to conserve water and sodium when the serum sodium level is low.

13. _______________ is a genetic disease that causes people to lose abnormal amounts of sodium and chloride in the sweat, which puts them at risk for hyponatremia.

14. True or False: Atrial natriuretic peptide (ANP) is a cardiovascular hormone that suppresses the effects of aldosterone on the kidney, thereby decreasing the reabsorption of sodium and increasing its excretion.

15. True or False: Diuretics act by preventing resorption of sodium and water by the kidneys.

NCLEX® Review Answers

1. 2 Diuretics can result in dehydration with a hypovolemic hyponatremia. Furosemide (Lasix) does not commonly cause confusion or nausea or vomiting.

2. 3 The neurocells are highly sensitive to fluid shifts. Although hypertonic solutions can cause hypernatremia, this is not always the case and can be avoided by close monitoring by a medical-surgical or long-term care nursing unit. The dextrose in the hypertonic solution is not enough to cause hyperglycemia.

3. 4 Patients who are on diuretics and have fluid loss are at risk for developing dehydration. Signs of dehydration may include an increased pulse, low blood pressure, confusion, and dry oral mucosa.

4. 1 Some malignancies can produce antidiuretic hormones, resulting SIADH. (2, 3, and 4 are conditions that can cause hypernatremia.)

5. 1 SIADH is a paraneoplastic syndrome associated with many malignancies, but it occurs more frequently in small cell lung cancer than it does in other types.

6. Serum creatinine. The serum creatinine reflects renal function. Many IV antibiotics, especially the aminoglycosides, are nephrotoxic. Because this patient has a known history of renal failure, assessing the renal status by monitoring the creatinine level is an important part of the fluid and electrolyte assessment process.

7. 4 Sodium tends to cause fluid retention, which is contraindicated for patients with heart failure. A high-fiber diet causes bulky stools. A soft diet would cause runny stools.

8. 1 Osmotic demyelination. When sodium is replaced too rapidly, the neurologic cells swell, which causes severe neurologic complications, such as cerebral edema.

9. 3 Canned vegetables and processed meats are high in sodium. Fresh fruits, whole grains, and dairy products are low in sodium.

10. 4 Young man with fever and severe vomiting and diarrhea, because of the significant loss of sodium and water in the body fluids.

11. Impulses.

12. Aldosterone.

13. Cystic fibrosis.

14. True.

15. True.

Notes

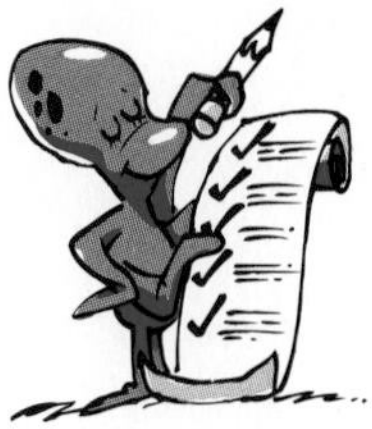

Chapter

4

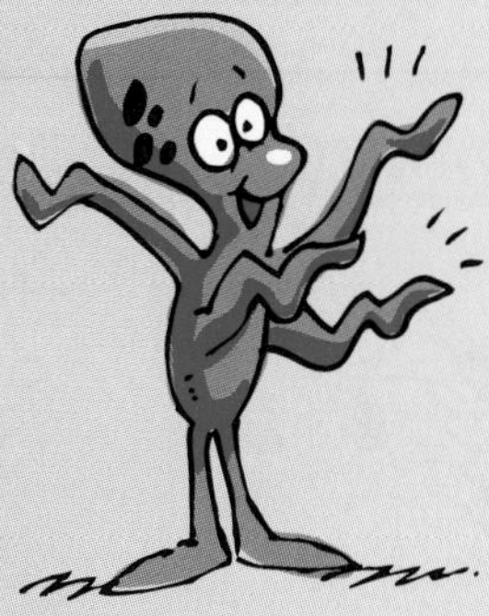

Chloride

What You WILL LEARN

After reading this chapter, you will know how to do the following:

- ✔ Describe the role of chloride in maintaining homeostasis.
- ✔ Define hyperchloremia.
- ✔ Differentiate hypochloremia from hyperchloremia.

What IS Chloride?

Serum *chloride* (Cl^-) is the most abundant extracellular anion and makes up two thirds of the plasma anions. Although often viewed as the least important electrolyte to measure for routine screening, chloride plays a major role in maintaining the metabolic acid-base balance and in assessing the anion gap. In the body, chloride combines with cations to form sodium chloride, potassium chloride, calcium chloride, and hydrochloric acid. Chloride provides electroneutrality, especially in relation to sodium and potassium. Chloride works with sodium to maintain osmotic pressure.

Normal Serum Chloride Values

- Newborn 98-104 mEq/L
- Infant 95-110 mEq/L
- Child 101-105mEq/L
- Adult 95-110 mEq/L
- Critical level: < 80 mEq/L or > 115 mEq/L

Approximately 80% of the total body chloride is found in the extracellular fluid (ECF), with the greatest concentration in lymph and interstitial fluid. The cerebrospinal fluid is made up of sodium chloride (NaCl). The intracellular chloride level is minimal; however, it is essential because it is found in specialized cells, such as nerve cells.

What You NEED TO KNOW

Sources of Chloride

Chloride is derived solely from exogenous sources that include ingested foods and drugs. The major dietary source of chloride is table salt (½ teaspoon equals 750 mg of chloride). Other sources of sodium chloride include meat, dairy products, and processed foods. Foods high in sodium (Na^+) are also high in chloride.

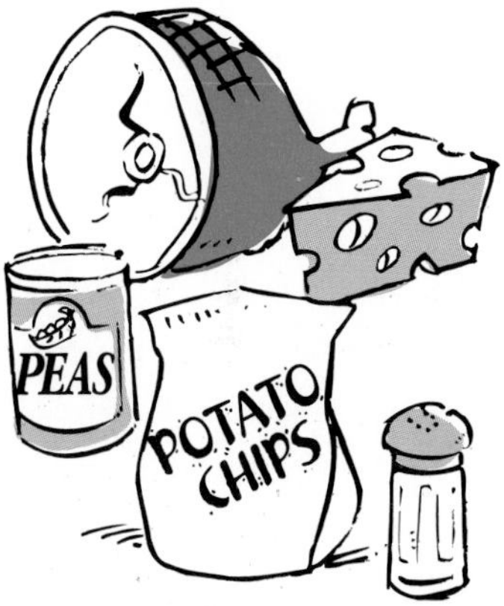

Table salt is the largest dietary source of chloride. Other sources include meat, dairy products, and processed foods.

Control of Chloride

Ingested chloride is almost totally absorbed by the colon, with small amounts absorbed by the ileum in exchange for bicarbonate. Chloride absorption from the colon exceeds sodium absorption. The stomach produces chloride in the form of hydrochloric acid.

Approximately 90% of chloride is excreted in the urine; the rest is excreted in feces and sweat. Excretion depends on the amount of chloride ingested and the presence of adequate fluid.

Reabsorption of chloride occurs in the renal tubules in response to the pH of the ECF to maintain normal acid-base balance. Chloride competes with bicarbonate for sodium to maintain an acid-base balance. When body fluids are acidic, chloride and sodium are excreted by the kidneys and bicarbonate is reabsorbed. Conversely, when the body fluids are basic (**alkalotic**), more sodium chloride is reabsorbed by the kidneys. The concentration of chloride varies inversely with changes in the bicarbonate level.

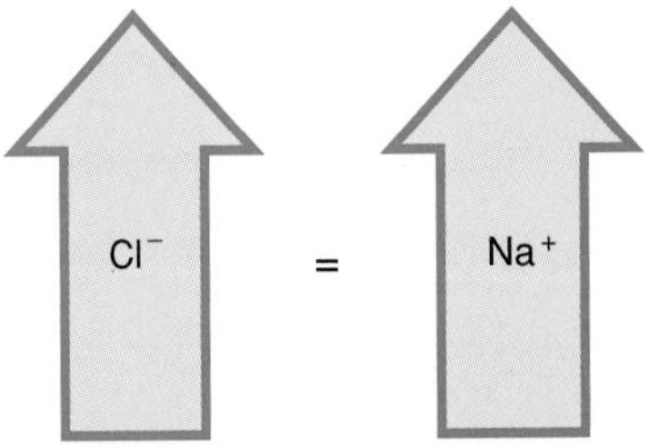

When body fluids are alkalotic, more chloride and sodium is reabsorbed by the kidneys.

Cystic fibrosis, an autosomal recessive genetic disease, causes abnormal chloride transport, resulting in a lack of sodium chloride in the secretions of the exocrine glands, such as the pancreas, intestine, and bronchi. The pancreas and bronchi become obstructed with the thick mucus, causing malabsorption, steatorrhea, chronic pancreatitis, abnormal sweat (high chloride content), and respiratory infections.

Functions of Chloride

The principle role of chloride in the body, along with sodium, is the regulation of osmotic pressure and water balance, and the maintenance of electroneutrality.

Chloride plays a vital role in the production of hydrochloric acid in the stomach, which is necessary for digestion. It serves as a buffer and enzyme activator for gastric hydrochloric acid. Alterations of gastric juices from vomiting and suctioning can affect chloride levels.

Chloride plays a role in acid-base balance. Maintenance of a constant pH in the body occurs through a process known as the *chloride shift.* Low-blood pH causes the diffusion of bicarbonate, a weak acid ion, from the red cells to the plasma in exchange for chloride, a strong acid ion, from the plasma to the red cells.

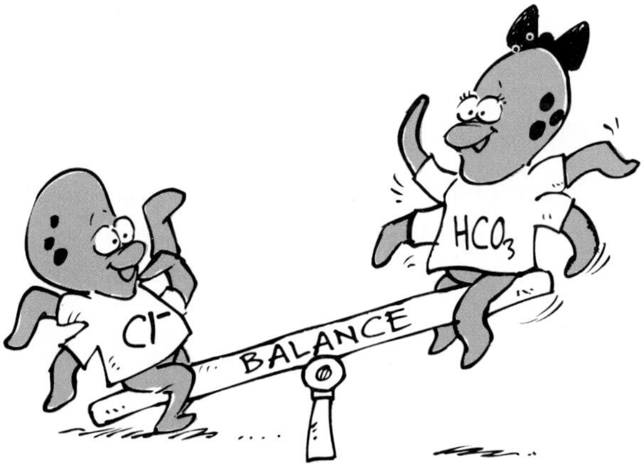

Do You UNDERSTAND?

DIRECTIONS: **Unscramble the italicized words to complete the statements.**

1. One quarter teaspoon of ________________________ equals 750 mg of chloride. *(batel lats)*
2. Eighty percent of chloride is found in the ECF, and ____________ percent of anions are chloride. *(tixsy-vesen)*
3. Chloride regulates ________________________. *(micotso reseuspr nad tware alneabc)*

Answers: 1. table salt; 2. sixty-seven; 3. osmotic pressure and water balance.

What IS Hyperchloremia?

A serum chloride level greater than 110 milliequivalents per liter (mEq/L) is called *hyperchloremia.*

What You NEED TO KNOW

A high serum chloride level is rare, but it may occur with intravascular fluid decreases and dehydration, bicarbonate deficiency, hypernatremia, decreased ventilation, shock, starvation, diabetic ketoacidosis, or metabolic acidosis secondary to ingestion of acid precursors, such as salicylate, ethylene glycol, or methanol. Medications can cause hyperchloremia by absorption of the chloride in the agent or from the drug causing chloride retention.

Chloride and bicarbonate have an inverse relationship. When chloride levels are high, the kidneys excrete bicarbonate to compensate, which can lead to acidosis. Bicarbonate deficiency occurs when the body's alkaline buffers titrate organic acids. Organic anions and carbon dioxide (CO_2) are formed when the organic acids react with bicarbonate. Normally, retained anions metabolize and produce bicarbonate. When the anions are excreted by the kidneys to compensate for low-serum pH, hyperchloremic acidosis occurs.

Hyperchloremia can lead to hyperchloremic metabolic acidosis, which occurs when bicarbonate ions are lost through the kidneys or the gastrointestinal (GI) tract. Acidosis from an accumulation of chloride ions in acidifying salts with decrease in bicarbonate ions also occurs. The chloride level is high, and the bicarbonate level is low, but the unmeasured anions are unchanged. To verify that metabolic acidosis is the cause of the acidotic state, a laboratory test called the anion gap is calculated. If the anion gap is normal, it is likely that the cause of acidosis is metabolic in nature. The anion gap indirectly measures the relationship between the cations and anions. Because sodium is the major cation, and chloride and bicarbonate are the major anions, the difference or gap between these two major cations and anions indirectly measures the anions that are not routinely measured, such as lactic acid, ketone acids, sulfates, phosphates, and proteins. To calculate the anion gap, add the serum chloride and bicarbonate, and subtract this number from the serum sodium level (chloride + bicarbonate) – (sodium) = Anion Gap. Remember the anion gap is the amount of the other anions (sulfates, phosphates, proteins, lactic acid, and ketone acids), and this remains unchanged in metabolic acidosis.

Chloride works closely with sodium, and therefore it is important to note that hyperchloremia often occurs with hypernatremia and other imbalances, such as hypervolemia, and metabolic acidosis.

Medications can cause hyperchloremia. Ammonium chloride, used as an acidifier in metabolic alkalosis, a urinary acidifier, or an expectorant, can raise chloride levels from the additional ingestion of chloride. Sodium polystyrene sulfonate (Kayexalate), a potassium-removing resin, exchanges the cations potassium and chloride causing potassium to be excreted and chloride to be absorbed in the colon.

TAKE HOME POINTS

Loss of anions in the urine produces loss of bicarbonates.

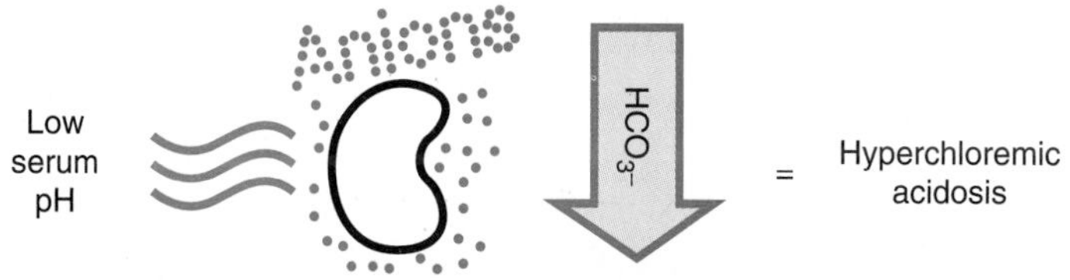

When retained anions are excreted by the kidneys to compensate for low serum pH, hyperchloremia acidosis occurs.

Signs and Symptoms of Hyperchloremia

- Hyperventilation (tachypnea). Respiratory compensation in an attempt to blow off carbon dioxide; excess carbon dioxide combines with water to form carbonic acid (H_2CO_3).
- Decreased cardiac output
- Peripheral vasodilatation
- Compensation for decreased fluid balance
- Headache
- Lethargy
- Hypotension, decreased cardiac output, volume depletion (headache, lethargy)
- Associated laboratory data: Elevated serum chloride, sodium, low pH, and elevated bicarbonate
- Hyperchloremia is often associated with metabolic acidosis and with a decreased level of consciousness, Kussmaul's respirations, and weakness. Hyperchloremia is also associated with hypernatremia, and therefore the health care worker should watch for signs of agitation, tachypnea, tachycardia, hypertension, and edema.

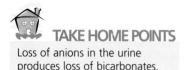

What You DO

The goals of hyperchloremic management are to correct fluid imbalance, increase blood pH, and increase bicarbonate levels. The registered nurse should do the following:

- Assess laboratory values for elevated chloride and sodium.
- Assess laboratory values for low serum pH (acidotic) and low bicarbonate level.
- Assess laboratory values for anion gap (normal anion gap with a low pH and bicarbonate level indicate metabolic acidosis).
- Administer intravenous (IV) hydration.
- Replace bicarbonate with sodium bicarbonate to increase blood pH.
- Continually monitor the levels of consciousness and respiratory status.

A rapid increase in the blood pH and the bicarbonate should be avoided. It may cause a paradoxical cerebrospinal fluid acidosis.

Do You UNDERSTAND?

DIRECTIONS: **Indicate in the spaces provided whether the following statements are *true* or *false*.**

1. _____ Chloride helps regulate osmotic pressure.
2. _____ A major dietary source of chloride is black pepper.
3. _____ The majority of total body chloride is found in the ECF.
4. _____ Excess ingestion of salicylates may lead to hyperchloremia.

What IS Hypochloremia?

Hypochloremia is defined as a serum level below 95 mEq/L. Hypochloremia may be caused by several factors. Chloride is excreted in perspiration, the GI tract, and kidneys. Because chloride is a negative ion (anion) and is usually attached to a positive ion (cation), such as calcium or potassium, these levels usually drop along with chloride in hypochloremia. Any condition that causes a decrease in sodium and potassium will also reduce the chloride level.

Answers: 1. True; 2. False; 3. True; 4. True.

What You NEED TO KNOW

Diarrhea, profuse perspiration, excessive loss of gastric acid from (GI) suctioning, vomiting, or fistula drainage may also lead to hypochloremia. People with cystic fibrosis lose abnormal amounts of sodium and chloride through perspiration and are at risk for dehydration secondary to electrolyte imbalance. Diabetic ketoacidosis and Addison's disease, which alter the acid-base and electrolyte balance, can lead to hypochloremia. Conditions such as emphysema, pneumonia, pulmonary edema, or hypoventilation may lead to respiratory acidosis. The renal tubules compensate for increased acid by increasing renal excretion of acid in the form of hydrogen ions, thereby leading to hypochloremia. Increased renal excretion of acid also occurs with the administration of loop, osmotic, or thiazide diuretics.

Decreased intake of dietary chloride is often observed with low sodium (sodium chloride) diets in the treatment of cardiac, renal, or hepatic disorders. Infant formulas deficient in chloride may result in hypochloremia, but this is rare. Postoperative patients on IV solutions without electrolytes are at risk for hypochloremia (usually seen in conjunction with hyponatremia). Any condition that alters the fluid balance, such as congestive heart failure and fluid overload, can cause a relative decrease in chloride. Removal of large amounts of ascitic fluid can cause a loss of chloride.

Excessive administration of bicarbonate or bicarbonate precursors, such as sodium lactate or sodium citrate, may increase levels of bicarbonate and decrease levels of chloride.

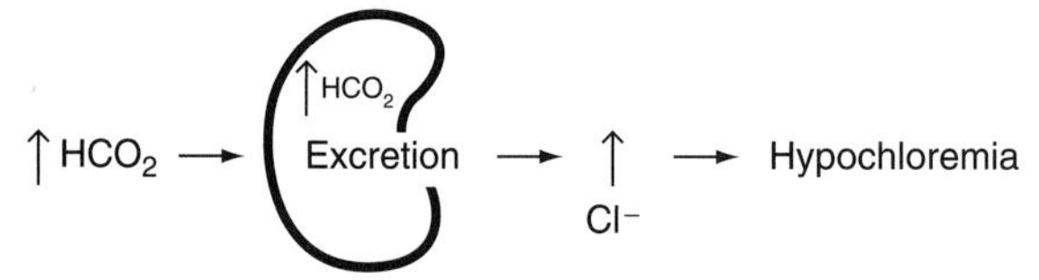

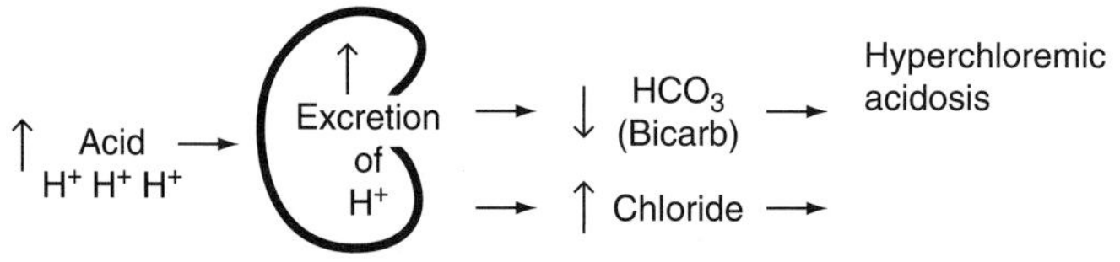

Signs and Symptoms of Hypochloremia

- Hypoventilation, caused by increased serum bicarbonate with compensatory excretion of chloride
- Tetany
- Hyperactive deep tendon reflexes
- Muscle cramps
- Paresthesia of extremities
- Restlessness/agitation
- Confusion
- Convulsions

It is important to note that tetany, paresthesia of the extremities, restlessness, confusion, and convulsions can be the result of metabolic alkalotic states that cause hypocalcemia from the binding of calcium to protein. Decreased calcium causes alterations in the calcium pump necessary for muscle contraction and relaxation and leads to muscle irritability. This often accompanies hypochloremia.

What You DO

Management of hypochloremia includes treating the underlying cause and replacing chloride with IV fluids and oral intake. Factors to consider are diet, IV fluid solutions, emesis control, GI suctioning reduction, and correction of metabolic alkalosis or electrolyte imbalance.

The health care provider should do the following:

- Assess laboratory values of chloride, sodium, and calcium, as well as creatinine for renal function.
- Assess laboratory values of pH and bicarbonate (elevated pH and decreased bicarbonate indicates metabolic alkalosis).
- Encourage the patient to consume salty, high-sodium chloride foods if oral intake is possible.
- Teach the patient and family about foods that contain chloride by providing a list.
- Administer acid inhibitors or institute treatment for nausea, vomiting, or diarrhea to correct GI acid loss.
- Discontinue diuretic therapy to decrease renal excretion of acid.

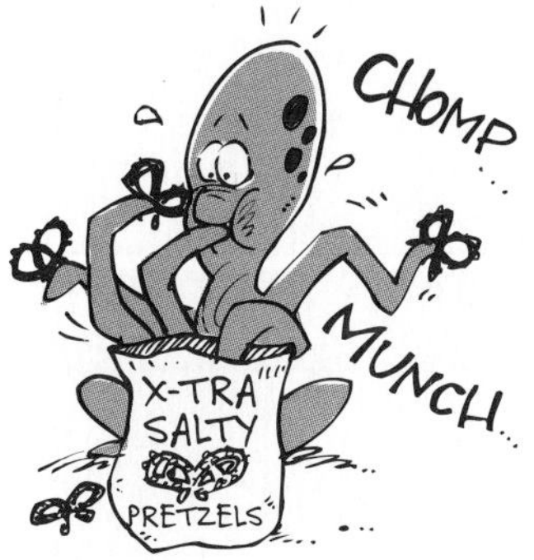

For treatment of hypochloremia, it is helpful to encourage the patient to consume salty, high-sodium foods.

TAKE HOME POINTS

Types of fluid solutions containing chloride are Na^+Cl^- and K^+Cl^-.

- Assess for seizures, and institute safety precautions as hypochloremia causes stimulation of the central nervous system.
- Ammonium chloride IV may be ordered in severe cases of metabolic alkalosis.

Do You UNDERSTAND?

DIRECTIONS: **Indicate whether the following symptoms indicate *hyperchloremia* or *hypochloremia.***

1. ______________________ Tetany
2. ______________________ Restlessness
3. ______________________ Lethargy
4. ______________________ Hypotension
5. ______________________ Hypoventilation
6. ______________________ Hyperventilation

References

Evans D, Evans C, Evans R: *Special tests: the procedure and meaning of common tests in hospital,* St Louis, 2003, Mosby.

Huether S: The cellular environment: fluids and electrolytes, acids and bases. In McCance K, Huether S, editors: *Pathophysiology: the biologic basis for disease in adults and children,* St Louis, 2002, Mosby.

McMullen AH, Bryson EA: Cystic fibrosis. In Allen PJ, Vess JA, editors: *Primary care of the child with a chronic condition,* St Louis, 2004, Mosby.

Oh MS, Uribarri J: Electrolytes, water, and acid-base balance. In Shils ME et al, editors: *Modern nutrition in health and disease,* Baltimore, 1999, Williams & Wilkins.

Skidmore-Roth L: *Mosby's 2004 nursing drug reference,* St Louis, 2004, Mosby.

Terry J: The major electrolytes: sodium, potassium, and chloride, *J Intraven Nurs* 17(5):240, 1994.

Whitney EN, Cataldo CB, Rolfes SR: *Understanding normal and clinical nutrition,* Belmont, CA, 1998, Wadsworth.

Answers: **1. hypochloremia; 2. hypochloremia; 3. hyperchloremia; 4. hyperchloremia; 5. hypochloremia; 6. hyperchloremia.**

NCLEX® Review

1. JJ, age 30, has a history of irritable bowel syndrome with chronic diarrhea. His chloride level is 93. You are to give him dietary instructions about foods high in chloride. This list would include all of the following *except:*
   1 Cheese
   2 Potato chips
   3 Broccoli
   4 Baked ham

2. TJ, age 22, is found unconscious in her apartment. Her respiratory rate is 42 with a blood pressure of 60/40 mm Hg. An empty bottle of aspirin is found on the floor. She is diagnosed with salicylate poisoning. What would you expect her bicarbonate level to be?
   1 Above normal
   2 Normal
   3 Below normal
   4 Very high

3. KZ, age 35, is a construction worker who is working on a new high-rise building in Florida. His boss brings him to your clinic because of KZ's intermittent confusion and complaints of muscle cramps, as well as numbness and tingling of his hands and legs. KZ's blood pressure on admission is 80/46 mm Hg. You suspect KZ is exhibiting symptoms of which of the following?
   1 Decreased chloride level
   2 Increased chloride level
   3 Decreased bicarbonate level
   4 Increased sodium level

4. Hypochloremia is caused by all of the following *except:*
   1 Vomiting
   2 Diarrhea
   3 Diuretic therapy
   4 Salicylate poisoning

5. PZ, age 16, has swallowed 38 tablets of a salicylate medication in an attempted suicide. Her serum chloride is 118 mEq/L. What would you expect her apical pulse and blood pressure to be?
   1 Bradycardia, hypotension
   2 Bradycardia, hypertension
   3 Tachycardia, hypotension
   4 Tachycardia, hypertension

6. You are caring for a 36-year-old woman, admitted with pancreatitis, who is being treated with continuous nasogastric suction and pain medication. The patient now complains of weakness, agitation, and muscle cramps. Which electrolyte imbalance would you suspect?

7. Chloride, the most abundant negatively charged ion (anion), binds with which cation?
   1 Magnesium
   2 Sodium
   3 Potassium
   4 Calcium

8. Most diets provide adequate amounts of chloride in the common source of:
   1 Table salt
   2 Drinking water
   3 Red meats
   4 Seafood

9. Acid-base balance involves the regulation of chloride and which other anion?
   1 Bicarbonate
   2 Iron
   3 Phosphorus
   4 Potassium

10. A common cause of hypochloremia in the hospitalized patient is:
    1 Gastric suctioning
    2 Diarrhea

3 Fever
4 Diuretics

11. Chloride (Cl) and bicarbonate (HCO_3) have a(n) ________________ relationship.

12. What is the formula for calculating the anion gap?

13. True or False: The anion gap is elevated in hyperchloremic metabolic acidosis.

14. True or False: A newborn with cystic fibrosis, who is being breast-fed, is at risk for hypernatremia or hyperchloremia.

15. True or False: Jane, a 48-year-old woman, underwent a partial gastrectomy for cancer, has a nasogastric tube to suction, and on the third postoperative day developed hypochloremia. This places her at risk for developing metabolic alkalosis.

NCLEX® Review Answers

1. 3 All of the foods listed (cheese, potato chips, baked ham) are high in sodium chloride except broccoli.

2. 3 The salicylate poisoning creates an acidic state. The bicarbonate level is decreased below normal.

3. 1 KZ is exhibiting signs and symptoms of decreased chloride level related to profuse sweating while working in a hot climate.

4. 4 Salicylate poisoning would cause hyperchloremia.

5. 1 Because of a decreased cardiac output in salicylate toxicity, you have a decreased pulse and low blood pressure.

6. Hypochloremia. Gastric and gastrointestinal track fluid loss causes a loss of chloride. Weakness, agitation, and muscle cramps are signs and symptoms of hypochloremia.

7. 2 Sodium and chloride work together to maintain serum osmolality and water balance. Potassium, calcium, and magnesium do not bind to chloride.

8. 1 Table salt, also known as sodium chloride, usually provides a sufficient amount of chloride. Drinking water, red meats, and seafood do not contain chloride.

9. 1 Bicarbonate. The body maintains the acid-base level through an inverse relationship between chloride and bicarbonate. When the chloride levels decrease, the kidneys retain bicarbonate. When the chloride levels rise, the kidneys excrete bicarbonate. Iron and phosphorus do not interact with chloride. Potassium is a cation.

10. 1 Gastric suctioning. Chloride is concentrated in the gastric, bile, and pancreatic fluids; therefore, removal of these fluids over a period may result in decreased chloride levels.

11. Inverse.

12. (Chloride + Bicarbonate) − Sodium = Anion Gap

13. False. The anion gap remains normal in metabolic acidosis, indicating that the acidosis is likely caused by a loss of bicarbonate ions through the kidneys.

14. False. People with cystic fibrosis have abnormal sodium and chloride loss in their sweat and are at risk for hyponatremia/hypochloremia and dehydration.

15. True. Nasogastric suction causes a loss of hydrochloric acid, causing hypochloremia, which can result in metabolic alkalosis.

Notes

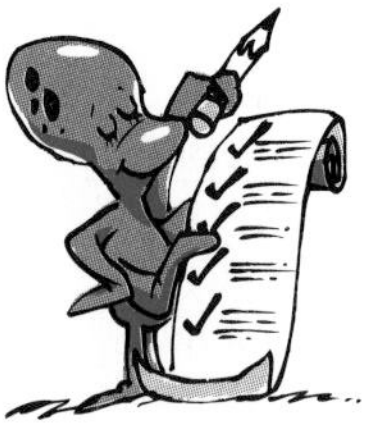

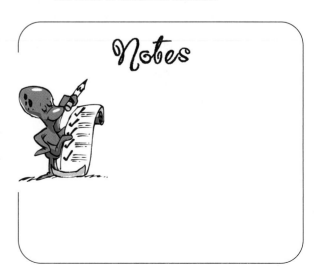

Potassium

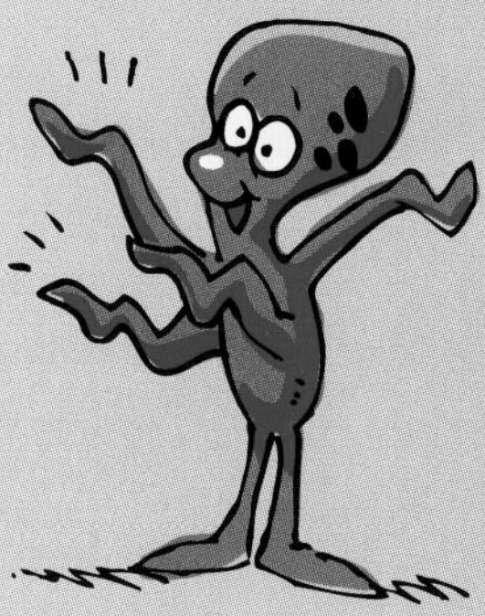

Chapter

5

What You WILL LEARN

After reading this chapter, you will know how to do the following:

✔ State two roles that potassium plays in the function of the human body.

✔ Define hyperkalemia.

✔ Identify two causes of hypokalemia.

What IS Potassium?

Potassium (K^+) is the major positively charged ion **(cation)** in the intracellular fluid (ICF). Of the body's potassium, 98% is found inside the cell (40 to 50 mEq/kg body weight). The remaining 2% is located outside the cell in the extracellular fluid (ECF) (1 mmol/kg of body weight). The ratio is 40:1 ICF to ECF. Normal serum level will fall between 3.5 and 5 mEq/L.

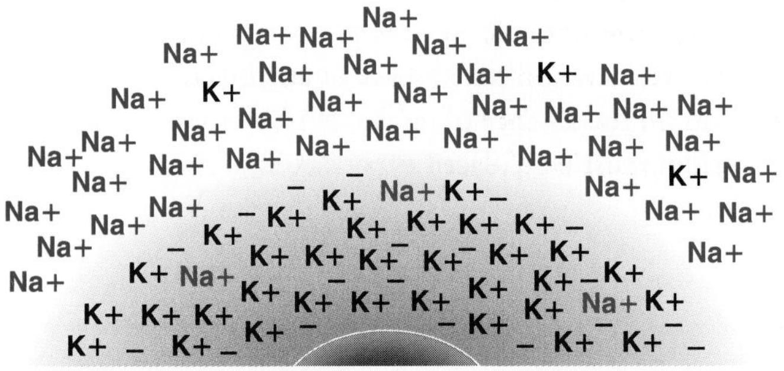

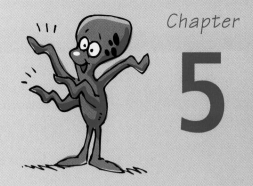

Potassium is constantly moving in and out of the cell. This movement is controlled by the sodium-potassium pump. Nerve–cell communication and the initiation of muscle contraction is dependent on this movement of potassium in and out of the cell. Potassium affects the depolarization and repolarization phases of the cardiac cycle.

TAKE HOME POINTS

Normal laboratory values are found on all laboratory slips or computer results.

Potassium Distribution

Enhances Movement into the Cells	Impairs Movement into the Cells
Insulin	Glucagon
Beta-adrenergic stimuli	Beta-blocking drugs, alpha-adrenergic stimuli
Alkalosis	Acidosis
Acute increase in osmolality	Acute cell-tissue breakdown

What You NEED TO KNOW

TAKE HOME POINTS

- 98% potassium is in the ICF.
- Normal serum level falls between 3.5 and 5.0 mEq/L.
- Nerve–cell communication and the initiation of muscle contraction are dependent on the ability of potassium to move in and out of the cell.
- Potassium affects the depolarization and repolarization phases of the cardiac cycle.

Sources of Potassium

The body needs 40 to 60 mEq/day of potassium. Foods high in potassium include meats; lentils; fruits such as bananas, cantaloupe, avocados, and dried fruit (e.g., apricots, dates, raisins, peaches, figs); green leafy vegetables; bran cereal; and molasses.

Control of Potassium

Insulin, catecholamines (increased renin-angiotensin leads to increased aldosterone), and aldosterone (promotes potassium excretion) affect the distribution of potassium between the ICF and ECF and help regulate total-body potassium. The kidneys excrete approximately 90% of potassium. Approximately 40 to 80 mEq of potassium is excreted in the urine every day. Approximately 10% of potassium is excreted through the bowel and sweat glands.

The kidneys are not able to conserve potassium efficiently and continue to excrete it even in the absence of any intake. The minimum loss of potassium (in the absence of intake) is 10 to 15 mEq/day. This means that potassium must be replaced every day.

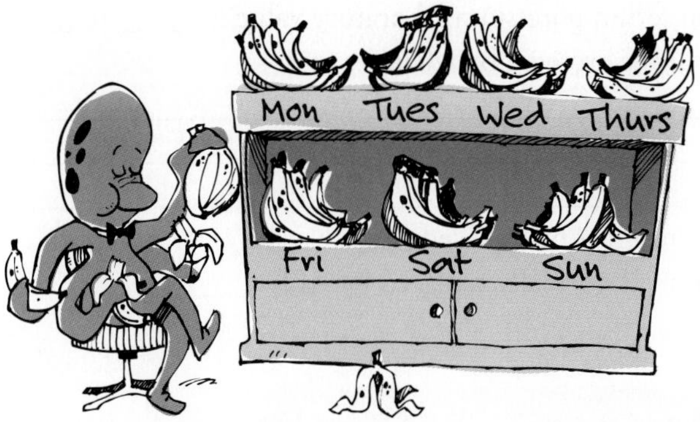

Potassium must be replaced every day.

Potassium Homeostasis

Excretion Increased	Excretion Decreased
Aldosterone	Absence of aldosterone
Diuretics	Low sodium delivery to the kidney
High urine output (osmotic diuresis)	Low unine output
High serum potassium level	Low serum potassium level
	Renal failure

Functions of Potassium

Potassium is found in high concentrations in organs and muscles. Potassium plays an important role in the following:

1. Maintenance of the volume of fluid within the cell
2. Cardiac, skeletal, and smooth muscle contractions and nerve impulse conduction
3. Metabolism of carbohydrates and proteins (Insulin and potassium are necessary to move glucose into ICF.)
4. Correction of imbalances of acid-base metabolism by maintaining the hydrogen ion concentration in the plasma

CULTURE

A Western diet contains an average of 50 to 100 mEq/day of potassium.

TAKE HOME POINTS

- Potassium must be replaced every day.
- Normally, a daily diet replaces potassium.
- Potassium moves into the ECF in times of stress or cell death.
- Potassium moves into the ICF with glucose metabolism by the cell.
- Approximately 80% of potassium is excreted in urine by the kidneys.
- A laboratory test result for potassium reports the level of potassium found in the ECF.

Do You UNDERSTAND?

DIRECTIONS: Fill in the blanks.

1. Ninety-eight percent of potassium is found in the ______________.
2. Two percent of potassium is found in the ____________________.

Answers: 1. ICF; 2. ECF.

3. Normal serum potassium laboratory value is _____ to _____ mEq/L.
4. Potassium is excreted by what organs?

____

____

____

5. Potassium must be replaced _____.
6. Potassium is normally replaced by daily _____.

What IS Hyperkalemia?

When the serum potassium level rises above 5.3 mEq/L, the imbalance is known as *hyperkalemia.* Hyperkalemia can also be seen with a blood pH less than 7.35 **(acidosis)**. Hyperkalemia is less common than hypokalemia, but it can be life threatening to the patient.

Hyperkalemia is diagnosed in up to 8% of hospitalized patients. Death can be as high as 67% if severe hyperkalemia is not treated quickly. Drugs are an underlying cause in 75% of inpatient cases.

Causes of Hyperkalemia

Decreased Excretion	Excessive Ingestion	Shift from ICF to ECF
• Renal failure (creatinine 10 mL/min or less)—most common cause • Adrenal insufficiency (Addison's disease)—decreased aldosterone secretion • Use of potassium-sparing diuretics • Drugs that cause inflammation of the kidney tissue (interstitial nephritis) (e.g., NSAIDs, methicillin)	• Too rapid administration of IV potassium • Excessive administration of IV potassium • Administration of any potassium supplements (e.g., food, salt substitutes, oral supplements, IV supplements) to patients with renal failure • Administration of potassium to patients with metabolic acidosis	• Metabolic acidosis from sodium bicarbonate loss (hydrogen moves into cell; potassium moves out of cell) • Lack of insulin (diabetic ketoacidosis) (water moves out of cell, taking potassium with it) • Antihypertensive beta-adrenergic blockers (propranolol)

Answers: 3. 3.5, 5.0; 4. kidneys, bowel, sweat glands; 5. daily; 6. diet.

Causes of Hyperkalemia—cont'd

Decreased Excretion	Excessive Ingestion	Shift from ICF to ECF
• Sickle cell disease • Systemic lupus erythematosus • Drugs that decrease aldosterone activity • Infection that causes interstitial nephritis • Interstitial nephritis as the result of diabetes mellitus	• Improper mixing of potassium to IV fluid • Cell destruction, as found with burns, major trauma, serious infections, and chemotherapy (when cells are destroyed, potassium inside the cells is released)	• Succinylcholine (depolarizing muscle) • Acute digoxin intoxication or overdose • Arginine hydrochloride

ECF, Extracellular fluid; *ICF,* intracellular fluid; *IV,* intravenous; *NSAIDs,* nonsteroidal antiinflammatory drugs.

What You NEED TO KNOW

The most common causes of hyperkalemia are acute or chronic renal failure (especially in patients on dialysis), diabetic ketoacidosis, trauma, burns, and secondary to medications such as nonsteroidal antiinflammatory drugs (NSAIDs), beta-blockers, cyclosporine and angiotensin-converting enzyme (ACE) inhibitors (e.g., captopril), digoxin, potassium supplements, and potassium-sparing diuretics

With improper blood-drawing techniques, sometimes a potassium laboratory result can be high even though the patient's actual serum potassium level is normal. This phenomenon is referred to as *pseudohyperkalemia* and can occur when the tourniquet is left in place too long before the blood is drawn; the patient has clenched the fist too excessively; the blood is hemolyzed; or the blood is drawn too close to an intravenous (IV) infusion containing potassium.

TAKE HOME POINTS

Serum potassium levels above 5.1 mEq/L = hyperkalemia

Causes of hyperkalemia are related to decreased excretion, excess ingestion or movement from the ICF to the ECF or any combination.

Improper blood drawing techniques can lead to misleadingly elevated potassium results.

Signs and Symptoms of Hyperkalemia

Hyperkalemia is usually only apparent with extremely elevated serum potassium levels. Rapid change in serum potassium level has the greatest effect on the appearance of symptoms. The patient with chronically elevated potassium may be asymptomatic, whereas the patient with the same serum value that occurred rapidly will be symptomatic. Often, hyperkalemia is found with a routine serum electrolyte laboratory test in

A high level of potassium in the blood is life-threatening. Critically high level of potassium is 6.4 mEq/L.

the patient who does not report any symptoms. The most common symptom is muscle weakness. The elevated potassium muscle cells are more excitable. As hyperkalemia worsens, muscle cells are unable to contract. Muscle weakness mirrors symptoms observed in those with hypokalemia, but the cause is different, which often makes it difficult to identify potassium imbalances on clinical symptoms alone. Serum levels and electrocardiographic (ECG) tracings are needed. Hyperkalemia causes dangerous arrhythmias in patients. The serum potassium level at which these arrythmias may occur varies from patient to patient. Common signs and symptoms of hyperkalemia are presented in the following box.

Signs and Symptoms of Hyperkalemia

MUSCLE WEAKNESS

Skeletal muscle (most common symptoms)

- Muscle cramps (early or mild)
- Weakness, usually starting in the lower extremities (late or severe)

Smooth muscle (most common symptoms)

- Nausea
- Diarrhea
- Hyperactive bowel sounds
- Intermittent colic

Cardiac muscle (most life-threatening symptoms)

- Low blood pressure
- Slow rate (bradycardia): regular or irregular
- Electrocardiographic changes (occur as the potassium level rises); more pronounced symptoms, with sudden rises rather than slow increases in the serum potassium level
  - With early hyperkalemia, the T wave becomes tall and narrow.

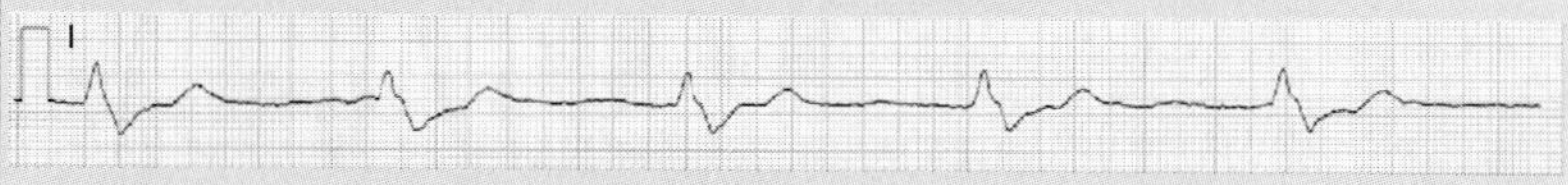

- As the serum potassium rises, the R wave becomes shorter, the S-T segment depresses, and the P wave disappears.

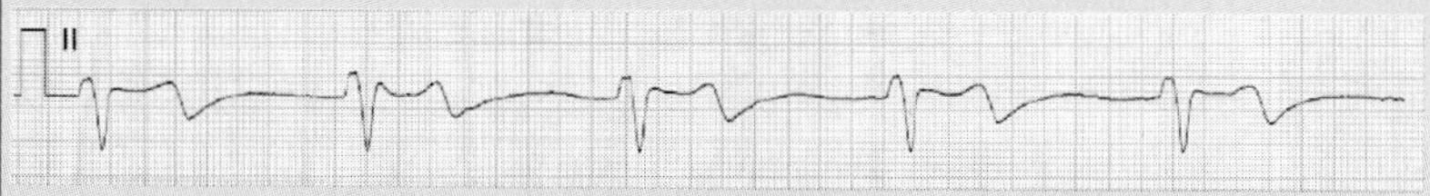

Signs and Symptoms of Hyperkalemia—cont'd

- As the potassium continues to rise, the P-R, QRS, and Q-T intervals become prolonged, leading to cardiac arrest.

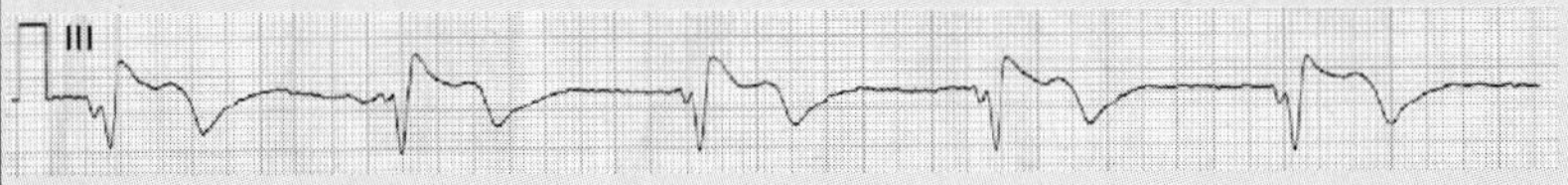

NEUROLOGIC PROBLEMS

- Numbness or tingling of the face, tongue, feet, or hands (can occur with a serum level of 6 mEq/L)
- Fatigue, drowsiness
- Irritability, mental confusion

TAKE HOME POINTS

With mild hyperkalemia, symptoms are related to increased excitability of muscles and nerves. As hyperkalemia worsens, symptoms are related to the inability of muscles to contract and nerves to communicate.

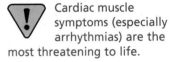

Cardiac muscle symptoms (especially arrhythmias) are the most threatening to life.

What You DO

Because patient complaints are often vague, diagnosis can be difficult. It is important to assess your patient's potential for hyperkalemia. If you can identify patients at risk, you can often prevent the imbalance from occurring or identify it in the early stage when it is easier to correct. Very premature infants and the elderly are in a high-risk population. Renal function deterioration is normal and renal blood flow decreases with advancing age. The fluid intake in the elderly is often diminished, resulting in poor renal perfusion. In addition, the elderly are often taking drugs that can potentiate the shift of potassium into the ECF.

It is important to assess a patient's potassium intake when renal function is impaired and urine output is low or absent. Even a small amount of potassium intake in the presence of renal failure can lead to hyperkalemia. To determine hydration versus renal failure, check the creatinine and blood urea nitrogen (BUN) laboratory levels. When the creatinine level is normal, dehydration should be considered. However, when the BUN and the creatinine levels are both elevated, renal failure should be considered.

Patients receiving chemotherapy, especially for the treatment of leukemia, lymphoma, or myeloma, or patients with a massive crushing injury or serious burns will have periods of rapid cell destruction, releasing a large amount of potassium into the ECF. Ask the following questions:

1. What is my patient's intake of potassium? Does the patient have a diet that includes many foods that are high in potassium? Is the patient on a diet (cardiac disease, hypertension, diabetes) that requires low sodium and higher potassium intake? Does the patient use over-the-counter salt substitutes or herbal supplements?
2. What medications is my patient taking? You need to be very familiar with drugs that impair renal potassium excretion:
   - Aminoglycosides (gentamicin, kanamycin, tobramycin)
   - Antibiotics/antiinfectives (amphotericin B, vancomycin, rifampin, methicillin, sulfonamides, tetracycline hydrochloride, pentamidine, ketoconazole)
   - Antineoplasics (cisplatin, methotrexate, cyclophosphamide)
   - NSAIDs (acetaminophen, indomethacin), cyclosporine, captopril
   - Cyclosporine or tacrolimus
   - ACE inhibitors: Capoten, Vasotec, Lotensin
   - Angiotensin receptor blockers (ARBs): Cozaar, Diovan, Hyzaar, Atacand, Benicar, Micardis, Avapro, Teveten
   - Potassium-sparing diuretics such as with cirrhosis, heart failure: amiloride (Midamor) hydrochlorothiazide and triamterene (Dyazide, Maxzide)
   - Heparin
3. Is my patient's potential elimination of potassium lower than the amount being replaced, such as with poor renal function?
4. Does my patient have a preexisting disease that makes normal serum potassium difficult to maintain, such as diabetes mellitus, sickle cell disease, lower urinary tract obstruction, polycystic kidney disease, or hypoaldosteronism?

- Tourniquet application times that are longer than 1 minute cause potassium to leak from the cells and may result in an inaccurate serum level.
- Avoid breaking red blood cells because the cell contents will leak into the plasma (hemolysis). Hemolysis can occur if specimen tubes are vigorously shaken instead of gently rocked, if too little blood is collected in relation to the additives, or if too rapid a draw causes enough turbulence for red cell destruction.

Because a false-positive blood test result is a possibility in the absence of any symptoms or potential risk factors, repeat the blood test to confirm hyperkalemia. When drawing blood from a peripheral vein, you should apply the tourniquet immediately before the venipuncture. The tourniquet should not be left in place longer than 1 minute before the venipuncture. Repeated opening and closing or clenching of the fist should be avoided because this muscle action releases potassium from the cell.

Treatment

Treating hyperkalemia is based on preventing cardiac arrhythmias and lowering the serum potassium level. The goal of the treatment is to decrease potassium intake, move the potassium from the ECF into the ICF, and increase excretion. Treatment depends on the severity of the imbalance and the urgency of the need for a response, the presence of symptoms, or the potential for life-threatening symptoms. In the absence of cardiac involvement, the intake of potassium is limited and urine output is increased.

1. Determine if life-threatening toxicity is present first.
   - Perform ECG.
   - Administer intravenous calcium to minimize cardiac toxicity if necessary. Calcium increases cardiac excitability and myocardial contractility, which is the opposite action of potassium on the heart muscle. Its action occurs within minutes and lasts approximately 1 hour. Calcium gluconate administration will increase digitalis toxicity. Its effects are potentiated by thiazide diuretics (Diuril, HydroDiuril). Because calcium gluconate can cause vein dilation, keep the patient lying down after administration to prevent postural hypotension. Also, monitor the patient's pulse rate. A slow rate (bradycardia) is a signal to stop the infusion.
2. Identify and remove sources (oral and parenteral) of potassium intake.
   - Eliminate foods high in potassium; potassium-containing salt substitutes.
   - Stop medications that are high in potassium (e.g., some penicillins, alkalizing salts).
3. Increase movement of potassium from ECF into ICF.
   - Administer insulin with hypertonic dextrose to enable the body to metabolize glucose. The response time is much shorter than those methods previously discussed (20 to 30 minutes), and the effects can last 2 to 6 hours. For a patient with diabetes who has an elevated blood glucose level, only insulin needs to be administered. Measure serum glucose and potassium every 2 hours.
   - Administer bicarbonate to correct metabolic acidosis. This raises the pH of the blood and shifts the potassium back into the cell. Sodium bicarbonate may be given via IV push, or 90 mEq can be added to 500 mL of $D_{10}W$ and administered by continuous IV infusion. The effects can be observed in 30 minutes to 1 hour and can last for 1 to 2 hours.
4. Promote the excretion of potassium.
   - Renal excretion: Increased flow in the urine can be achieved by administering normal saline IV and potassium-losing diuretic medications (e.g., thiazides, furosemide).
   - Gastrointestinal excretion: Administer sodium polystyrene sulfonate (Kayexalate) by retention enema (1 hour). The enemas may be repeated every 2 to 4 hours. Some lowering of serum potassium can be achieved in 1 to 4 hours. Because the Kayexalate must travel

TAKE HOME POINTS

- Assess the patient's potassium intake, including a diet history.
- Assess the patient's renal function. Decreased renal function increases the risk for hyperkalemia.
- Assess the patient's disease process in relation to its influence on the movement of potassium from the ICF to the ECF. Potassium moving into the ECF causes hyperkalemia.
- Review all of the medications the patient is taking, including over-the-counter and herbal.

LIFE SPAN

Remember, renal function decreases with age. You need to be very familiar with drugs that are toxic to the kidneys (e.g., nephrotoxic medications).

through the entire GI tract, response time is slower (longer than 6 hours) when using the oral route of administration. When administering Kayexalate by mouth (suspended in 70% sorbitol), remember that additional osmotic laxatives should be avoided unless indicated. Keep an accurate intake and output record, including the number and consistency of bowel movements.

5. Begin dialysis if patient is unresponsive to treatment or shows signs of lethal hyperkalemia.
   - A 4-hour dialysis treatment removes 40% to 50% of the serum potassium. Hemodialysis is more effective than peritoneal dialysis. When dialysis is begun, other treatments that have been started that move potassium into the ICF should be stopped. The potassium needs to be in the plasma so it can be removed by the dialysis.

TAKE HOME POINTS

- The first step in treatment is to determine whether life-threatening cardiac toxicity is present and treat if required.
- Treatment is based on eliminating or decreasing potassium intake, shifting potassium from the ECF to the ICF, and improving renal and gastrointestinal potassium excretion.
- With cardiac arrhythmias or changes in the ECG, IV calcium gluconate is given first, then insulin or sodium bicarbonate is administered. If output is not improved, dialysis is begun.

Treatment Overview

Mechanism	Onset of Action
Minimize cardiac toxicity. IV calcium	Minutes; effect lasts about 1 hour
Identify and remove sources of portassium. Oral and parenteral	
Increase potassium movement into ICF. Insulin and glucose Sodium bicarbonate	30-60 minutes; effect lasts several hours
Promote excretion. Diuretics Gastrointestinal (Kayexalate)	Several hours, sometimes does not work 2-3 hours
Begin dialysis.	Several hours

Do You UNDERSTAND?

DIRECTIONS: **Fill in the blanks.**

1. Hyperkalemia is present when the level of potassium in the blood is higher than __________ mEq/L.
2. You can suspect that hyperkalemia is present if the patient's pH is less than ______________.

Answers: 1. 5.1; 2. 7.35.

3. Select one of these words—*high, normal, low*—to complete this equation:
   High-normal intake + ______________ output = hyperkalemia.

DIRECTIONS: Match the reason for hyperkalemia in column A with the appropriate cause in column B.

Column A	Column B
4. _____ Renal failure	a. Cell destruction
5. _____ Chemotherapy	b. Excretion
6. _____ Amphotericin B	c. Ingestion
7. _____ K-salt	d. Nephrotoxic

DIRECTIONS: Unscramble the symptoms of hyperkalemia.

8. ______________________________ *(guatife)*
9. ______________________________ *(clemus pracms)*
10. ______________________________ *(ceariepvthy lebow donuss)*
11. ______________________________ *(mithayrar)*
12. ______________________________ *(steyopnhion)*
13. ______________________________ *(crabridaayd)*
14. ______________________________ *(senbmuns)*

DIRECTIONS: Fill in the squares on p. 90 to form the words that are the missing link to connect the words provided.

15. — — — — — — —
    — — — — — — — — — —

DIRECTIONS: Indicate in the spaces provided whether the following statements are *true* or *false.*

To distend the vein when drawing blood for potassium:

16. _______ Leave the tourniquet on the patient's extremity at least 2 minutes.
17. _______ Ask the patient to clinch the fist.
18. _______ Shake the blood tube to completely mix the blood.

The administration of calcium gluconate:

19. _______ Can cause tissue sloughing through infiltration.
20. _______ Causes elevation of the blood pressure.
21. _______ Increases the pulse rate.
22. _______ May lead to cardiac arrest.

Calcium gluconate and sodium bicarbonate are very irritating to veins and can cause phlebitis and tissue damage with infiltration.

Answers: **3. low; 4. c; 5. b; 6. e; 7. d; 8. fatigue; 9. muscle cramps; 10. hyperactive bowel sounds; 11. arrhythmia; 12. hypotension; 13. bradycardia; 14. numbness; 15. cardiac arrhythmia; 16. false. 17. false; 18. false; 19. true; 20. false; 21. false; 22. true.**

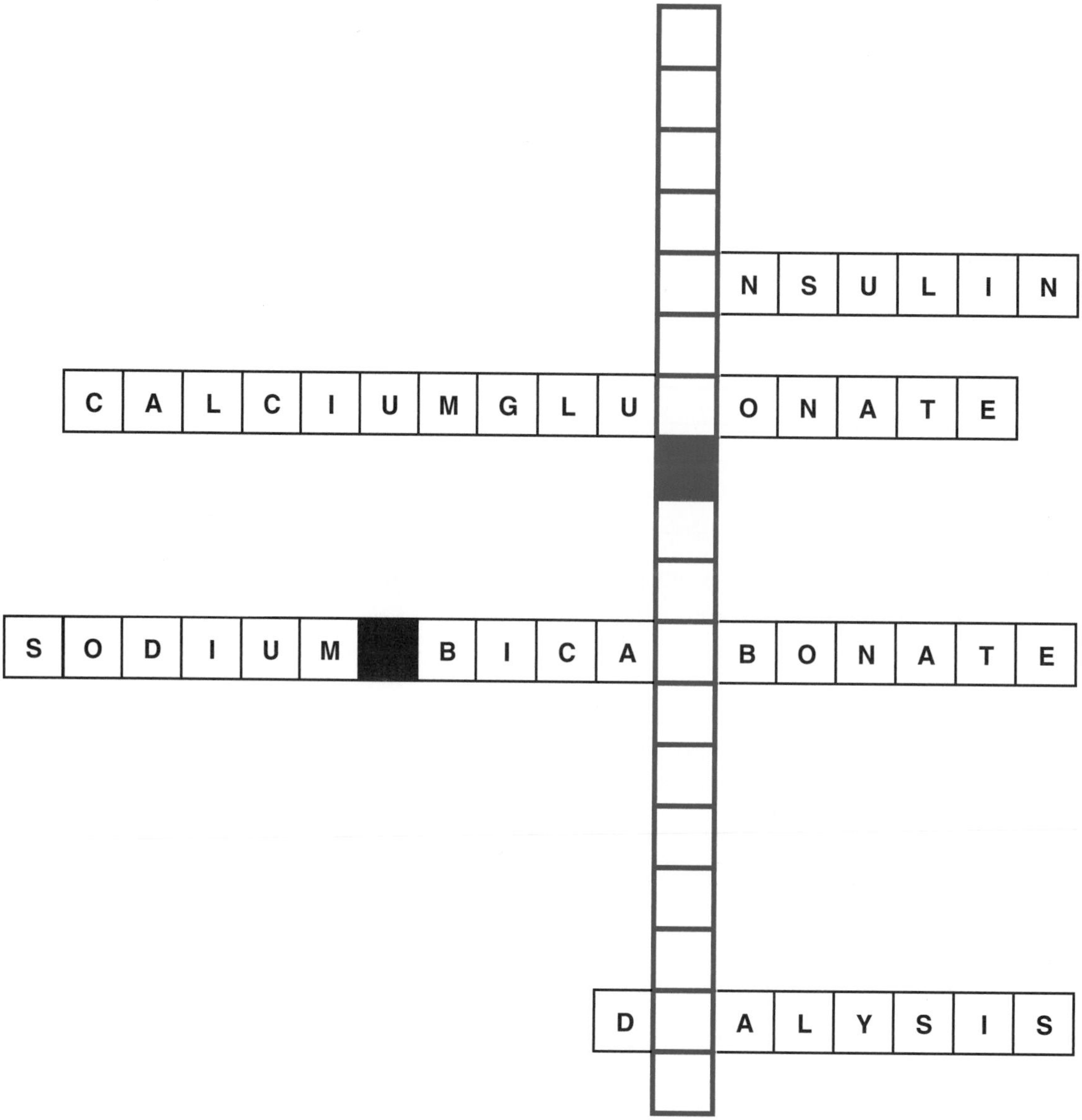
N S U L I N
C A L C I U M G L U O N A T E
S O D I U M B I C A B O N A T E
D A L Y S I S

What IS Hypokalemia?

When the serum potassium level falls below 3.5 mEq/L, the imbalance is known as *hypokalemia.* Moderate hypokalemia is 2.5 to 3 mEq/L. Severe hypokalemia is less than 2.5 mEq/L and is relatively uncommon. Hypokalemia occurs in 20% of hospitalized patients. Eighty percent of patients taking diuretics become hypokalemic. Hypokalemia is usually caused by either renal or GI disturbances (see table below). Causes of hypokalemia include the following:

- Decreased potassium intake (malnutrition or decreased dietary intake, parenteral nutrition)
- Increased renal excretion (hyperaldosteronism, magnesium depletion, leukemia)
- Increased GI or sweat-gland excretion (vomiting, nasogastric suctioning, diarrhea, enemas, or laxative use)
- Drugs (potassium-wasting diuretics, steroids, beta-adrenergic agonists, theophylline, aminoglycosides)
- Shift of potassium from the ECF to the ICF (insulin, alkalosis)

When potassium shifts from the ECF to the ICF, the total body store of potassium is normal, but the amount in the plasma (i.e., ECF) is low.

TAKE HOME POINTS

- Serum level < 3.5 mEq/L = hypokalemia.
- Common causes of hypokalemia are diuretics, vomiting, nasogastric suction, and diarrhea.
- When potassium is forced into the cell, as with metabolic acidosis, the total amount of potassium in the body may be close to normal, but the concentration in the ECF is low.

Causes of Hypokalemia

Increased Kidney Excretion	Increased Gastrointestinal/Sweat Gland Excretion (Loss/L)	Potassium Shift from ECF into ICF	Low Potassium Intake
• Diuretics—thiazides, furosemide (Lasix), ethacrynic acid • Large doses of steroids • Prolonged infusion of potassium-free IV fluids • Increased diuresis (glucosuria) associated with uncontrolled diabetes mellitus • Hyperaldosteronism—tumor of the adrenal cortex	• Diarrhea (40-60 mEq/L) • Diarrhea associated with villous adenoma of the rectum (80-180 mEq/L) • Laxative abuse • Vomiting (5-10 mEq/L) • Gastric suctioning • Fistulas	• Metabolic alkalosis • Hydrogen moves out of the cell to lower the pH, potassium moves into the cell • Prolonged administration of sodium carbenicillin or sodium penicillin (causes metabolic alkalosis) • Recovery from severe malnourishment	• Anorexia • Alcoholism • Improper oral or IV replacement

Continued

Causes of Hypokalemia—cont'd

Increased Kidney Excretion	Increased Gastrointestinal/Sweat Gland Excretion (Loss/L)	Potassium Shift from ECF into ICF	Low Potassium Intake
• Acute myeloid leukemia • Hypomagnesemia • Cushing's syndrome • Drugs such as sodium penicillin, amphotericin B, carbenicillin • Stress causes adrenal cortex to excrete aldosterone	• Excessive diaphoresis, such as with heatstroke	• Recovery from diabetic ketoacidosis • High serum insulin levels • Severe exertion • Epinephrine infusions	

IV, Intravenous.

What You NEED TO KNOW

If potassium is lost slowly, the body has time to adjust to the loss, and it takes longer for clinical signs and symptoms to appear. If the loss is rapid, the body cannot adjust, and the symptoms may be severe.

Signs and Symptoms of Hypokalemia

Clinical signs and symptoms are usually not present until the potassium serum level is below 3 mEq/L. With metabolic alkalosis, arterial blood gases will show an elevated pH and bicarbonate. Urine analysis will show a decreased potassium level. With hypokalemia, muscle and nerve cells are less excitable. Muscle cells are less likely to contract, causing muscle weakness, and nerve cells are slower to communicate, causing neurologic changes. Signs and symptoms of hypokalemia are presented in the following box.

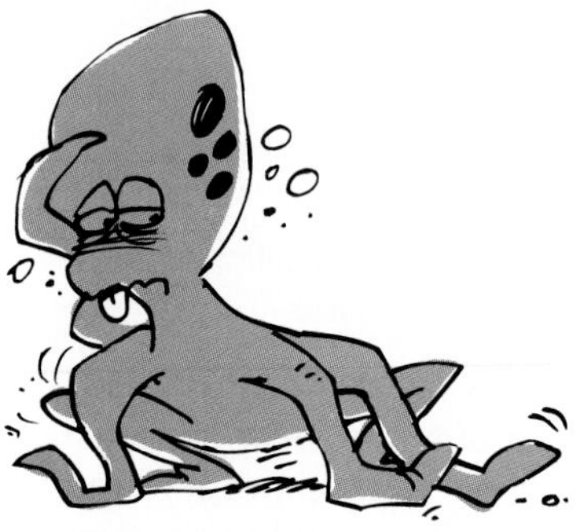

Fatigue, weakness, and heaviness in the legs are some clinical manifestations of hypokalemia.

Signs and Symptoms of Hypokalemia

MUSCLE WEAKNESS

Skeletal muscle

- Fatigue
- Weakness
- Heaviness in legs

Signs and Symptoms of Hypokalemia—cont'd

Smooth muscle

- Decreased bowel motility
- Nausea and vomiting secondary to the abdominal distention
- Constipation
- Possible ileus
- Postural hypotension

Cardiac muscle

- Postural hypotension
- Irregular pulse with extra or early beats, especially with a patient taking digitalis
- Digitalis sensitivity
- Electrocardiographic changes:
  - ST depression
  - Flatter or inverted T waves
  - Enlarged U wave, which may be superimposed on the T wave, giving the appearance of a prolonged Q-T interval

Respiratory muscle

- Shallow, ineffective respirations **(hypoventilation)**

RENAL PROBLEMS

- Frequent urination **(polyuria)**
- Urination at night **(nocturia)**

NEUROLOGIC PROBLEMS

- Decreased deep tendon reflexes
- Drowsiness
- Confusion
- Mental depression

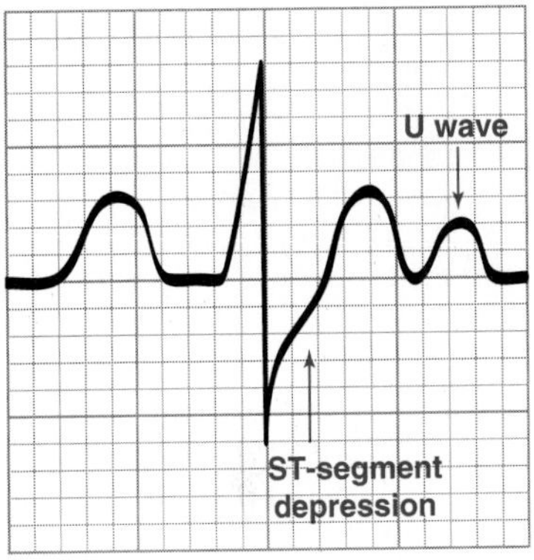

If hypokalemia is left undiagnosed and allowed to progress, you can see the following:
1. Kidney damage
2. Absent bowel sounds (paralytic ileus)
3. Paralysis
4. Death secondary to cardiac or respiratory arrest (muscles cease to contract)

What You DO

It is important to assess your patient for the possibility of hypokalemia. If you can identify patients at risk, you can often prevent the imbalance from occurring or identify it very early when it is easier to correct.

Because potassium must be replaced daily, it is important to assess a patient's potassium intake if renal function and output are normal. An inadequate intake of potassium in the presence of normal renal function will lead to hypokalemia.

Patients with GI disorders are excreting large amounts of potassium and will need more potassium intake daily. Patients taking diuretics for hypertension or congestive heart failure (CHF) will also excrete large amounts of potassium. Most of your patients will be under some level of stress, will have altered fluid intake, and will be on a variety of medications.

Ask the following questions:

- What is my patient's intake of potassium?
- Is my patient's potential elimination of potassium higher than the amount being replaced?
- Does my patient have a preexisting disease that makes normal serum potassium difficult to maintain?

Perform a complete assessment to identify all symptoms. The most organized way to complete a thorough assessment is to follow a head-to-toe system. Quick assessment for potassium problems should include the following:

- Identify changes in the level of consciousness. You can ask the patient to solve a simple problem or ask, "Where are you?"
- Take apical pulse.
- Take lying, sitting, and standing blood pressure readings and compare them. If there is a 20 mm Hg decrease in the systolic pressure or a 10 mm Hg decrease in diastolic pressure, postural hypotension is present.
- Monitor ECG for changes.
- Breathing sounds will be diminished. Monitor depth and rate of respiration. Can the patient talk and breathe at the same time?
- Maintain intake and output records.
- Check for bowel sounds.
- Check deep tendon reflexes and handgrips.
- Plan for patient safety.

Treatment

Treatment for hypokalemia should be twofold. Replacement therapy must be considered, as well as the identification of the cause for the underlying deficit. The need for potassium replacement and the speed by which this replacement must occur is based on the following:

TAKE HOME POINTS

- Hypokalemia symptoms vary from patient to patient.
- Symptoms are related to decreased functionality of the muscles (heart, lungs, GI tract) and nerve impulse conduction.
- Assess potassium intake and output and excretion to identify risk.

LIFE SPAN

Older adults are at risk for hypokalemia secondary to chronic illness, medications, and potential poor intake.

TAKE HOME POINTS

- Treatment includes potassium replacement and identification of the underlying cause for the deficiency.
- Replacement and the urgency for replacement are based on the severity of symptoms, the potential for cardiac arrhythmia or hyperventilation, treatment of ketoacidosis, and the serum blood level.

Impaired renal function or adrenal insufficiency can cause potassium excess.

- Potential for cardiac arrhythmia, such as a patient on digitalis
- Presence of weakness and metabolic acidosis, increasing the potential for hyperventilation
- Potential for a rapid shift of potassium into the cell, such as in the recovery phase of diabetic ketoacidosis (potassium shifts into the cell with insulin)
- Potential for continuing loss
- Serum blood level

Oral replacement is the easiest, most cost effective, and safest method for administering potassium. When the patient exhibits no symptoms but has a slightly low serum potassium level (3 to 3.5 mEq/L), an oral supplement replacement is the first choice. These are available in liquids, tablets, powders, and effervescent tablets.

- When administering oral potassium supplements, instruct the patient on the importance of taking potassium supplements and the need to report any side effects. The major side effects of taking oral potassium supplements are nausea, vomiting, and diarrhea. These effects can be minimized by diluting medications, increasing fluid intake with the tablets, or taking medications with or after meals. Medications should be taken with a full glass of water. Effervescent tablets should be allowed to dissolve completely before ingesting. The patient should drink effervescent medications slowly, over 5 to 10 minutes.
- Perform routine blood tests to identify whether the serum potassium is becoming too high **(hyperkalemia)** in patients taking potassium supplements.
- Monitor the output and be alert to any decrease in urinary output. Monitoring should include the number of bowel movements and their consistency, which is especially important if the patient has renal impairment.
- Add potassium to the patient's diet, which is especially helpful with patients who are taking prolonged diuretic therapy and who are also sodium restricted. Salt substitutes (Co-Salt, Morton's Lite Salt) contain potassium. When patients are at risk for potassium depletion (e.g., those taking diuretic or corticosteroid medications, those with diabetes), or when patients require digitalis, foods high in potassium are important in preventing hypokalemia.

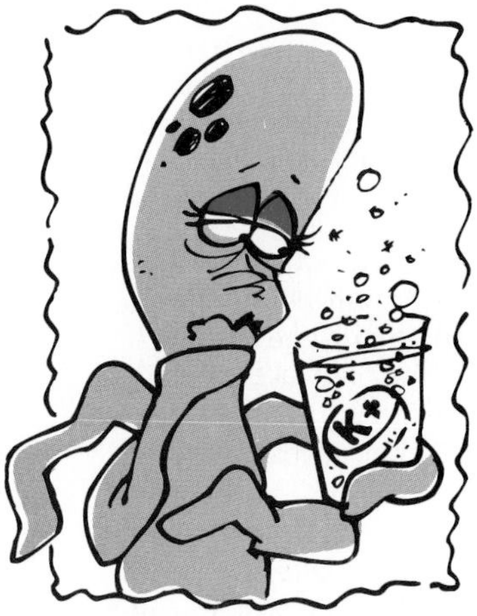

Oral replacement is the safest method for administering potassium in non-urgent hypokalemia.

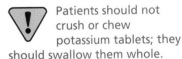

Patients should not crush or chew potassium tablets; they should swallow them whole.

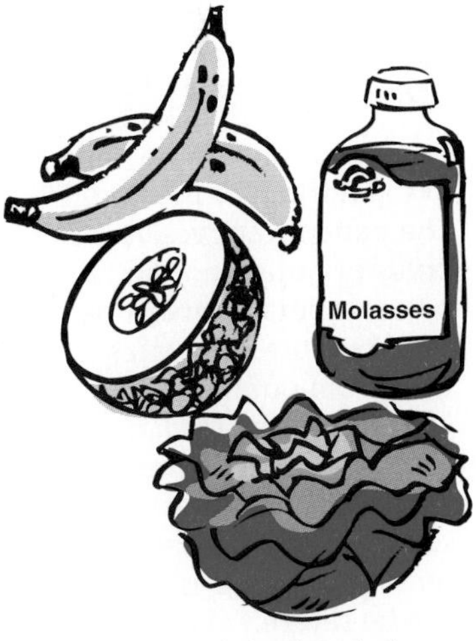

Potassium-rich foods include: bananas, cantaloupe, green leafy vegetables, and molasses.

TAKE HOME POINTS

Patients who require digitalis or are given diuretic medications must include foods high in potassium in their diets.
- Monitor serum potassium levels.
- Patients should take their entire prescribed potassium supplement.
- Potassium supplements should be taken with or after meals to minimize side effects.
- Monitor intake and output.

- Direct IV push potassium can be instantly fatal.
- High doses should be administered through a central vein with continuous cardiac monitoring. Watch for increased sensitivity to digitalis. Digitalis toxicity can occur even when the patient is taking a low dose.

- Adding potassium to a hanging bag will result in a high concentration of potassium in the bottom of the bag. The patient can receive a bolus of potassium. An IV bolus of potassium can be fatal because it elevates the serum potassium too rapidly, causing cardiac arrest.
- When peripheral infusions are used, the patient may complain of a burning sensation. This sensation can be severe.

- Instruct patients about the importance of including potassium-rich foods in their diet. Foods rich in potassium include bananas, cantaloupe, green leafy vegetables, avocados, dried fruit (e.g., apricots, dates, raisins, peaches, figs), bran cereal, molasses, and lentils.

Intravenous Replacement

When a patient is unable to eat, unable to absorb nutrients through the GI tract, has symptoms such as muscle weakness, is being treated for diabetic ketoacidosis, is receiving digitalis, or has a serum potassium level below 3.1 mEq/L, IV potassium replacement is the method of choice. The goal with this type of therapy is to improve the patient's immediate condition and to return the serum potassium to a normal level slowly.

There are three potassium IV preparations. Potassium chloride is the most common. Potassium acetate and potassium phosphates are also available.

- **Usual dosage**
  20 to 60 mEq/24 hours
  200 mEq/24 hours is usually not exceeded
- **Dilution**
  Usually diluted in dextrose-free solutions, such as 0.9% saline (Dextrose can cause potassium to move into the cell and therefore lower the serum level.)
  40 mEq/L is the preferred dilution.
  80 mEq/L is the usual maximum dilution.
  10 mEq/100 mL of normal saline is administered at 100 mL/hr.
- **Incompatible medications**
  Amikacin, amphotericin B, blood or blood products, diazepam, dobutamine, ergotamine, fat emulsion 10%, mannitol, methylprednisolone, penicillin G sodium, phenytoin, promethazine.
- **Rate of administration**
  Maximum 10 mEq/hr (no matter the dilution) should not be exceeded. In extreme situations, 20 to 40 mEq/hr have been given. Rapid infusion should not be performed. Large potassium deficits should be corrected over a few days, not a few hours.
- **Precautions**
  Impaired renal function or adrenal insufficiency can cause potassium intoxication.

- **Drug interactions**

  Supplements are contraindicated with patients receiving potassium-sparing diuretics (spironolactone, hydrochlorothiazide [Dyazide]), potentiated by captopril, enalapril, and lisinopril (Capoten, Vasotec, Prinivil, Zestril).

Potassium phosphate is used to keep potassium in the ICF during periods of tissue regeneration as during hyperalimentation administration or when treating diabetic ketoacidosis.

When adding potassium to IV fluid, it is important to hold the bag downward and inject the potassium down into the solution. The bag should then be held upright and agitated back and forth to distribute the potassium throughout the solution.

The use of an infusion pump is recommended in all situations and is required with any dose exceeding 60 mEq/24 hr. Potassium is very irritating to veins. Use the largest vein and the smallest catheter possible to promote hemodilution. Apply a warm compress above the insertion site along the vein track throughout the infusion.

Because a burning sensation is common with potassium infusions, it is important to monitor the site closely for infiltration. Monitor the IV site for any signs of swelling, redness, or inability to maintain prescribed flow rate.

If the prescribed rate slows or the infusion pump alarm indicates occlusion, infiltration should be considered, and infusion should be stopped.

A burning sensation along the vein path is common with the administration of IV potassium. Whenever signs or symptoms, such as difficulty maintaining a flow rate or skin above the distal venous site that feels taut, the IV infusion should be discontinued. The patient should be instructed to report any stinging or burning sensations.

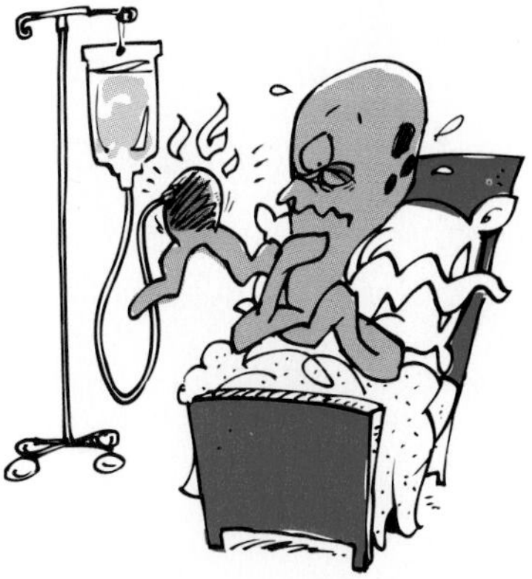

Intravenous potassium is an irritant that may cause swelling, redness, and burning pain at, near, or above the IV site.

- If any swelling is noted over the tip of the catheter, stop infusion immediately.
- If you have any question about patency, the infusion should be stopped, and a new IV site should be found.

TAKE HOME POINTS

A blood return is not a true indicator of vein integrity. The ability to flush is also not an indicator of vein integrity. If infiltration occurs, discontinue the IV, apply a cold compress to the site, and notify the health care provider.

Do You UNDERSTAND?

DIRECTIONS: Unscramble each word to identify common causes of hypokalemia.

1. imtivogn
2. asnosactirg custon
3. rehaidra
4. riduecits

DIRECTIONS: Choose the appropriate word to complete the equation: high, normal, low.

5. Normal intake + _______ output = hypokalemia.
6. _______ intake + normal output = hypokalemia.

DIRECTIONS: Unscramble the italicized words.

7. Symptoms *yrva.*
8. With hypokalemia, muscle functionality is *creddease.*
9. Hypokalemia can cause *draciac strare.*

DIRECTIONS: Fill in the squares to form a word that is the missing link to connect the words provided.

10. ____________________________________

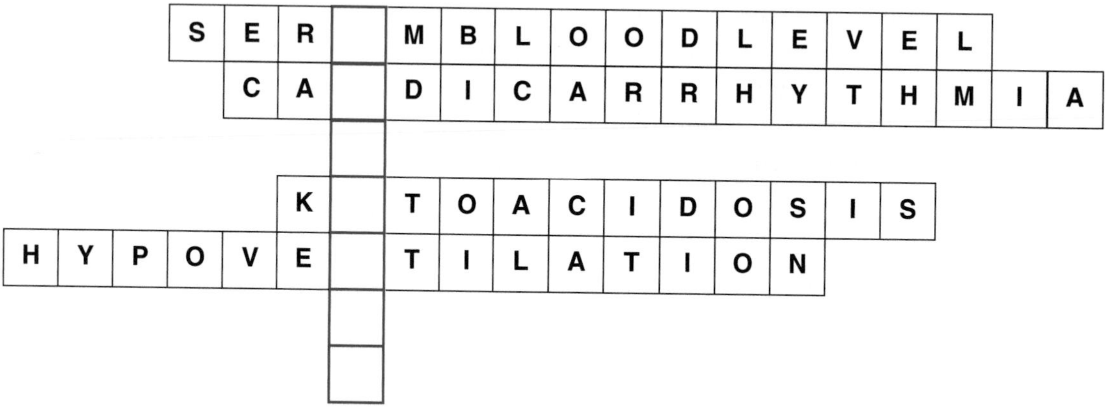

Answers: 1. vomiting; 2. nasogastric suctions; 3. diarrhea; 4. diuretics; 5. high; 6. Low; 7. vary; 8. decreased; 9. cardiac arrest; 10. urgency.

Crossword Puzzles

Across

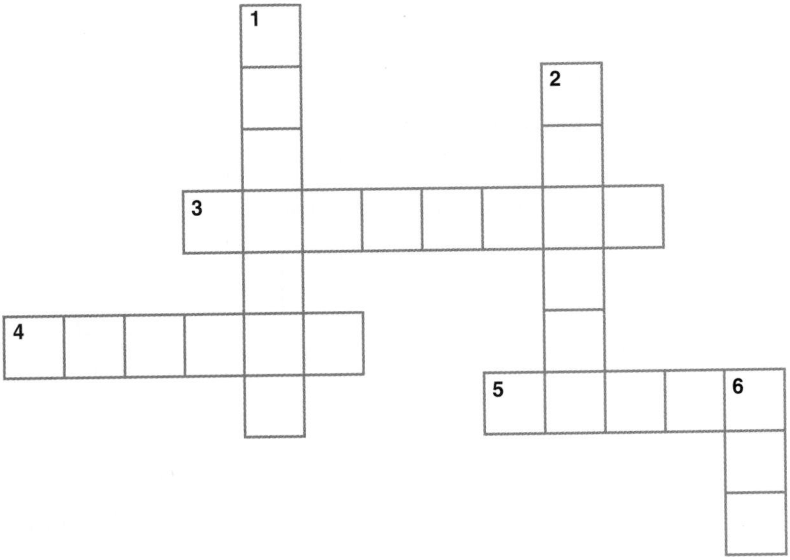

3. Potassium is important in correcting these imbalances
4. Potassium moves into the ECF during this
5. Potassium plays an important role in what kind of conduction

Down

1. Potassium moves into the ICF during the metabolism of this by the cell
2. Potassium plays an important role in the contraction of this
6. Short for extracellular fluid

TAKE HOME POINTS

- Use a central venous catheter with high doses.
- Continuous cardiac monitoring is preferable for any potassium infusion over 10 mEq/hr.

When treating a patient for hypokalemia, it is very important to monitor serum potassium levels. IV potassium is a vesicant and can cause tissue damage if infiltration occurs. Cold compresses, not heat, are used for the treatment of infiltration.

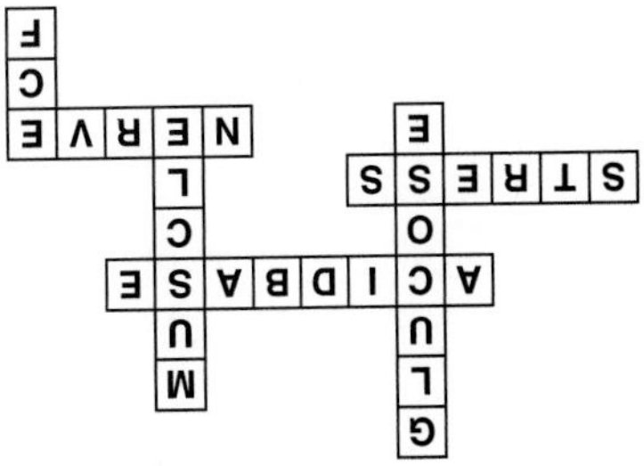

Answers:

Words that pertain to complications with IV potassium

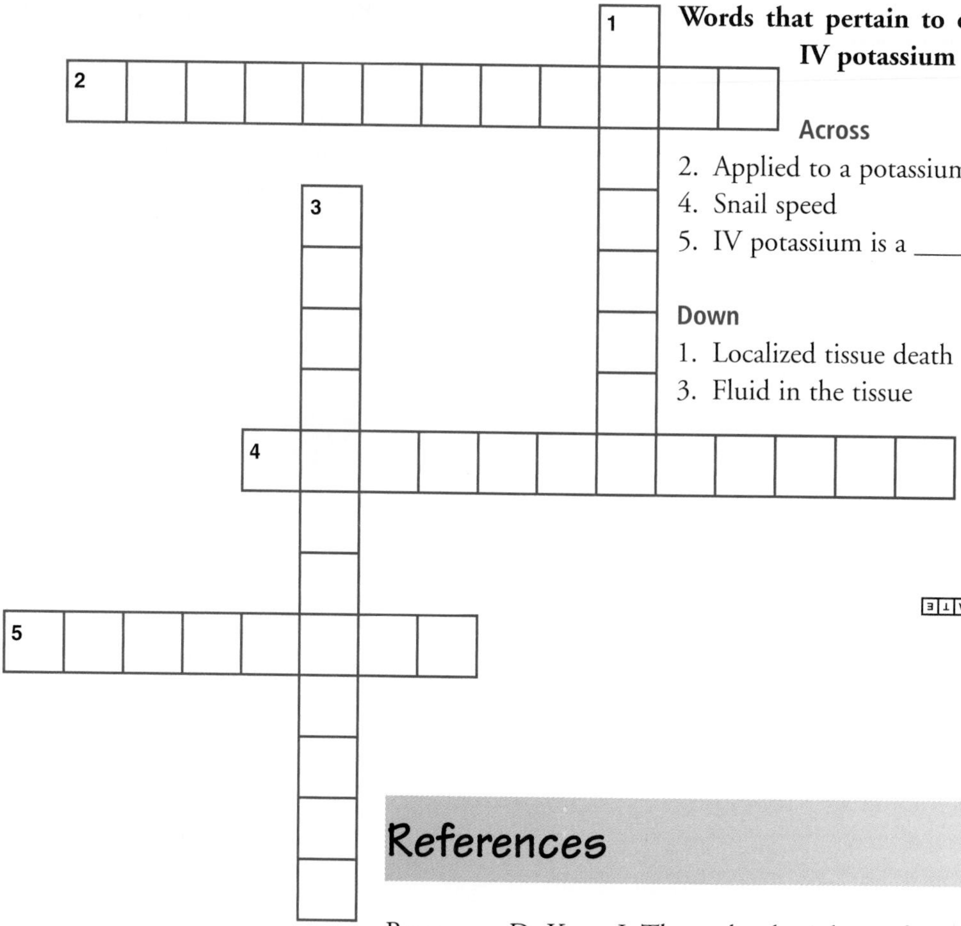

Across

2. Applied to a potassium infiltration
4. Snail speed
5. IV potassium is a ________

Down

1. Localized tissue death
3. Fluid in the tissue

Answer:

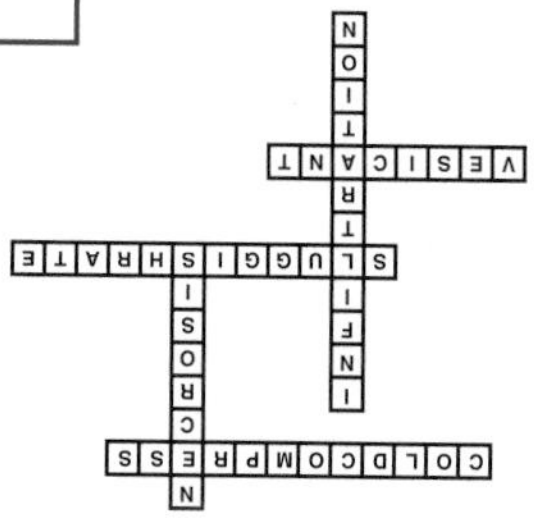

References

Braxmeyer D, Keyes J: The pathophysiology of potassium balance, *Crit Care Nurse* 16(5):59, 1996.

Cohn JN, Kowey PR, Whelton PK: New guidelines for potassium replacement in clinical contemporary review by the National Council on Potassium in Clinical Practice, *Arch Intern Med* 160(16):2429-2436 2000.

Forbes GB: Potassium: the story of an element, *Biol Med* 38:554, 1995.

Gahart BL, Nazareno AR: *Intravenous medications,* ed 21, St Louis, 2005, Mosby.

Garth D: *Hyperkalemia,* 2001. Available online at www.emedicine.com.

Garth D: *Hypokalemia,* 2001. Available online at www.emedicine.com.

Halperin ML, Goldstein MB: *Fluid, electrolyte, and acid-base physiology: a problem based approach,* ed 3, Philadelphia, 1999, Saunders.

Jones E: Hypokalemia, *N Engl J Med* 349(22):2116, 2003.

Josephson DL: *Intravenous infusion therapy for nurses principles and practices,* Albany, NY, 2004, Delmar.

Metheny NM: *Fluid and electrolyte balance: nursing considerations,* ed 4, Philadelphia, 2000, Lippincott Williams & Wilkins.

NCLEX® Review

1. A patient admitted for diabetic ketoacidosis is now hydrated and has a normal blood sugar. During assessment, the patient presents with a weak pulse, shallow breathing, and an ashen color. Which of the following imbalances is the cause?
   1 Hypokalemia
   2 Hyperkalemia
   3 Hypoglycemia
   4 Hyperglycemia

2. During continuous IV administration of potassium, the infusion pump signals occlusion. The most appropriate health care provider action is to:
   1 Get a new infusion pump.
   2 Continue the infusion.
   3 Assess the IV site, and restart if vein patency is in question.
   4 Apply a warm compress.

3. When assessing a postoperative patient who had a bowel resection, the total urinary output was 50 mL for the last 3 hours. It is time to hang the next IV of D_5.45 NaCl with 20 mEq/L. The most appropriate action is to:
   1 Hang the IV as ordered.
   2 Call the health care provider to report the low output.
   3 Increase the IV rate to improve output.
   4 Slow the IV to keep veins open (KVO).

4. The patient with an ileus has a nasogastric tube to suction. As the health care practitioner assists the patient up to the bedside chair, the patient complains that his legs feel very heavy, and it is difficult to walk. The most appropriate action for the health care practitioner is to:
   1 Check the laboratory value for hyperkalemia.
   2 Put the patient in bed, and check when the last laboratory test for serum potassium was done.
   3 Set the patient in a chair with legs elevated.
   4 Apply warm compresses to the legs.

5. When reviewing the patient's laboratory test, the health care practitioner notices that the blood urea nitrogen (BUN) level is elevated, the creatinine is normal, and the potassium is slightly elevated. The patient is most likely:
   1 In early renal failure
   2 Dehydrated
   3 Overhydrated
   4 Suffering from diabetes

6. Which of the following actions is contraindicated when administering potassium chloride intravenously?
   1 Central venous access use
   2 Electrocardiographic (ECG) monitoring use
   3 Infusion control device use
   4 IV push method of administration

7. Patients who are receiving oral replacements of potassium should be taught to:
   1 Limit fluid intake.
   2 Report episodes of nausea, vomiting, or diarrhea.
   3 Test urine for potassium loss.
   4 Schedule potassium replacements before meals.

8. When teaching the patient to include potassium-rich foods in his or her diet, what three foods could the health care practitioner provide as examples?

9. The most important action the health care practitioner should do when administering Kayexalate to a patient with hyperkalemia is to:
   1 Monitor bowel movements.
   2 Monitor ECG.
   3 Premedicate with insulin.
   4 Restrict fluids.

10. Select the ECG tracing characteristic that the health care practitioner should recognize as an early indication of hyperkalemia.
    1 T waves are tall and peaked.
    2 Q-T interval is lengthened.
    3 P wave is heightened.
    4 P-R interval is shortened.

11. The most common cause of hyperkalemia is ___________ combined with ___________.

12. True or False: Muscles are usually flaccid with mild hyperkalemia.

13. What route of administration is the safest for replacing potassium?

14. To determine hydration versus renal failure, __________ and __________ should be checked.

15. True or False: The serum potassium level at which arrhythmias occur with hyperkalemia varies from patient to patient.

NCLEX® Review Answers

1. 1 The normal plasma potassium was the result of the dehydrated state. Once hydration was achieved, the potassium was extremely low. Also, potassium shifted into the cells with the insulin. Low potassium is fatal, and this patient would die of cardiac arrest unless the hypokalemia was corrected. Hypoglycemia has headache, rapid respirations, and pounding pulse with polydipsia, polyuria, and polyphagia.

2. 3 If the prescribed flow rate slows or the infusion pump alarms occlusion, infiltration could be the cause. The site should be closely examined, and a new IV site should be started if there is any question about the vein patency. When infiltration occurs, tissue damage will occur. The infusion pump is highly sensitive to changes of resistance. A broken pump is unusual. The health care practitioner should look for other causes first and get a new pump only as a last resort. The occlusion alarm signals a problem; this situation should be investigated, and a solution should be found before continuing the infusion. Warm compresses improve venous dilatation, which will aggravate an infiltration. Potassium is a vesicant. You do not want to increase vasodilatation. You would apply a cold compress to an infiltrated site.

3. 2 Potassium is contraindicated in the patient with urinary output less than 30 mL/hr. Potassium replacement should not be administered in the absence of normal urinary output because potassium intake cannot be excreted sufficiently and hyperkalemia may result. There is a danger of tubular necrosis secondary to prerenal deficiency. With low urinary output, continued infusion of IV fluids can cause circulatory overload. Slowing the IV to KVO will further increase serum potassium, causing potentially lethal cardiac arrhythmias.

4. 2 Checking the value is an appropriate safety measure. Hypokalemia is a life-threatening complication. The classic symptom for hypokalemia is skeletal muscle fatigue or weakness, because potassium is necessary for muscle contraction and impulse conduction. Early diagnosis will prevent serious complications from occurring. Hypokalemia is a life-threatening complication, but patient safety comes first. Putting the patient in bed is the safest option. After patient safety is ensured, check when the last laboratory test was performed. The cause of the weakness is hypokalemia. Warm compresses will not alleviate the symptoms.

5. 2 An elevated BUN level with a normal creatinine is a classic sign of dehydration. The volume of blood is more concentrated, resulting in a false increase in serum potassium. The hyperkalemia is a result of fluid loss rather than an increase of potassium. With renal failure, the BUN and the creatinine levels are both elevated. The BUN level would be normal or low and is not affected with diabetes.

6. 4 An IV push/bolus of potassium chloride can be fatal because it elevates the serum potassium level too rapidly, leading to cardiac arrest. Potassium chloride is irritating to the venous system, and the patient usually feels a burning sensation during administration, especially with high-dose administration. Infiltration of potassium chloride

into the surrounding tissue may cause severe tissue damage. Cardiac monitoring is recommended, especially with high-dose administration. Changes in ECG tracings may be the first sign of overdosing. An infusion-controlling device provides a consistent rate of infusion, which helps prevent too rapid an infusion.

7. 2 Nausea, vomiting, or diarrhea are the major side effects of oral potassium supplements and may also contribute to increased loss of potassium. These symptoms should be reported. Oral potassium replacements should be taken with a full glass of water. A blood serum analysis is required for evaluation of potassium levels. Potassium replacements should be taken during or after meals to minimize gastrointestinal side effects.

8. Potassium-rich foods identified in the text include bananas, cantaloupe, green leafy vegetables, avocado, dried fruit, all-bran cereal, molasses, and dry lentils.

9. 1 Most potassium is absorbed in the colon. Kayexalate binds with potassium, thus preventing absorption with fecal excretion. Although ECG changes may be observed with changes in serum potassium, Kayexalate enemas correct potassium imbalance over a period of hours and may need to be administered twice. Although insulin administration may facilitate the movement of potassium, it is critical that fecal excretion is obtained with Kayexalate enemas. Fluids may enhance the excretion of feces, thereby increasing the amount of potassium available to be bound to the Kayexalate; therefore, fluids should not be restricted.

10. 1 The ECG changes in hyperkalemia include spiked T waves, widened QRS complex, and shortened Q-T interval. The Q-T interval is shortened with hyperkalemia. The P wave is flattened and may disappear with hyperkalemia. The P-R interval becomes prolonged with hyperkalemia.

11. A normal to excessive intake combined with a diminished ability of the body to remove potassium.

12. False. Muscle cramps occur in early or mild hyperkalemia.

13. Oral route of administration. Potassium is absorbed well through the GI tract.

14. BUN and creatinine. If both are elevated, renal failure should be suspected. When the creatinine level is normal, dehydration should be suspected.

15. True. Arrhythmias are more pronounced with sudden rises (such as with cell destruction) rather than slow increases.

Notes

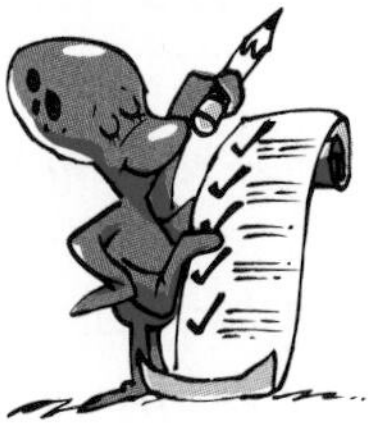

Chapter

6 Phosphorus

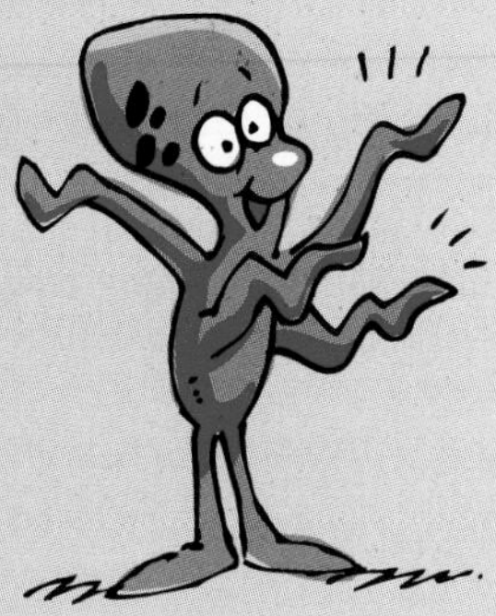

What You WILL LEARN

After reading this chapter, you will know how to do the following:

- ✔ Define phosphorus and name two uses by the human body.
- ✔ Define hyperphosphatemia.
- ✔ Name two potential causes of hypophosphatemia.

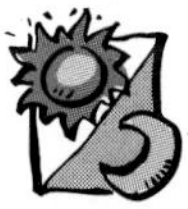

LIFE SPAN

Blood levels in older adults: the normal level of phosphorus is 2.3 to 3.7 mg/dL for men and 2.8 to 4.1 mg/dL for women. Levels are 50% higher in infants and 30% higher in children (effect of growth hormone). Adequate intake of phosphorus is 0.9 to 1.5 g/day.

What IS Phosphorus?

Phosphorus (P^-) is the most abundant negatively charged ion **(anion)** in the intracellular fluid (ICF). Approximately 85% of all phosphorus in the body is combined with calcium in the bones and teeth, with 10% in muscle, 1% in nerve tissue, and 1% in the blood as inorganic and organic phosphates. The normal blood level of phosphorus is 2.7 to 4.5 mg/dL.

What You NEED TO KNOW

Sources of Phosphorus

Phosphorus is present in most foods. Food sources that are high in phosphorus include milk, cheese, egg yolk, meat, fish, fowl, and nuts.

Control of Phosphorus

Calcium and phosphate ions have an interdependent relationship. When one is increased, the other is decreased.

Similar to calcium, phosphorus needs vitamin D for absorption in the gastrointestinal (GI) tract. Phosphorus is found in the body in a substance called adenosine triphosphate (ATP). ATP is required for substances to move into or out of a cell. ATP is used as an energy storage medium in the body.

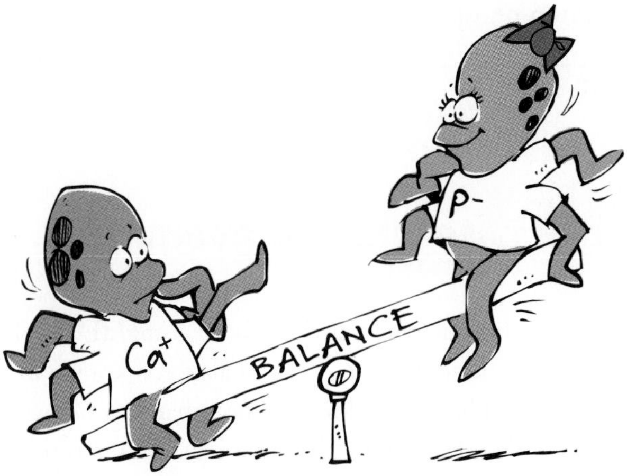

Calcium and phosphate ions have an interdependent relationship. When one is increased, the other is decreased.

Phosphorus is excreted in urine and the intestine (33% in feces). Parathyroid hormone (PTH) is important in maintaining the normal serum levels of phosphorus by altering the kidney's reabsorption of phosphorus and the shift of phosphorus from the bones to the plasma.

TAKE HOME POINTS

- Normal blood level of phosphorus is 2.7 to 4.5 mg/dL.
- ATP is important in the active transport of substances in and out of the cell.
- Calcium and phosphate ions have an interdependent and inverse relationship. When one is increased, the other is decreased.

Functions of Phosphorus

Phosphorus is important in the following:

1. Metabolism of protein, calcium, and glucose.
2. Muscle contraction.
3. Conversion of glycogen to glucose.
4. Transport of fatty acids.
5. Maintaining acid-based balance. Phosphorus can bind with hydrogen, which occurs mostly in the urine, making phosphorus the primary urinary buffer.
6. Acidification of urine. It is the acidic nature of urine that minimizes urinary tract infections and helps prevent stone formation.
7. Proper function of red blood cells. Proper function affects the ability to deliver oxygen to the tissues.
8. Use of B vitamins that are effective only when combined with phosphorus. B vitamins help the body release energy, carbon dioxide, and water as the end products of metabolism.

Do You UNDERSTAND?

DIRECTIONS: **Fill in the blanks.**

1. If phosphorus is increased, then calcium is ____________________.
2. Normal serum phosphorus level is ____________________ mEq/L.
3. ____________________ is essential for substances to move into and out of cells.

What IS Hyperphosphatemia?

When the serum phosphorus level rises above 5 mg/dL in adults and 7 mg/dL in children and adolescents, the imbalance is known as *hyperphosphatemia.* Hyperphosphatemia is less common than low phosphorus levels (**hypophosphatemia**). Hyperphosphatemia is associated most commonly with patients with renal failure (acute or chronic) (see Chapter 14).

What You NEED TO KNOW

TAKE HOME POINTS

- Hyperphosphatemia is most commonly observed with renal failure.
- Hyperphosphatemia is caused by excessive intake of products containing phosphorus, a shift of phosphorus from the ICF to the ECF, and conditions leading to a decreased excretion of phosphorus.

Hyperphosphatemia is caused by many factors, most commonly by decreased excretion in relation to phosphorus intake or absorption rate. This condition is usually the result of renal insufficiency from any cause. Seventy percent of patients with either chronic or acute renal failure encounter hyperphosphatemia. Increased intake and excessive use of laxatives or enemas containing phosphate (Fleet's enema) also cause an excess of serum phosphorus.

The shift of phosphorus from the ICF to the ECF causes the phosphorus serum level to increase, although the total amount of phosphorus in the body is not altered. This shift occurs with cell destruction, trauma, heat stroke, infections, myelogenous leukemia, lymphoma, and respiratory acidosis.

Answers: 1. decreased; 2. 2.7 to 4.5 mEq/dL; 3. ATP.

Overview of Causes of Hyperphosphatemia

- Renal insufficiency (acute or chronic)
- Increased cell breakdown or cellular injury
  - Rhabdomyolysis
  - Trauma, burns, crush injuries, shock
  - Exhaustive exercise
  - Prolonged immobilization
  - Heat-related illnesses
  - Malignant hyperthermia
  - Hypothermia
  - Massive hemolysis
  - Severe infections
  - Ischemic bowel
- Diseases of the endocrine system
  - Hypoparathyroidism
  - Pseudohypoparathyroidism
  - Abnormal parathyroid hormone
  - Acromegaly and other causes of growth hormone excess
  - Glucocorticoid withdrawal or deficiency
- Excessive intake or administration
  - Bisphosphonate therapy
  - Vitamin D intoxication or other causes of increased vitamin D (sarcoidosis)
  - Ingestion or administration of phosphate salts (e.g., oral/rectal laxatives, enemas, intravenous phosphate)
  - Hyperalimentation (including lipid administration)
  - Transfusion of outdated blood
- Cancer
  - Leukemia
  - Lymphoma
  - Bone tumors
  - Tumor lysis after chemotherapy
- Acidosis
  - Acute respiratory acidosis
  - Lactic acidosis
  - Diabetic ketoacidosis
  - Alcoholic ketoacidosis

LIFE SPAN

Vitamin D excess, which can be observed with bottle-fed infants, also causes high serum phosphorus.

Causes of Hyperphosphatemia

Increased Intake	Decreased Excretion	Shift from ICF to ECF
• Excessive oral or rectal use of Phospho-soda • Excessive parenteral administration of phosphate • Vitamin D intoxication • Hyperalimentation	• Acute or chronic renal failure • Hypoparathyroidism • Severe hypomagnesemia	• Acute hemolysis • Acute respiratory acidosis • Diabetic ketoacidosis • Alcoholic ketoacidosis • Alkalosis • Tumor lysis (chemotherapy) • Crushing trauma • Burns

Signs and Symptoms of Hyperphosphatemia

Although hyperphosphatemia is usually asymptomatic, signs and symptoms are usually related to hypocalcemia, which will be present with hyperphosphatemia (see Chapter 8). Symptoms of hypocalcemia include tetany, seizure, and delirium. Tingling, numbness, cramps, twitching of muscles, especially of the hands and feet, are the leading characteristics of tetany. Typically noticed signs include sharp flexion of the wrist and extreme extension of the feet. Nervousness, irritability, and apprehension may also be present. The deposit of calcium phosphate in soft tissue, connective tissue, lung, myocardium, and arteries usually occurs with prolonged hyperphosphatemia caused by chronic renal failure. This can cause joint pain, loss of movement, conjunctivitis, and vascular calcifications (calciphylaxis). Calciphylaxis leads to ulceration and gangrene in the affected extremity.

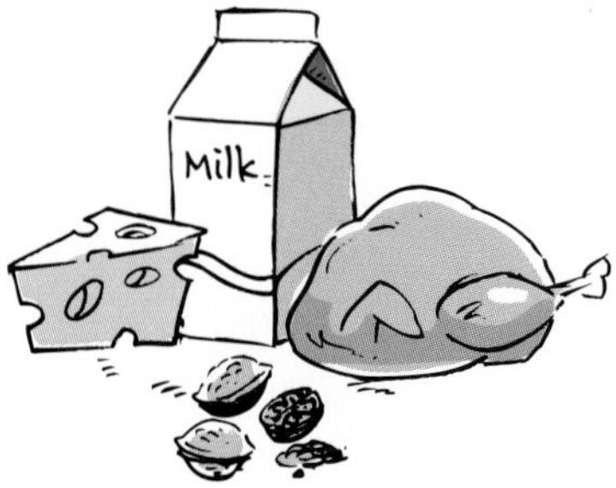

Foods rich in phosphorus include milk, cheese, egg yolk, meat, fish, fowl, and nuts.

What You DO

Treatment of hyperphosphatemia should be twofold: the identification of the cause for the elevation and actions to reduce serum levels.

Because a false-positive blood test result is a possibility, in the absence of any symptoms or potential risk factors, the blood test should be repeated for accuracy. If the patient is receiving an intravenous (IV) fluid containing glucose, the IV should be held for 4 to 8 hours before the blood specimen is drawn. Remember, phosphorus moves into the cell with the glucose; thus, the serum level will be lower than normal.

Once hyperphosphatemia has been confirmed, the provider should do the following:

- Aim initial care at management and correction of the hypocalcemia.
- For toxic ingestions, give gastric lavage and oral phosphate binders to prevent further absorption.
- Limit phosphorus intake with the restriction of foods that are high in phosphorus, including milk, cheese, egg yolk, meat, fish, fowl, and nuts.
- Remember that vegetables and fruits are low in phosphorus. Spinach, rhubarb, bran, and whole grain foods may decrease the absorption of phosphates. A low-protein diet restricts phosphorus intake.
- Administer aluminum-based antacids such as Amphojel, Basaljel, Dialume, Alternagel, Alu-Tab, or Aluminet to bind with phosphorus in the gastrointestinal (GI) tract. The phosphorus will be eliminated in the feces.
- Administer diuretics such as acetazolamide to increase urine output.
- Monitor laboratory tests for serum phosphate, calcium, and uric acid levels.
- Administer glucose and insulin to move phosphorus from ECF to ICF.
- With severe hyperphosphatemia, dialysis might be necessary.
- When administering glucose-containing fluids, stop the infusion for 4 to 8 hours before obtaining a blood specimen for serum phosphorus level.

Because antacids can decrease the absorption of oral medications, patients should allow 1 to 2 hours between the ingestion of antacids and the ingestion of oral medications. Tablets should be completely chewed before swallowing, followed by a full glass of water or fruit juice. Liquid antacids should be shaken before being ingested and should also be followed with a full glass of water or juice.

Do You UNDERSTAND?

DIRECTIONS: Fill in the blanks.

1. What major cause of hyperphosphatemia is demonstrated by the following equation?
   Normal or high intake + low or absent output = ______________
2. Symptoms of hyperphosphatemia are most commonly related to ______________________.
3. The most common symptom of hyperphosphatemia is _________.

Answers: 1. renal failure; 2. hypocalcemia; 3. tetany.

TAKE HOME POINTS

Remember, antacids decrease the absorption of tetracyclines, chlorpromazine, iron salts, isoniazid, digoxin, fluoroquinolones; may increase salicylate excretion, causing lower blood levels; and may decrease the effects of methenamine and the excretion of quinidine and anticholinergics. Aluminum-based antacids promote the elimination of phosphorus from the GI tract.

- Because the purpose of antacids is to bind with the phosphorus in the small intestine and then be expelled, constipation must be avoided.
- Antacids and oral medications should not be administered at the same time.

4. Monitor ______________________ daily, because this is how phosphorus is eliminated.
5. ______________________ bind with phosphorus in the GI tract.
6. ______________________ and ______________________ are foods low in phosphorus.
7. In the absence of any symptoms or potential risk factors, ______________________ ______________________ should be repeated to check for accuracy.

DIRECTIONS: **Indicate in the spaces provided whether the following statements are *true* or *false*.**

8. _____ Amphojel blocks the excretion of phosphorus.
9. _____ Whole milk is recommended for patients with hyperphosphatemia.
10. _____ Antacids decrease the absorption of digoxin.
11. _____ A low-protein diet restricts phosphorus intake.

What IS Hypophosphatemia?

When serum phosphorus falls below 2.7 mEq/dL, the imbalance is known as *hypophosphatemia.* Hypophosphatemia is caused by many factors, the most common of which is hyperventilation (respiratory alkalosis). Any cause of hyperventilation (e.g., sepsis, anxiety, pain, heatstroke, alcohol withdrawal, diabetic ketoacidosis [DKA], hepatic encephalopathy, salicylate poisoning gram-negative bacteremia) may cause hypophosphatemia. In patients with alcoholism, diabetic ketoacidosis, or sepsis, the frequency of hypophosphatemia may be 40% to 80%. Increased excretion of phosphorus is relation hyperparathyroidism (stimulates the kidneys to excrete phosphate) or acute volume expansion, osmotic diuresis, carbonic anhydrase inhibition (e.g., acetazolamide), and some malignancies can result in hypophosphatemia. Patients with transplanted kidneys or Fanconi syndrome (proximal tubule dysfunction) may also excrete excess phosphorus because of the increased urinary output.

Another cause of low serum phosphorus level is decreased absorption of phosphorus. Conditions that can alter intake or absorption are vitamin D

Answers: 4. bowel movements; 5. Aluminum-based antacids; 6. Fruits, vegetables; 7. blood test; 8. False; 9. False; 10. True; 11. True.

deficiency, vomiting, diarrhea, overuse of aluminum hydroxide antacids (e.g., Amphojel, Basaljel, Dialume, Alternajel, Alu-Tab, Aluminet), alcohol withdrawal, anorexia, and inadequate replacement in total parenteral nutrition (TPN).

Causes of Hypophosphatemia

Inadequate Intake	Increased Excretion	Decreased Absorption	Shift from ICF to ECF
• Alcoholism • Hyperalimentation • Eating disorders	• Hyperparathyroidism • Saline diuresis • Heavy metal intoxication • Drugs: loop diuretics, cisplatin, pamidronate, and acetazolamide	• Dietary restriction • Chronic diarrhea • Chronic use of phosphate-binding antacids • Intestinal disorders (Crohn) • Vitamin D deficiency	• Diabetic ketoacidosis • Refeeding • Respiratory alkalosis

TAKE HOME POINTS

- A serum level of less than 2.7 mEq/dL = hypophosphatemia.
- Hypophosphatemia occurs most commonly with hyperventilation.
- Other causes include increased excretion, such as hyperparathyroidism, and decreased gastrointestinal absorption, either because of vomiting and/or diarrhea or ingestion of aluminum hydroxide antacids.

What You NEED TO KNOW

Because phosphorus is essential for the production of cell energy, low stores of phosphorus contribute to cell malfunction. The severity and number of clinical signs and symptoms present with hypophosphatemia are related to whether the depletion occurred suddenly or gradually and how low the serum level is when first identified. Remember, when an imbalance occurs gradually, the body has time to adjust; when the imbalance occurs rapidly, the body has no time to adjust.

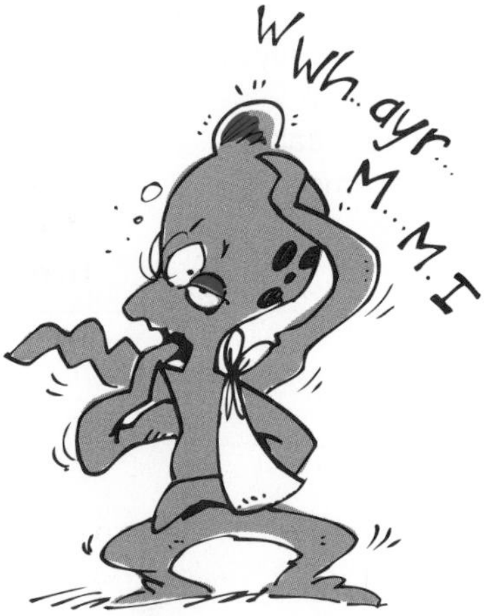

Disorientation can be a symptom of hypophosphatemia.

Signs and Symptoms of Hypophosphatemia

Neurologic	Musculoskeletal	Hematologic	Other
Numbness or tingling **(paresthesia)** often an early symptom Staggering gait **(ataxia)** Tremor Disorientation Confusion Convulsive seizures Difficulty speaking **(dysarthria)** Difficulty swallowing **(dysphagia)** Unequal pupils or involuntary eye movements **(nystagmus)** Coma Peripheral neuropathy and ascending motor paralysis, (similar to Guillain-Barré syndrome)	Weakness of skeletal or smooth muscle (most common) Rhabdomyolysis (acute sometimes fatal disease marked by destruction of skeletal muscle) because of ATP depletion and the subsequent inability of muscle cells to maintain membrane integrity Respiratory insufficiency (rate and tidal volume), particularly when the underlying cause is malnourishment Impaired cardiac contractility leading to generalized signs of myocardial depression Decreased GI motility (nausea, vomiting, and ileus) Hypotension	Hemolytic anemia (inability of erythrocytes to maintain integrity of cell membranes) Bruising GI bleeding Poor leukocyte function	Hyperglycemia Metabolic acidosis Congestive cardiomyopathy

What You DO

It is important to assess your patient for the possibility of hypophosphatemia. If you can identify patients who are at risk, then you can often prevent the imbalance from occurring by identifying hypophosphatemia early when it is more easily treated. Any patient with prolonged hyperventilation is at risk for hypophosphatemia. Patients with a history of alcoholism or liver disease, admitted with diabetic ketosis, suffering from malnutrition, or receiving TPN are candidates for hypophosphatemia. Ask the following questions:

- What is my patient's intake of phosphorus?

- Is the potential use of phosphorus by the body higher than the amount being replaced?
- Does the patient have a preexisting disease that makes a normal serum phosphorus level difficult to maintain? Patients who are healing from or fighting an infection are examples of patients who need to build proteins. Building proteins requires nitrogen. For each gram of nitrogen, the body must also have 4 mEq of phosphate.
- Does the patient's condition predispose him or her to poor absorption of phosphorus? Carefully assess the patient's use of over-the-counter antacids, including quantity and frequency.

Treatment is based on identification of the hypophosphatemia and replacement therapy. The need for phosphorus replacement and the speed with which this replacement must occur are based on how low the serum phosphorus is and the presence of symptoms. There are different treatments for different severities of phosphorus deficiency.

TAKE HOME POINTS

Early identification of hypophosphatemia = early resolution.

Mild Deficiency

- Increase dietary sources of phosphorus. Food sources high in phosphorus include milk, cheese, egg yolk, meat, fish, fowl, and nuts. Vegetables and fruits are low in phosphorus. Spinach, rhubarb, bran, and whole grain foods may decrease the absorption of phosphates.
- A quart of cow's milk provides 1 mg phosphorus/mL. Dairy products have an additional advantage of supplying absorbable calcium, which can help avoid the hypocalcemia that may result with more aggressive replacement regimens.
- Administer oral supplements such as K-Phosphate, Neutra-Phos K, and Phospha-Soda. Phosphorus preparations with sodium and potassium have disadvantages, including causing osmotic diarrhea, volume overload, or hyperkalemia.

- Tablets or capsules should not be swallowed whole.
- Potassium phosphate may cause hyperkalemia when the patient is taking potassium-sparing diuretics or angiotensin-converting enzyme (ACE) inhibitors. Sodium phosphate may cause hypernatremia when the patient is taking glucocorticoids.
- Antacids containing aluminum, magnesium, or calcium should not be taken with potassium-sparing diuretic medications, ACE inhibitors, or glucocorticoids.

Severe Deficiency

- Administer potassium phosphate or sodium phosphate intravenously (IV) using an extremely dilute concentration. An electronic pump should be used to administer IV phosphorus.

The health care provider should monitor the patient to identify improvement in symptoms with treatment. These may include the following:

- Assessing level of consciousness or disorientation
- Assessing neurologic changes, which might include unequal pupils or involuntary movement of the eyeball **(nystagmus)**

- Assessing motor strength weakness by checking handgrip strength and observing any difficulty swallowing
- Monitoring vital signs routinely, every 4 hours
- Assessing respirations and breathing sounds, which may be diminished and shallow
- Assessing the skin routinely for signs of bruising and petechiae
- Monitoring intake and output; patients must drink at least 8 ounces of water each hour to prevent the formation of kidney stones
- Monitoring daily weight
- Routine lab testing; when patients are on TPN, it is extremely important to monitor the phosphorus level
- Instituting safety measures (essential), such as seizure precautions, side rails in the up position, and assistance with ambulating
- Avoiding antacids containing aluminum, magnesium, or calcium

- Phosphorus is incompatible with Ringer's or lactated Ringer's solution, D10/0.9% Na^+Cl^-, or D5 lactated Ringer's solution. Remember, potassium or sodium is also being administered.
- Use caution when administering sodium phosphate to a patient with edema, congestive heart failure, or renal or liver impairment.
- Remember, there is an inverse relationship between phosphorus and calcium. As phosphorus rises, calcium falls.
- If calcium falls too rapidly, tetany can occur. Phosphorus must NOT be administered intramuscularly.

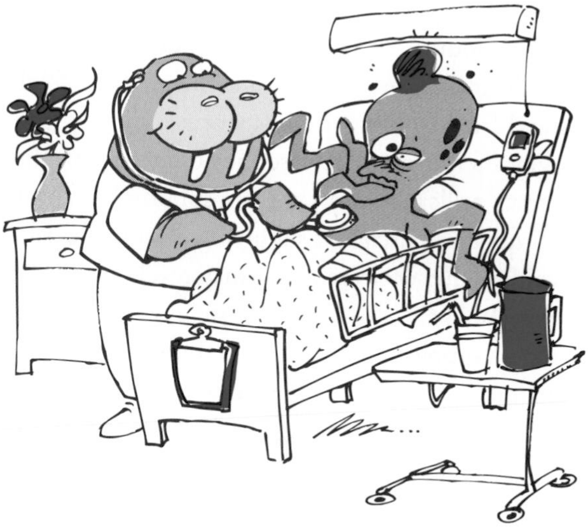

The health care provider should routinely monitor vital signs every 4 hours in a patient with severe phosphate deficiency.

TAKE HOME POINTS

- Patients predisposed to hypophosphatemia require frequent monitoring of vital signs and head-to-toe assessment.
- Instituting safety measures is essential.
- One quart of cow's milk supplies the required daily amount of phosphorus and provides the necessary vitamin D to enhance absorption.

Do You UNDERSTAND?

DIRECTIONS: Fill in the missing letters in each word to reveal a word that is related to all the words.

1.

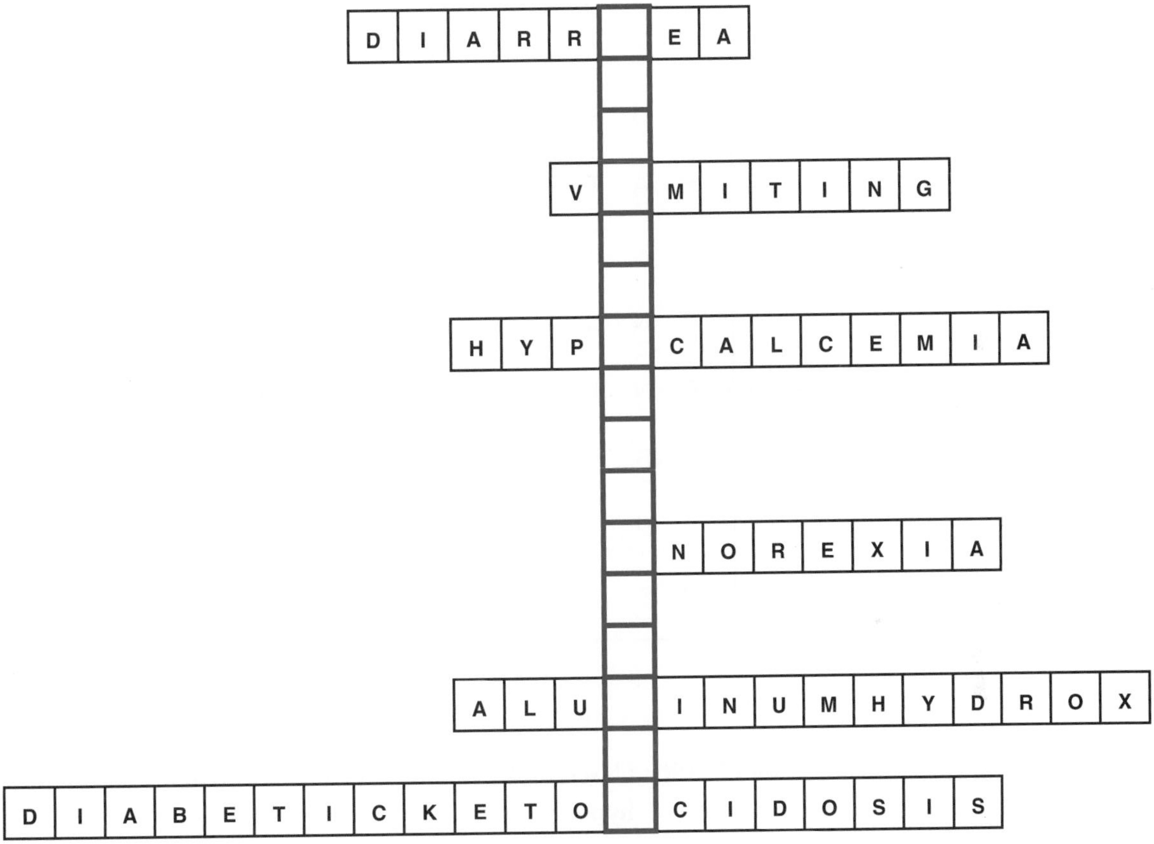

DIRECTIONS: Choose words to complete the following equations.

2. ________________ intake or ________________ absorption + normal output = hypophosphatemia.

3. Low intake + _______ _______ output = hypophosphatemia.

Answers: 1. hypophosphatemia; 2. Low, poor; 3. high, normal.

DIRECTIONS: Circle four symptoms of hypophosphatemia.

4.

O	N	W	E	R	Q	X	V	B	M	M	O	P	L
I	V	C	D	I	S	H	J	D	K	M	N	C	N
T	Z	X	W	B	O	N	E	P	A	I	N	A	U
M	U	S	C	L	E	W	E	N	Y	U	E	M	M
H	A	T	N	E	I	E	E	P	A	I	N	S	B
L	K	J	L	M	E	I	A	A	S	A	E	I	N
G	N	C	T	L	R	I	K	K	K	V	X	S	E
G	N	I	S	S	E	N	B	M	U	N	E	S	S
B	R	S	S	U	M	V	C	D	S	E	E	J	S
F	U	I	B	R	U	I	S	I	N	G	S	S	B
M	D	I	S	P	R	I	E	N	T	E	D	S	S

DIRECTIONS: Unscramble nursing measures for patients experiencing hypophosphatemia.

5. ______________________________ *(danhsrigp)*
6. ______________________________ *(trebah donsus)*
7. ______________________________ *(sedi lirsa)*
8. ______________________________ *(tival gisns)*

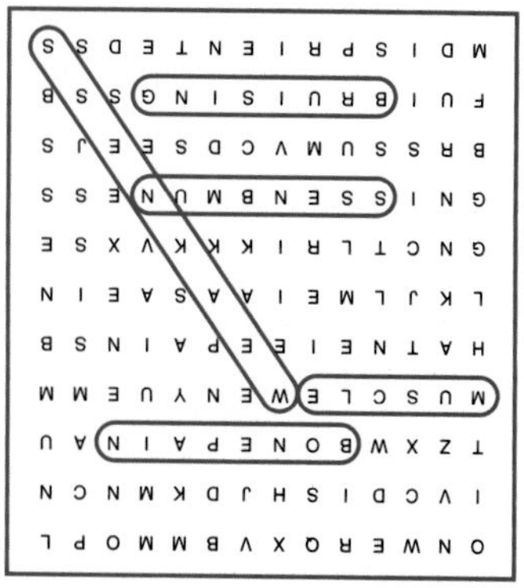

Answers: 4. bruising, bone pain, muscle weakness, numbness; 5. handgrips; 6. breath sounds; 7. side rails; 8. vital signs.

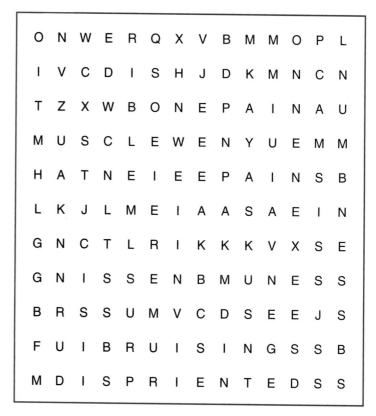

References

Bove L: Restoring electrolyte balance: calcium and phosphorus, *RN* 59(3):47, 1996.

Deglin JH, Vallerand AH: *Davis's drug guide for nurses,* ed 9, Philadelphia, 2004, FA Davis.

Ignatavicius DD, Workman ML, Mishler MA: *Medical-surgical nursing critical thinking for collaborative care,* ed 4, Philadelphia, 2002, Saunders.

Lederer E: *Hyperphosphatemia,* 2003. Available online at www.emedicine.com.

Lederer E: *Hypophosphatemia,* 2003. Available online at www.emedicine.com.

Metheny NM: *Fluid and electrolyte balance: nursing considerations,* ed 4, Philadelphia, 2000, Lippincott Williams & Wilkins.

Notes

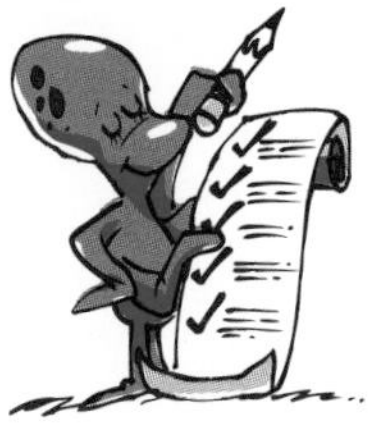

NCLEX® Review

1. On the second day of total parenteral nutrition (TPN) administration, the patient's serum phosphorus has dropped from 3.1 to 2.6 mg/dL. Which of the following rationales best describes this occurrence?
   1 The high-glucose content of TPN causes phosphorus to shift into the cells.
   2 The high-glucose content of TPN causes phosphorus to shift out of the cells.
   3 The lipid content of TPN causes phosphorus to shift into the cells.
   4 The lipid content of TPN causes phosphorus to shift out of the cells.

2. During a physical assessment of the patient with a renal condition, the patient complains of numbness around the lips. When reviewing the laboratory results, the health care practitioner would expect to see:
   1 Elevated phosphorus and decreased calcium
   2 Decreased phosphorus and increased calcium
   3 Normal phosphorus and increased calcium
   4 Normal calcium and increased phosphorus

3. The patient who takes furosemide daily is admitted with congestive heart failure. The patient demonstrates weak grip pressure and complains of bone pain. The most appropriate nursing measure is to:
   1 Instruct the patient to eat fruits and vegetables.
   2 Instruct the patient to eat dairy and meat products.
   3 Withhold the furosemide (Lasix).
   4 Administer Amphojel.

4. The health care practitioner has to perform a venipuncture for drawing a blood specimen for serum phosphorus level. The most appropriate nursing measure for the health care practitioner is to:
   1 Have the patient open and close his or her fist.
   2 Withdraw the blood within 1 minute of tourniquet application.
   3 Apply the tourniquet for a minimum of 3 minutes.
   4 Pat the vein with quick snaps.

5. When the nurse administers the 8:00 PM dose of Amphojel to a patient with a serum phosphorus level of 4.8 mg/dL, she is told that the patient has not had a bowel movement since yesterday morning. The most appropriate measure is to:
   1 Administer the laxative as prescribed.
   2 Call the physician.
   3 Tell the patient to eat foods high in fiber.
   4 Withhold the Amphojel.

6. A patient is admitted with a diagnosis of congestive heart failure. Paresthesia, particularly around the mouth, is observed. The physician's order includes potassium phosphate (15 μmol) intramuscularly for the patient whose serum phosphorus level is 1.4 mEq/dL. Which of the following factors best describes the basis of the nurse's action to question the physician's written prescription?
   1 Dose is too high.
   2 Potassium may cause hypokalemia.
   3 Route is contraindicated.
   4 Serum level may be inaccurate.

7. Which of the following interventions should the health care provider include in teaching the patient to reduce serum phosphorus levels?
   1 Take an antacid with oral medications.
   2 Avoid aluminum-based antacids such as Amphojel.
   3 Include dairy products, fish, and nuts in the diet.
   4 Include spinach and whole grain foods in the diet.

8. Symptoms of hyperphosphatemia are most commonly associated with which of the following electrolyte imbalances?
   1 Hypocalcemia
   2 Hypercalcemia
   3 Hypokalemia
   4 Hyperkalemia

9. The patient is receiving continuous hyperglucose intravenous fluids. Before obtaining a serum specimen for phosphorus levels, the health care provider must:
   1 Infuse IV 0.9% NaCl for 2 hours.
   2 Obtain two separate blood specimens.
   3 Stop the current IV fluids for 4 to 8 hours.
   4 Use the opposite extremity from the IV site for the blood withdrawal.

10. What is the most common disorder associated with hyperphosphatemia?

11. Why is constipation to be avoided when treating hyperphosphatemia with antacids?

12. True or False: Antacids and oral medications should be administered at the same time.

13. How much water should a patient drink when taking Phospha-Soda for treating hypophosphatemia?

14. What are three dietary sources of phosphorus?

15. Tablets administered to treat hypophosphatemia should be __________ before swallowed.

NCLEX® Review Answers

1. 1 The phosphorus enters the cell with glucose during carbohydrate metabolism. The phosphorus enters the cell with insulin and carbohydrate during metabolism. Lipid content does not normally affect phosphorus. Phosphorus moves into the cell with metabolism.

2. 1 Numbness around the lips is a common sign of tetany, which is a result of hypocalcemia. Phosphorus and calcium are inversely related. Therefore, if calcium is increased, phosphorus will be decreased, not normal. Hyperphosphatemia would be present with hypocalcemia. Paresthesia and profound muscle weakness are early signs of hypophosphatemia.

3. 2 Loop diuretics increase the excretion of phosphorus through the kidneys. The patient presents with signs and symptoms of hypophosphatemia. Therefore, dietary replacement with foods high in phosphorus, such as dairy and meat products is necessary. Fruits and vegetables are low in phosphorus. Diuretics are necessary to manage the cardiac heart failure. Amphojel hinders the absorption of phosphorus.

4. 2 Serum phosphorus levels can be inaccurate if the blood specimen is obtained by altering the hemoconcentration or hemolysis. Leaving the tourniquet in place less than 1 minute will prevent this problem by increasing the movement of phosphorus into the cell with an increased requirement for energy during muscle contraction. The patient opening and closing the fist will cause a false result. Applying a tourniquet for more than 3 minutes and patting the vein with quick snaps causes cell lysis.

5. 1 Antacids may cause constipation. The purpose of Amphojel is to bind with the phosphorus in the small intestine and then be expelled. Therefore, daily bowel movements are necessary. First, use a laxative to correct constipation. Document. If no relief from the laxative is achieved, notify the health care provider. Although eating foods high in fiber is important in diet teaching, the patient needs quicker results than a high-fiber diet can produce. Administer the laxative, and instruct the patient to include fiber in the diet to prevent reoccurrence. Amphojel is ordered to lower phosphorus. Administer the medication, and monitor bowel movements. Administer laxatives as required.

6. 3 Phosphate must not be administered intramuscularly. The dose is within the general guidelines for parenteral administration. Although potassium phosphate may elevate the serum potassium level, sodium phosphate may lead to hypernatremia, especially in patients with congestive heart failure. Clinical findings of paresthesias, particularly around the mouth, support the serum level report.

7. 4 Foods such as spinach and whole grains decrease the absorption of phosphates. Antacids interfere with the absorption of oral medications. Patients should allow 1 to 2 hours between the ingestion of antacid and the ingestion of oral medications. Aluminum-based antacids bind with phosphorus in the gastrointestinal tract and the phosphorus will be eliminated in the feces. Dairy products, fish, and nuts are high in phosphorus.

8. 1 There is an inverse relationship between calcium and phosphorus. When phosphorus levels are elevated, calcium levels are lowered. Changes in serum potassium levels are usually a result of underlying disorders and not directly related to phosphorus levels.

9. 3 Phosphorus moves into the cell with the glucose; thus, the serum level will be lower than normal. Accuracy depends on the stoppage of the fluids containing glucose. IV fluids containing glucose should be held for 4 to 8 hours to ensure an accurate serum level. Separate blood specimens do not ensure accuracy of serum levels during the administration of intravenous glucose. The glucose effect is systemic; thus, either extremity will be affected.

10. Renal disease

11. Antacids bind with the phosphorus in the small intestine, and are then expelled in the feces.

12. False. Antacids decrease the absorption of oral medications. Patients should allow 1 to 2 hours between ingestion of antacids and the ingestion of oral medications.

13. 8-ounce glass every hour to prevent kidney stones.

14. Dairy products, egg yolk, meat

15. Dissolved in an 8-ounce glass of water. The solution should stand for 2 to 5 minutes to ensure that the medication is completely dissolved.

Notes

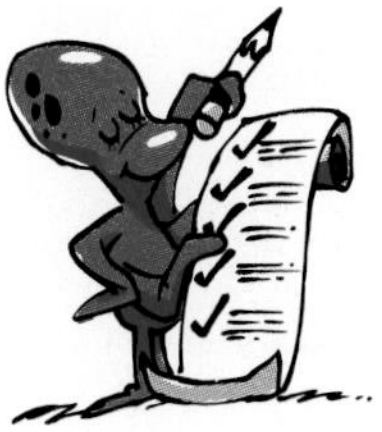

Chapter

7 Magnesium

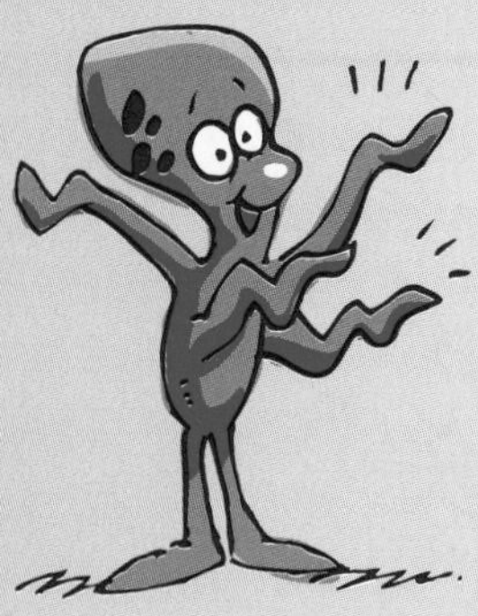

What You WILL LEARN

After reading this chapter, you will know how to do the following:

- ✔ Name one use of magnesium in the human body.
- ✔ Describe hypermagnesemia.
- ✔ List two outcomes of hypomagnesemia.

Magnesium (Mg) is the second most abundant positively charged ion (**cation**) in the intracellular fluid (ICF). Potassium (K^+) is the most abundant ICF cation (see Chapter 5). The basic functions of magnesium are similar to the functions of potassium and calcium, affecting action potentials, bone metabolism, and many other intracellular reactions. Magnesium imbalances are not as common as other electrolyte problems, and the serum levels do not correlate well with total body magnesium stores. Since magnesium plays a major role in cardiac electrophysiology, laboratory values are monitored in cardiac patients. Therefore it is important for the health care provider to understand who is at risk for imbalances and which signs and symptoms should be assessed.

What IS Magnesium?

Magnesium is a mineral element found abundantly in nature in a combined state. It is one of the most plentiful elements of the earth's crust and is an essential component of all living material as a constituent of chlorophyll. In the body, it is second only to potassium as the most abundant intracellular electrolyte and is essential as a cofactor for many enzymes, especially for enzymes using adenosine triphosphate (ATP).

Normal Serum Values

- Adult: 1.5 to 2.5 mEq/L or 1.8 to 3.0 mg/dL
- Critical level for adults: less than 0.5 mEq/L or more than 3.0 mEq/L or less than 1.2 mg/dL or greater than 5.0 mg/dL
- Child: 1.6 to 2.6 mEq/L or 1.7 to 2.1 mg/dL
- Newborn: 1.4 to 2.9 mEq/L or 1.5 to 2.2 mg/dL

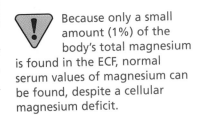

Because only a small amount (1%) of the body's total magnesium is found in the ECF, normal serum values of magnesium can be found, despite a cellular magnesium deficit.

Nearly all of the body's magnesium is found in the ICF. Approximately 40% to 60% of the body's magnesium is stored in bone, with the remainder in soft tissue and muscle cells. Only 1% of the total is in the extracellular fluid (ECF), with one third of this amount bound to plasma proteins.

What You NEED TO KNOW

Sources of Magnesium

Magnesium, present in the plant pigment chlorophyll, is ingested primarily through plant sources. Vegetables, particularly spinach, broccoli, squash, avocado, potato, and lima beans, are great sources of magnesium. Whole grains, notably wheat germ, rolled oats, nuts, and seeds, are other highly nutritional sources for magnesium. Meats that are high in magnesium include tuna, beef, pork, and chicken. Other common sources include raisins, milk, and yogurt. "Hard" tap water (well water) contains a high concentration of magnesium. Because magnesium is abundant in food and water, a magnesium deficiency caused by lack of ingestion is rare in healthy people.

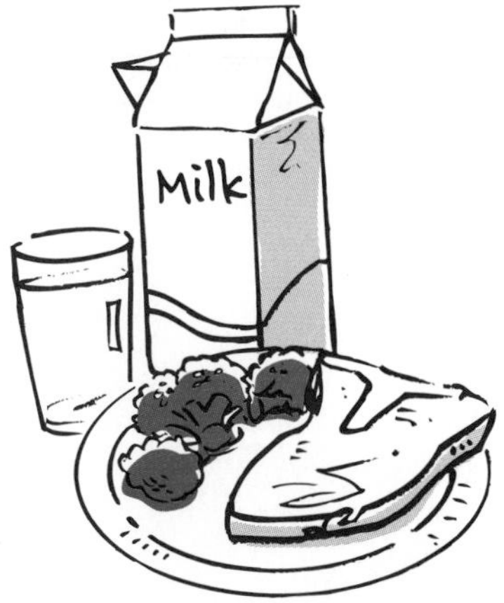

Foods rich in magnesium include: milk, broccoli, and tuna.

Recommended Daily Allowances for Magnesium

Infants: 40 to 60 mg
Children ages 1 to 3: 80 mg
Children ages 4 to 6: 120 mg
Children ages 7 to 10: 170 mg
Adults: ranges from 270 to 350 mg depending on age and gender
Pregnant women: 320 mg
Lactating women: 350 mg

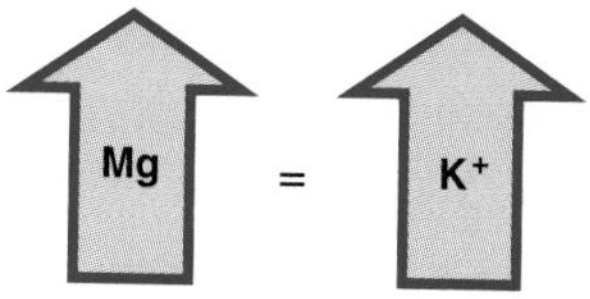

Control of Magnesium

The regulation of magnesium levels is not completely understood, and currently, there are no known hormones that are identified in the regulatory process. It is known, however, that magnesium and potassium levels increase and decrease together, and the regulation of calcium, potassium, and magnesium is interrelated.

Stability in the normal body states (**homeostasis**) of mineral balance depends on the amount of magnesium ingested, the amount absorbed in the intestine, and the amount excreted.

An increased intake of calcium or phosphorus can decrease the intestinal absorption of magnesium. Conversely, a decreased intake of calcium or phosphorus can increase the amount of magnesium absorbed in the intestines.

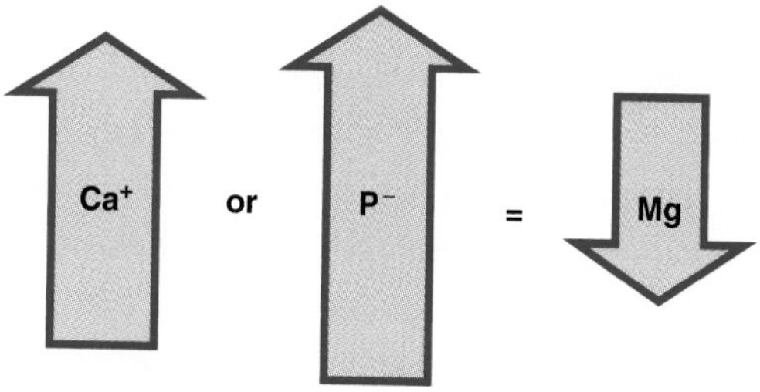

TAKE HOME POINTS

Only approximately one third of the magnesium ingested is absorbed in the ileum and colon; the remainder of the ingested magnesium is excreted in feces.

The kidneys help to regulate the magnesium level by excreting magnesium when the ECF levels are high and conserving it when the levels are low. When the serum magnesium level drops, absorption takes place at the proximal tubule and Henle's loop.

Functions of Magnesium

Most of the activities of magnesium are intracellular in nature because most of it is located in the ICF.

- Magnesium serves as an activating co-factor in more than 300 enzymes in the body.
- Magnesium acts directly on the myoneural junction, affecting neuromuscular irritability and contractions.

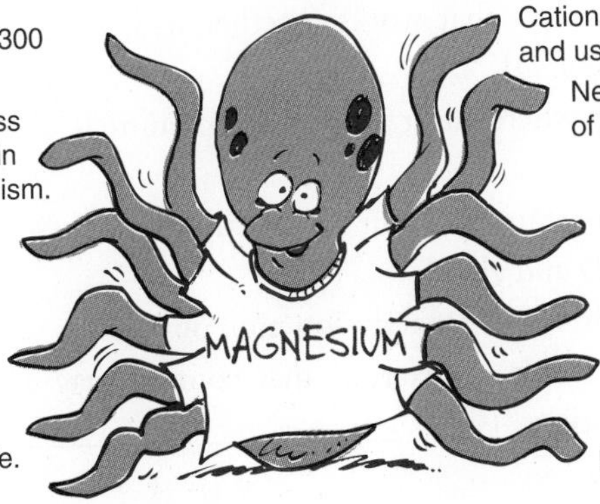
Activating co-factor > 300 enzymes.
Increases effectiveness of the enzymes used in carbohydrate metabolism.
Co-factor in DNA & RNA synthesis.
Activates many B-complex vitamins.
Co-factor in blood-clotting cascade.
Acts directly on the myoneural junction, affecting neuromuscular irritability and contractions.
MAGNESIUM
Cations activate ATP in the production and use of energy.
Necessary for formation & functions of healthy bones.
Influences the parathyroid hormone so calcium level is maintained.
Helps the process of vasodilation, contributing to cardiovascular regulation.
Transports sodium and potassium ions across cellular membranes.
Is an excitable membrane stabilizer.

- Magnesium is a co-factor in DNA and protein synthesis.
- Magnesium assists with RNA synthesis.
- Magnesium increases the effectiveness of many of the enzymes used in carbohydrate metabolism.
- Magnesium activates many of the B-complex vitamins.
- The ECF magnesium is a co-factor in the blood-clotting cascade.
- Magnesium cations provide a bridge between the second and third phosphate groups of the ATP molecule to activate ATP in the production and use of energy.
- Magnesium is necessary for the formation and functions of healthy bones.
- Magnesium influences the parathyroid hormone to maintain the calcium level.
- Magnesium helps the process of vasodilation, contributing to cardiovascular regulation.
- The sodium-potassium pump depends on the magnesium ions for the transportation of sodium (Na^+) and potassium ions across cellular membranes.
- Magnesium is an excitable membrane stabilizer.

Do You UNDERSTAND?

DIRECTIONS: Unscramble the italicized words in the spaces provided.

1. Plant source of magnesium. ______________________ *(lyprlchoohl)*
2. Place where most magnesium is stored. ______________________ *(nobe)*

Answers: 1. **chlorophyll**; 2. **bone.**

TAKE HOME POINTS

Magnesium is vital to the transmission and conduction of nerve impulses through the myoneural junction to skeletal, cardiac, and smooth muscle, which is essential for contraction.

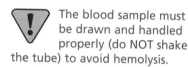

The blood sample must be drawn and handled properly (do NOT shake the tube) to avoid hemolysis.

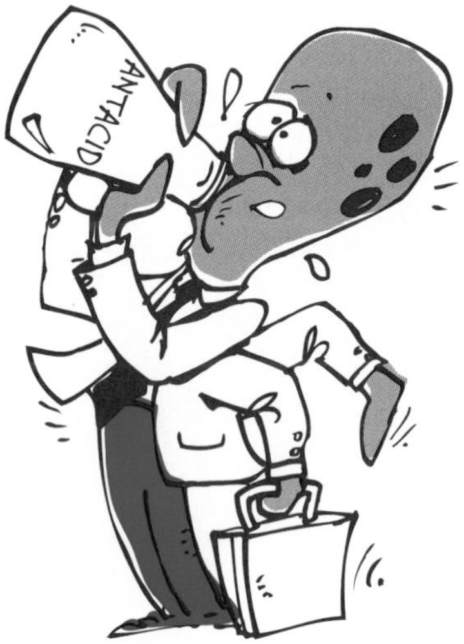

Patients who have renal dysfunction and take antacids or laxatives containing magnesium are at risk for hypermagnesemia.

LIFE SPAN

Women receiving intravenous (IV) magnesium sulfate for pregnancy-induced hypertension or for controlling premature labor are also at risk for hypermagnesemia. Neonates exposed to magnesium during labor are also at risk for hypermagnesemia.

3. Electrolyte that works together with magnesium. __________ *(mistpusao)*
4. Place where most of the magnesium is absorbed. __________ *(luime)*
5. Magnesium helps in the synthesis of these. __________ *(NAD* and *ARN)*
6. Patients with renal dysfunction or patients who use excessive amounts of antacids or laxatives that contain magnesium are at risk for this condition. __________ *(amsnarphyemgeei)*

What IS Hypermagnesemia?

Because the normal value is 1.5 to 2.5 milliequivalents per liter (mEq/L), a serum magnesium level greater than 2.5 mEq/L is called *hypermagnesemia.* Although rare, the most likely causes of hypermagnesemia are impaired magnesium excretion from renal failure or an excessive intake of magnesium.

What You NEED TO KNOW

Hemolyzed (destruction of red blood cells in the test tube) blood samples may provide a false elevated magnesium level.

Patients who have renal dysfunction and take antacids or laxatives containing magnesium are at risk for hypermagnesemia. Chronic and excessive users of antacids such as Maalox, Mylanta, Di-Gel, or laxatives such as milk of magnesia, citrate of magnesia, or **magnesium sulfate** (Epsom salts) may develop hypermagnesemia.

Hypermagnesemia may occur in patients with diabetes mellitus or diabetic ketoacidosis with renal insufficiency. Occasionally, hypermagnesemia occurs in lymphocytic and myelocytic leukemia. These patients are at risk for renal insufficiency from exposure to the nephrotoxic effects of certain chemotherapy and antibiotics. Also, when leukostasis occurs, the glomerular filtration rate decreases. During treatment, leukemic cells release uric acid, which may crystallize in the renal tubules, causing obstruction.

With hypermagnesemia, muscle cell activity is decreased as a result of the blockage of acetylcholine release at the myoneural junction where the nerve and muscle fibers meet. Respiratory paralysis may result if respira-

Answers: 3. **potassium;** 4. **ileum;** 5. **DNA and RNA;** 6. **hypermagnesemia.**

tory muscles are affected. Delayed conduction in the myocardium may result in heart block. With mild hypermagnesemia, a prolonged PR and QT interval may be indicated on the electrocardiogram (ECG), progressing to QRS complex widening, T-wave elevation, and eventual heart block as the serum level of magnesium rises.

Signs and Symptoms of Hypermagnesemia

- Flushing
- Increased perspiration
- Muscular weakness
- Diminished deep tendon reflexes
- Nausea and vomiting
- Hypotension
- Cardiac dysrhythmia
- Respiratory compromise

With severe hypermagnesemia (serum level greater than 9 mEq/L), sedation will be present, which can be followed by a decreased heart rate and falling blood pressure, culminating in coma and cardiac arrest.

What You DO

The goals of hypermagnesemia management are to speed the elimination of magnesium and to curtail its intake. Treatment is aimed at identifying and eliminating the cause.

- Maintain continuous cardiac monitoring in severe cases. Electrocardiogram (ECG) changes such as a prolonged PR interval, widened QRS complex, and tall T wave should be reported.
- Because calcium antagonizes magnesium, administer an IV solution containing calcium salts (calcium gluconate) when encountering extremely high levels of hypermagnesemia.
- Discontinue medications that contain magnesium such as Maalox, Mylanta, Di-Gel, milk of magnesium, citrate of magnesium, and Epsom salts.
- Institute renal hydration or administer diuretics for patients with normal renal function. Also, record intake and output.
- Watch for decreasing level of sensorium (magnesium has a sedative effect), and assess for muscular responsiveness.
- Monitor vital signs to assess for hypotension and decreased respiratory rate.
- Complete and document a neurologic assessment for mental status, reflexes, and muscle strength. Compare findings to patient's baseline, and report changes.

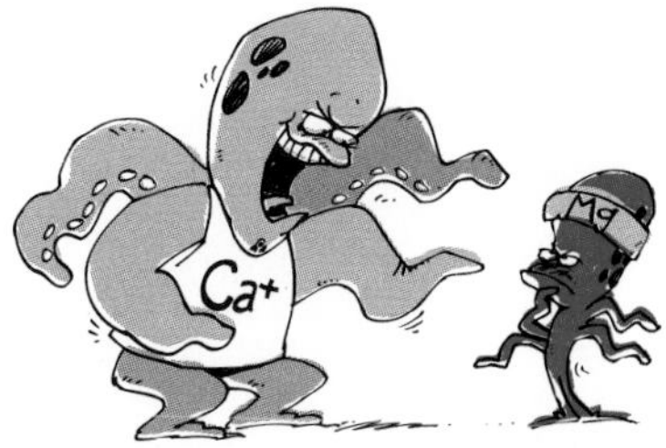

Because calcium antagonizes magnesium, administer an IV solution containing calcium salts when treating hypermagnesemia.

- Assess the skin for flushing and diaphoresis.
- Monitor laboratory data, including the serum magnesium level and renal function tests, for blood urea nitrogen (BUN) and creatinine levels.
- Review and provide a list of drugs (antacids and laxatives) that contain magnesium for patients who take large amounts of these agents or are renal compromised.
- Treat renal failure with dialysis.

Do You UNDERSTAND?

DIRECTIONS: Unscramble the following signs and symptoms of hypermagnesemia.

1. ______________________ *(smarlucu skawenes)*
2. ______________________ *(slugfinh)*
3. ______________________ *(aneasu dan gnovtimi)*
4. ______________________ *(taginwes)*
5. ______________________ *(poshneyniot)*
6. ______________________ *(recaddese prearroitys tear)*

What IS Hypomagnesemia?

Hypomagnesemia is defined as a serum level below 1.5 mEq/L or 1.8 mg/dL. Usually, magnesium deficiency occurs in the same conditions that lead to decreased potassium and calcium levels. The patient may be asymptomatic until the serum magnesium level is less than 1 mEq/L.

What You NEED TO KNOW

Magnesium depletion may be caused by an inadequate dietary intake, associated with alcoholism, or by malabsorption, as in inflammatory bowel disease or after a bowel resection.

Answers: 1. muscular weakness; 2. flushing; 3. nausea and vomiting; 4. sweating; 5. hypotension; 6. decreased respiratory rate.

Excessive gastric or intestinal drainage may lead to a significant loss of magnesium. Renal tubular disease, osmotic diuresis (caused by hyperglycemia), acidosis, or nephrotoxic drugs are common causes of renal loss of magnesium from excessive excretion. Hypomagnesemia can occur with some endocrine disorders, such as hypothyroidism, and with a rare genetic disorder known as primary idiopathic hypomagnesemia.

Decreased magnesium levels are often associated with certain clinical conditions, including decreased protein intake or absorption, cirrhosis of the liver, chronic diarrhea, bowel resection complications, prolonged administration of IV fluids that do not contain magnesium, hypoparathyroidism, hyperaldosteronism, and hypokalemia. Alcohol withdrawal may be associated with hypomagnesemia because magnesium shifts as glucose moves into the cell during the withdrawal period.

Drugs that have been found to sometimes decrease serum magnesium levels include diuretics, amphotericin B, aminoglycoside antibiotics (gentamicin, tobramycin, and neomycin), corticosteroids, calcium gluconate, insulin, and cisplatin.

Magnesium affects the central nervous, neuromuscular, cardiovascular, and gastrointestinal systems; therefore a wide variety of symptoms can be obsereved. A heightened reactivity is caused by the greater acetylcholine release, which triggers increased action potential transmissions from nerve to nerve and from nerve to cell. Cardiovascular effects result from myocardial irritation, causing cardiac arrhythmia, manifested as premature ventricular contractions that may predispose to ventricular or atrial fibrillation. The gastrointestinal effects, often observed with hypomagnesemia, are caused by decreased contractility of gut musculature.

TAKE HOME POINTS

The body usually has adequate stores of magnesium. Symptoms of magnesium deficiencies are not commonly observed until the serum level is less than 1 mEq/L.

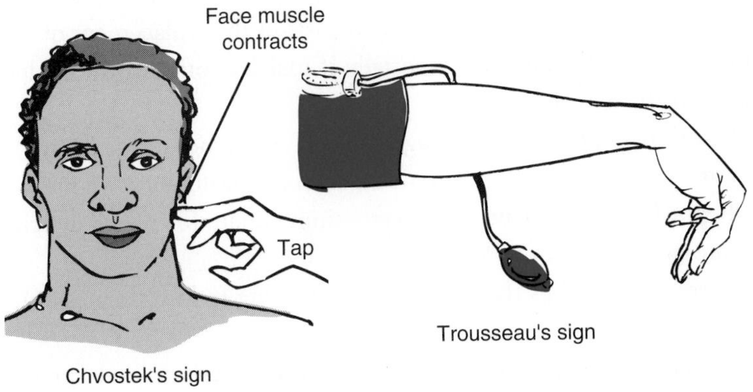

LIFE SPAN

Seizures, particularly in children with severely decreased levels, is a sign of hypomagnesemia.

Signs and Symptoms of Hypomagnesemia

- Increased neuromuscular irritability, twitches, tremors, and leg and feet cramping
- Behavioral disturbances, restlessness, or disorientation
- Hyperreflexia
- Muscle spasms and possible tetany
- Nystagmus
- Cardiac arrhythmia
- Electrocardiographic changes: prolonged QT interval, widened QRS complex, T-wave inversion, and depression of the ST segment
- Swallowing difficulties
- Anorexia
- Nausea and vomiting
- Paralytic ileus

Because of coexisting hypocalcemia, a positive Chvostek's sign (spasm of the muscles innervated by the facial nerve, elicited by tapping lightly over the facial nerve below the temple to produce a spasm of the face, lip, or nose) may be observed, as well as a positive Trousseau's sign (carpal spasm causing contraction of the fingers and hand when circulation is constricted for 1 to 4 minutes by inflating a blood pressure cuff on the upper arm).

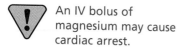

An IV bolus of magnesium may cause cardiac arrest.

What You DO

Management of hypomagnesemia consists of the replacement of magnesium orally or parenterally, especially if malabsorption is the underlying cause of the deficiency.

- Administer prescribed oral agents such as magnesium oxide tablets or antacids that contain magnesium, such as Maalox or Mylanta.
- Begin IV replacement with magnesium sulfate for severe deficits at a rate no faster than 150 mg/min.
- Discontinue drugs that may be contributing to low magnesium, such as diuretics.
- Check for digitalis toxicity when serum magnesium levels are low.

TAKE HOME POINTS

Most electrolyte imbalances do not occur in isolation. With hypomagnesemia, there is often a potassium or a calcium imbalance, which should be corrected simultaneously.

Do You UNDERSTAND?

DIRECTIONS: Match the sign or symptom of hypomagnesemia in column A with the description in column B.

Column A	Column B
1. _____ Positive Chvostek's sign	a. Carpal spasm
2. _____ Increased neuromuscular irritability	b. Serum magnesium level below 1.5 or 1.8 mEq/L
3. _____ Difficulty swallowing	c. Facial-nerve spasm
4. _____ Positive Trousseau's sign	d. Related to decreased contractility
5. _____ Hypomagnesemia	e. Caused by greater acetylcholine release that triggers increased action potential in nerve transmission

References

Brody T: *Mineral deficiency: Gale encyclopedia of medicine,* Detroit, 1999, Gale Research.

Glynn-Tucker EM: Hypomagnesemia. In Chernecky C, Berger B, editors: *Advanced and critical care oncology nursing: managing primary complications,* Philadelphia, 1998, Saunders.

Haggerty M: *Magnesium imbalance. Gale encyclopedia of medicine,* Detroit, 1999, Gale Research.

Kee JL: *Laboratory and diagnostic tests with nursing implications,* ed 6, Upper Saddle River, NJ, 2001, Prentice Hall.

Phipps WJ et al: *Medical-surgical nursing concepts and clinical practice,* ed 7, St Louis, 2003, Mosby.

Rosdahl CB, Kowalski MT, editors: *Textbook of basic nursing,* ed 8, Philadelphia, 2003, Lippincott Williams & Wilkins.

Answers: 1. c; 2. e; 3. d; 4. a; 5. b.

Notes

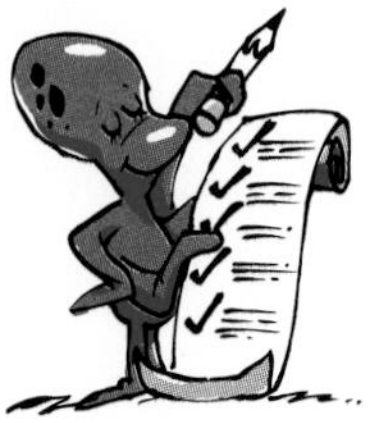

NCLEX® Review

1. Mr. GQ, the CEO of a large corporation, is having an endoscopy today for increased gastric distress, which included a feeling of fullness, nausea, and a burning pain. You note that he is extremely flushed, perspiring profusely, hypotensive, and weak. You recognize these as signs of hypermagnesemia. What would you ask this patient?
   1 "Do you take any diuretic medications?"
   2 "Have you has any surgery on your bowel"
   3 "What medications do you take to help the burning pain in your stomach?"
   4 "What have you eaten in the past 24 hours?"

2. Which of the following signs and symptoms would you observe with hypomagnesemia?
   1 Restlessness and confusion
   2 Twitching and tremors
   3 Anorexia, nausea, and vomiting
   4 All of the above

3. Miss PY, age 27, has had a bowel resection. You note that her magnesium level is 1.3 mg/dL. What would you expect her calcium and potassium levels to be?
   1 Within normal range
   2 Slightly elevated above normal range
   3 Below normal range
   4 Greatly elevated above normal range

4. RH, age 37, has a long history of alcoholism. He has a serum magnesium level of 1.2 mg/dL. You are to instruct him to eat food rich in magnesium. All of the following are rich in magnesium *except:*
   1 Spinach
   2 Wheat bran
   3 Milk chocolate
   4 Sunflower seeds

5. A patient with which of the following is at the greatest risk for hypermagnesemia?
   1 Renal failure and diabetes mellitus
   2 Pancreatitis and fever
   3 Hypotension and hyperchloremia
   4 History of colon cancer and glaucoma

6. The health care provider is caring for a 52-year-old man with lung cancer who was admitted with a low serum magnesium level (hypomagnesemia) after chemotherapy. The health care provider has established IV access and is about to administer magnesium sulfate 4 g IV piggyback over 2 to 6 hours when the patient starts to develop neuromuscular symptoms of irritability, spasticity, and tremors. Besides administering the magnesium, what is the next immediate nursing intervention?

7. Which of the following patients is at the greatest risk for hypomagnesemia?
   1 Alcoholic during withdrawal
   2 Athlete
   3 Premature infant
   4 Older adult on long-term diuretics

8. Which of the following signs and symptoms would be observed with hypermagnesemia?
   1 Flushing and muscular weakness
   2 Increased appetite
   3 Diarrhea
   4 Polyuria

9. Which of the following agents, if taken in excess, can lead to hypermagnesemia?
   1 Diuretics
   2 Potassium supplements
   3 Antidepressants
   4 Antacids

10. When administering IV magnesium, the health care provider should make certain that the rate is no more than 150 mg/min. Administration of magnesium in fast rate or bolus can cause which serious complication?
   1 Vein irritation
   2 Paralysis
   3 Mental confusion
   4 Cardiac arrest

NCLEX® Review Answers

1. **3** Antacids such as Mylanta, Maalox, and Di-Gel contain magnesium. It would be important to learn whether the patient is using an antacid, the type, and the amount. The rest of the choices do not account for a raised magnesium level.

2. **4** There is greater acetylcholine release in hypomagnesemia, which triggers increased action potential transmission from nerve to nerve and from nerve to cell.

3. **3** Potassium and calcium depletions are often caused by the same factors that cause magnesium depletion.

4. **3** The pigment chlorophyll in plant sources has the highest nutritional value for magnesium.

5. **1** Patients with renal failure and diabetes mellitus caused by renal insufficiency and diabetic ketoacidosis are at risk.

6. Initiate seizure precautions. Place suction equipment and an oral airway at the bedside. Central nervous system irritability and neuromuscular hyperexcitability demand safety precautions.

7. **1** Alcohol withdrawal cause a magnesium shift as glucose moves into the cell.

8. **1** Flushing and use of antacids that contain magnesium can lead to elevated serum levels.

9. **4** Excessive use of antacids that contain magnesium can lead to elevated serum levels. The remaining choices do not affect magnesium.

10. **4** IV replacement is reserved for severe deficits and should be given slowly because rapid infusion can cause cardiac arrest. Vein irritation can also occur with rapid infusion of many agents but is not a life-threatening complication.

Notes

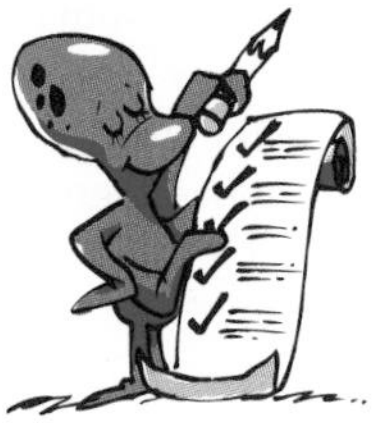

Calcium

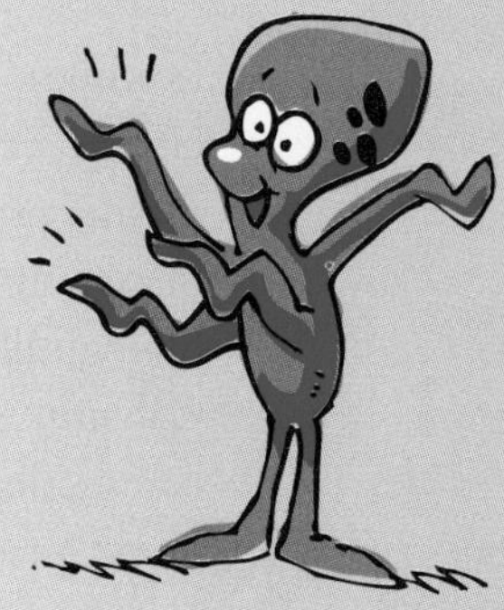

Chapter

8

What You WILL LEARN

After reading this chapter, you will know how to do the following:

- ✔ State two uses of calcium in maintaining homeostasis in the human body.
- ✔ Name two signs/symptoms of hypercalcemia.
- ✔ Describe two potential findings in a person with hypocalcemia.

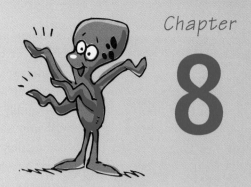

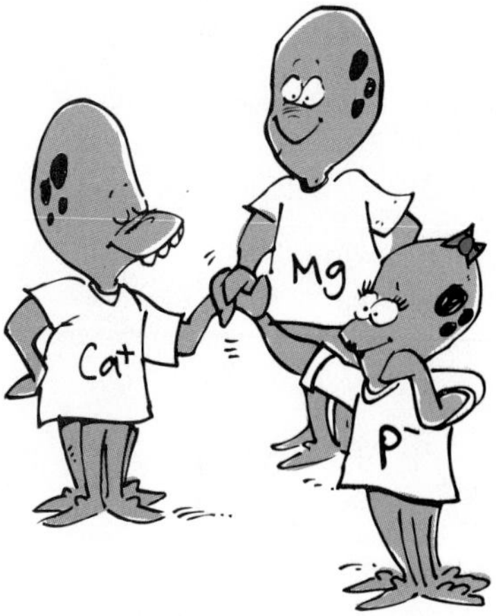

Calcium (Ca^{+}) works closely with phosphorus (P^{-}) and magnesium (Mg).

Calcium (Ca^{+}) is an ion with two positive charges **(divalent cation)** and works closely with phosphorus (P^{-}) and magnesium (Mg). It is the most abundant cation and the fifth most abundant substance after carbon, hydrogen, oxygen, and nitrogen. Most of the body's calcium is used to provide mass and strength to the bones and teeth. The small amount found in the body fluids is essential for maintaining many critical physiologic functions. Therefore it is important for the health care provider to identify and properly manage patients with a calcium imbalance.

What IS Calcium?

Calcium is the most abundant mineral in the body, accounting for approximately 40% of all body minerals and 2% of body weight. Most of the body's calcium is located in the bone as hydroxyapatite, an inorganic compound that provides bone rigidity; the remaining 1% is in the plasma and cells. The plasma calcium is found in three forms free (ionized), protein-bound (to albumin), and complexed with phosphate, citrate, or carbonate. In the plasma, half of the calcium is bound to plasma proteins, 10% complexed with another electrolyte, and approximately 40% is in the free or ionized form. The ionized calcium is the biologically active form that performs major physiologic functions. Calcium is necessary for the transmission of nerve impulses and normal contraction of skeletal and heart muscles, regulation of the heart and blood pressure, hormone secretion, maintenance of muscle tone, and formation of blood clots (serves as an enzymatic cofactor for blood clotting). Calcium is required for hormone secretion and the function of cell receptors. Calcium phosphorus forms the teeth and bone. The bones serve as an available store of calcium for the body when the plasma blood level is low. It is a common mineral in nature and is found in limestone, marble, coral, pearls, seashells, eggshells, and bones.

Normal Total Serum Values*

- Adults: 8.5 to 10 mg/dL
- Infants younger than 10 days old: 7.6 to 10.4 mg/dL
- Infants from 10 days to 2 years: 8.8 to 10.8 mg/dL
- Children from 2 to 12 years: 8.8 to 10.8 mg/dL
- Children from 12 to 18 years: 8.4 to 10.2 mg/dL

*This value includes both the free and protein-bound calcium and is the laboratory test most often prescribed. The serum calcium concentration remains constant in normal physiologic functioning.

Ionized Serum Calcium Values*

- Adults: 4.64 to 5.28 mg/dL
- Newborns: 2.24 to 2.46 mg/dL
- Children: 4.80 to 5.52 mg/dL

*This value measures the amount of calcium that is free and unbound to protein and therefore available; measured in low-protein states.

When a patient has a high calcium level with a low serum albumin, a correction factor can be used to calculate the true calcium value. Corrected serum calcium is calculated by the following formula:

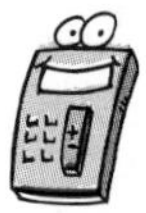

$$\text{serum calcium} + 0.8\,(4.0 - \text{serum albumin}) = \text{corrected serum calcium}$$

Approximately 99% of the body's calcium is found in bones and teeth. The remainder is found in plasma and extracellular fluid (ECF). The ECF concentration of calcium is relatively high compared with the intracellular fluid (ICF) level, with a ratio of 10,000:1. This large ratio demonstrates a steep concentration gradient between the ECF and ICF, which allows the movement of calcium into cells when the calcium channels are open.

Because calcium is a divalent cation (Ca^{2+} two positive charges), it is found in two forms: bound and unbound. The bound form is connected mostly to albumin, a serum protein, with a small amount bound to globulin.

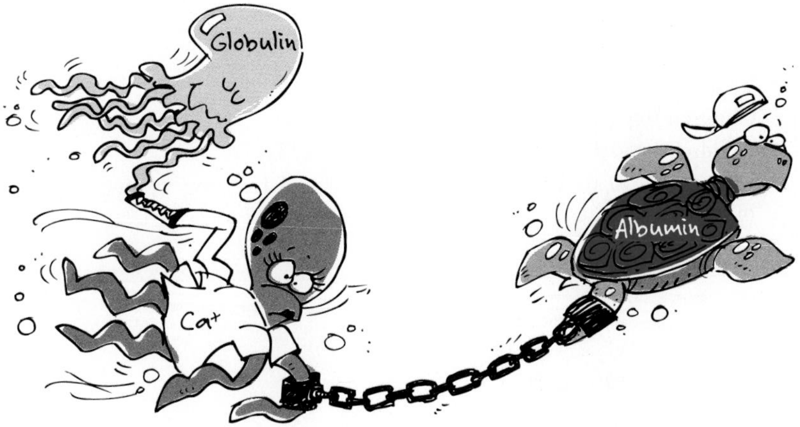

Calcium tends to float around bound to albumin.

The fact that calcium is bound to proteins is important to consider when caring for a patient who has low serum albumin, because less calcium will be protein bound, which causes a false low reading.

With hypoalbuminemic states, the serum calcium level may be low, but this does not necessarily indicate a decrease in biologically available calcium. Rather, it reflects that there is less protein available to bind with calcium. In these situations, a calculated or actual serum ionized calcium level is more helpful.

Free calcium (ionized calcium) is the biologically active form in the ECF and must be maintained within a narrow range for normal physiologic functioning. Approximately 50% of total serum calcium is ionized.

The laboratory serum calcium level measures both the bound and unbound forms.

TAKE HOME POINTS

Approximately 40% of the serum calcium is bound to proteins.

It is important to measure the serum ionized calcium for patients with low protein (hypoalbuminemia) because the ionized form indicates what amount of calcium is free and available.

What You NEED TO KNOW

Sources of Calcium

In the average diet, approximately 72% of calcium is derived from dairy products, with 11% from grain products and 6% from vegetables and fruits. Excellent food sources of calcium include milk, yogurt, cheese, sardines, canned salmon, egg yolks, cauliflower, and oysters. Other plant sources include soybeans, and dark green leafy vegetables such as kale, chard, spinach, collard greens, and rhubarb. Fortified orange juice also contains calcium.

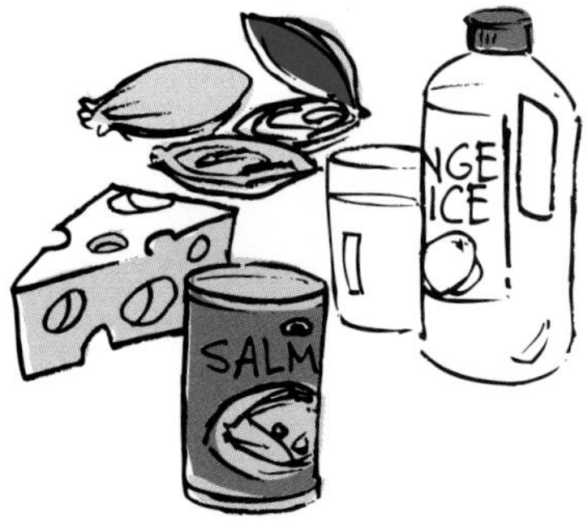

Foods high in calcium include: milk, yogurt, cheese, salmon, and oyster shells.

Recommended Daily Allowance (RDA) of Calcium

- Infants from 3 mo to 1 yr: 400 mg/day
- Infants from 6 mo to 1 yr: 600 mg/day
- Children from 1 to 10 yr: 800 to 1200 mg/day
- Children from 11 to 14 yr: 1200 to 1500 mg/day
- Women: 1200 to 1500 mg/day; pregnant and lactating women require more
- Men: 800 mg/day

Control of Calcium

The control of calcium is a complex process. Calcium concentration is controlled by four major factors: vitamin D, parathyroid hormone, calcitonin (thyrocalcitonin), and serum concentrations of calium and phosphate ions.

In the normal absorption process, calcium is removed from complexes in the diet during digestion and released in a soluble form for absorption. Calcium absorption occurs by transcellular and paracellular transfer. Transcellular or active transfer involves a calcium-binding protein called calbindin, which binds calcium on the cell surface, then fuses with the lysosomes. After the release of the bound calcium into the lysosomal interior, the calbindin returns to the cell surface, and the calcium ions exit the cell through the basolateral membrane. Paracellular calcium transport occurs between cells. The rate of transfer depends on calcium concentration and tightness of the junctions.

Calcium absorption is greatest in the ileum where the residence time is the greatest. Active absorption also occurs in the duodenum and the proximal jejunum where the pH is more acidic and calbindin is present. Only 20% to 30% of calcium is absorbed.

Calcium absorption requires vitamin D (cholecalciferol), which is a fat soluble steroid ingested from dairy products or synthesized in the skin after ultraviolet exposure. Many activation steps take place in the liver and kidney before vitamin D can act on target tissue. An inactive form of vitamin D is activated into the active form when photochemically stimulated by the ultraviolet light from the sun. A lack of sunlight resulting in vitamin D deficiency is known as rickets. Only a small amount of sunlight exposure is required to synthesize vitamin D. This active form of vitamin D is critical for the process of increasing serum calcium by enhancing absorption through the intestines, reabsorption of calcium in the kidneys, and resorption of calcium from the bone.

Absorption is affected by several physiologic factors. Decreased absorption occurs with vitamin D deficiency, menopause, old age, decreased stomach acid, and rapid intestinal transit time. Oxalic acid, found in spinach, rhubarb, sweet potatoes, and dried beans, inhibits calcium absorption. Calcium competes with zinc, manganese, magnesium, copper, and iron for absorption; thus, increased intake of any of these minerals may decrease absorption of others. Absorption of calcium supplements is improved when they are taken with food.

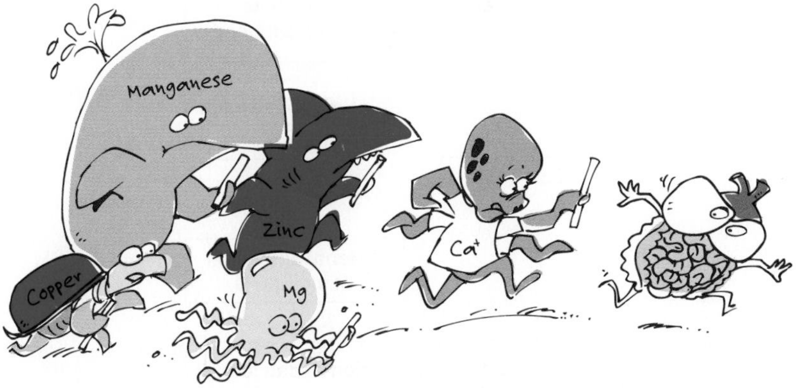

Calcium competes with zinc, manganese, copper, and iron for absorption; thus increased intake of any of these minerals may decrease absorption of others.

Calcium is excreted in the urine, feces, and perspiration. Approximately 100 to 120 mg/day is lost in urine and feces, and 15 to 25 mg/day is excreted in sweat.

The serum calcium level is normally maintained within a narrow range by several intricate processes. Calcium-sensing protein is a receptor-like protein that detects the extracellular calcium ion concentration in the parathyroid cells and kidney. In healthy states, the rate of bone formation and resorption is equal, and the amount of calcium reabsorbed from the gut is equal to the amount excreted by the kidney. Two hormones, parathyroid hormone (PTH) and thyrocalcitonin (TCT), along with vitamin D and the blood pH, play an extremely important role in maintaining the delicate serum calcium concentration. PTH is secreted in response to low serum calcium and acts to raise the level. TCT is secreted in response to high serum calcium and acts to reduce the calcium level.

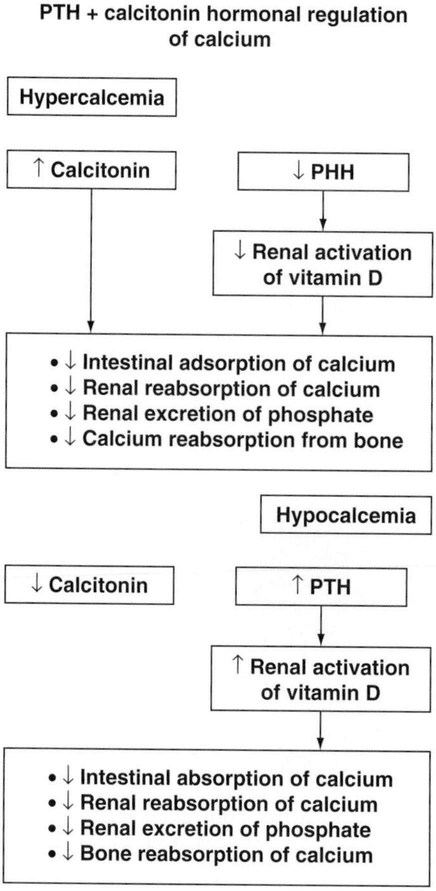

Initially, when the plasma calcium concentration decreases, the parathyroid gland stimulates the release of PTH, which raises ICF calcium levels in several ways. First, PTH acts on the kidneys by increasing the renal tubular reabsorption of calcium and stimulating phosphorus to be excreted. Second, PTH causes the kidneys to convert vitamin D to an active form, which increases the gastrointestinal (GI) absorption of calcium. Third, PTH releases calcium from bone storage by the process of resorption. When the calcium level is low, PTH is released, which stimulates osteoclasts (the cells in the bones that break down bone tissue). This osteoclastic process causes calcium and phosphorus to be transferred from the bone into the plasma. Once the extracellular calcium concentration is increased, a negative feedback loop occurs, and release of PTH is reduced.

Thyrocalcitonin, commonly known as *calcitonin,* is another important hormone that regulates serum calcium levels in several interesting ways. Calcitonin is a peptide hormone released by the thyroid gland in response to a high serum calcium level and has several binding sites or direct effects on the bone, kidney, GI tract, and central nervous system. Calcitonin secretion is stimulated by a high serum calcium level, and its function is to reduce calcium concentration. Its major effect is to inhibit bone resorption by slowing osteoclastic resorption, which stops the bones from releasing calcium. In addition, it causes an increase in bone uptake of calcium. Calcitonin acts directly on the GI tract by inhibiting the activation of vitamin D, which is necessary for calcium absorption, resulting in decreased calcium absorption in the gut. Calcitonin causes the kidneys to inhibit calcium reabsorption at the proximal convoluted tubule, resulting in an increased urinary excretion. See the PTH and calcitonin hormonal regulation of calcium figure.

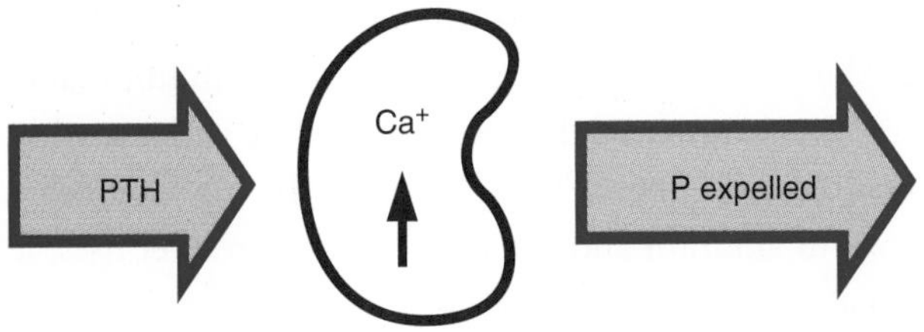

Parathyroid hormone acts on the kidney to reabsorb calcium and excrete phosphorus

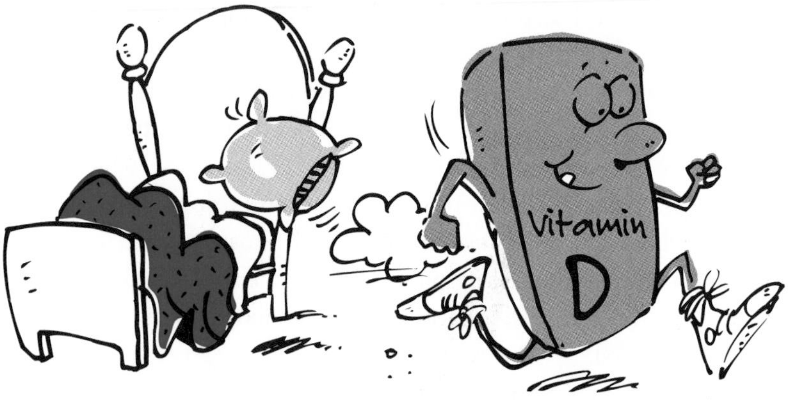

Parathyroid hormone causes the kidney to convert vitamin D into its active form so that calcium can be absorbed from the GI track.

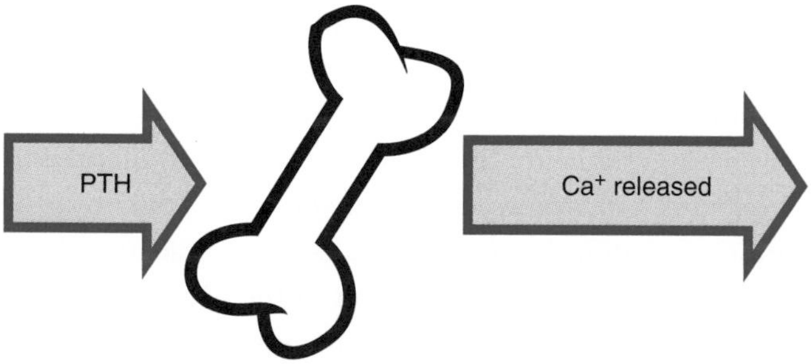

Parathyroid causes calcium to be released from the bone as part of the normal reabsorption process of bone tissue breakdown.

LIFE SPAN

Decreased absorption occurs with vitamin D deficiency, menopause, old age, decreased stomach acid, and rapid intestinal transit time.

The pH of the blood also affects the serum calcium level because both hydrogen and calcium compete for the binding sites on albumin. With alkalosis, as the pH is rising, calcium binds with albumin, and the ionized (free form) calcium level decreases. Therefore patients with alkalosis may become hypocalcemic. With acidosis, as the pH level decreases, less calcium binds to albumin and the ionized calcium level rises, leading to hypercalcemia.

Functions of Calcium

1. Most calcium is used for the development and maintenance of teeth and bones.
2. Calcium is a biochemical co-factor in several enzyme reactions necessary for metabolism.

HYPONATREMIA

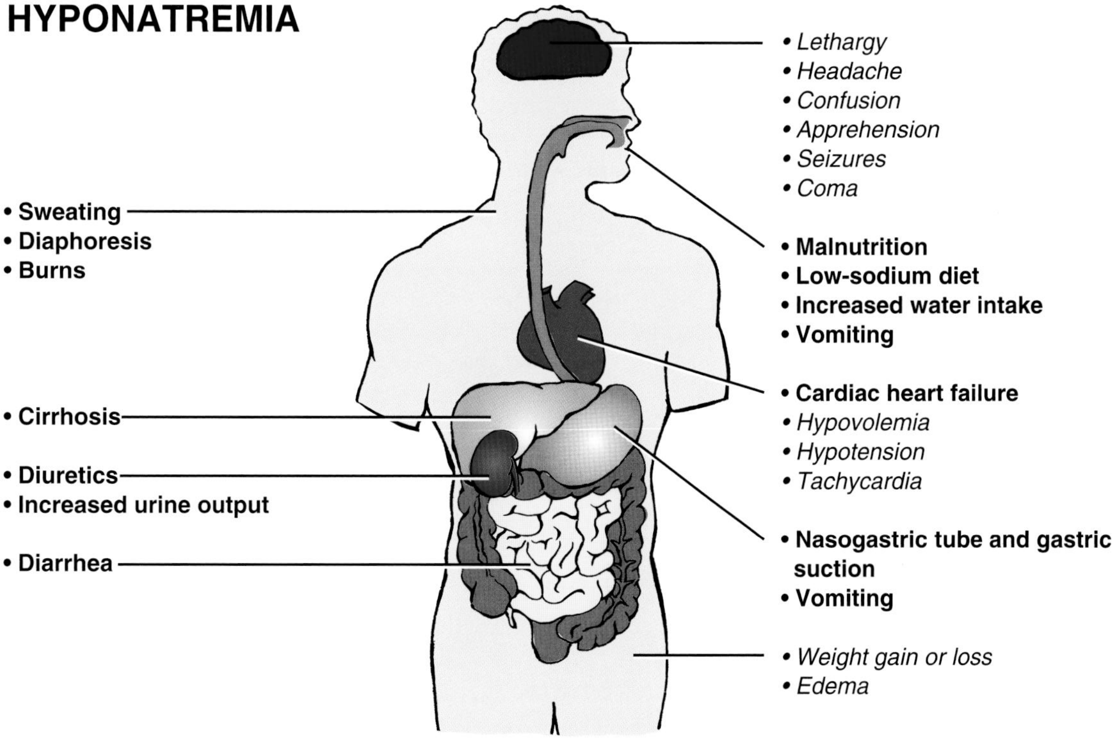

Pathophysiologic Effects

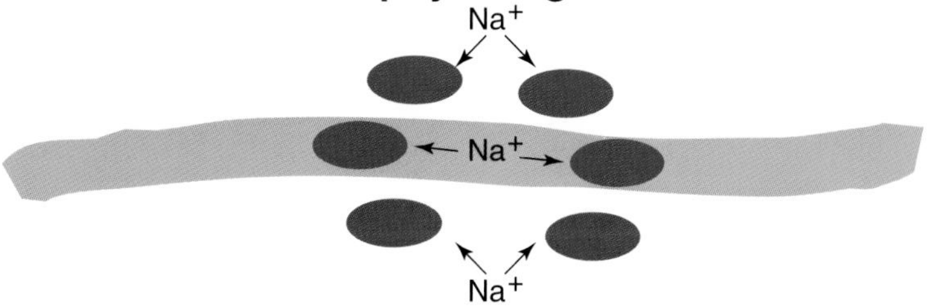

Sodium moves into the cell, causing water to move with it. Additionally, if plasma lipids, plasma proteins, or hyperglycemia increase, additional swelling of the cell occurs.

Associated signs and symptoms *(italics)* and causes of clinical syndromes **(bold)** are shown by organ systems.

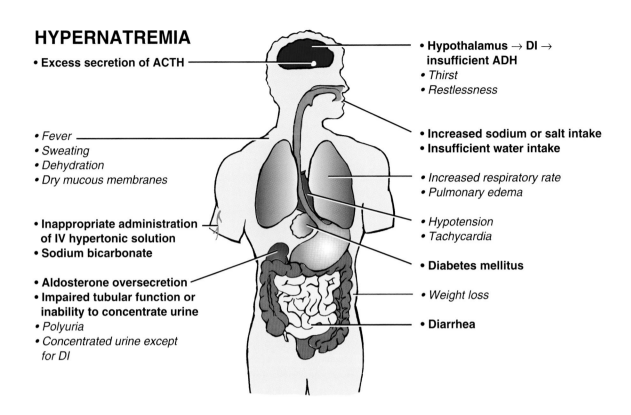

HYPERNATREMIA

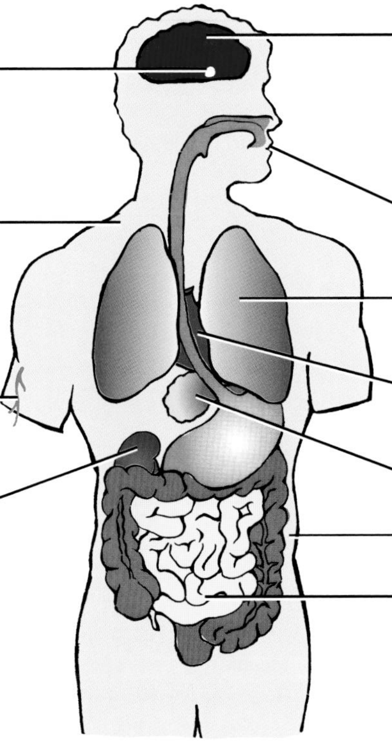

Pathophysiologic Effects

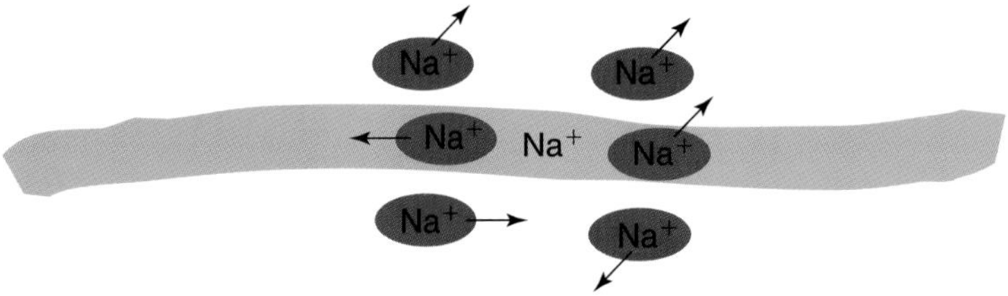

Sodium moves out of the cell, causing water to move with it.

Associated signs and symptoms *(italics)* and causes of clinical syndromes **(bold)** are shown by organ systems.

HYPOKALEMIA

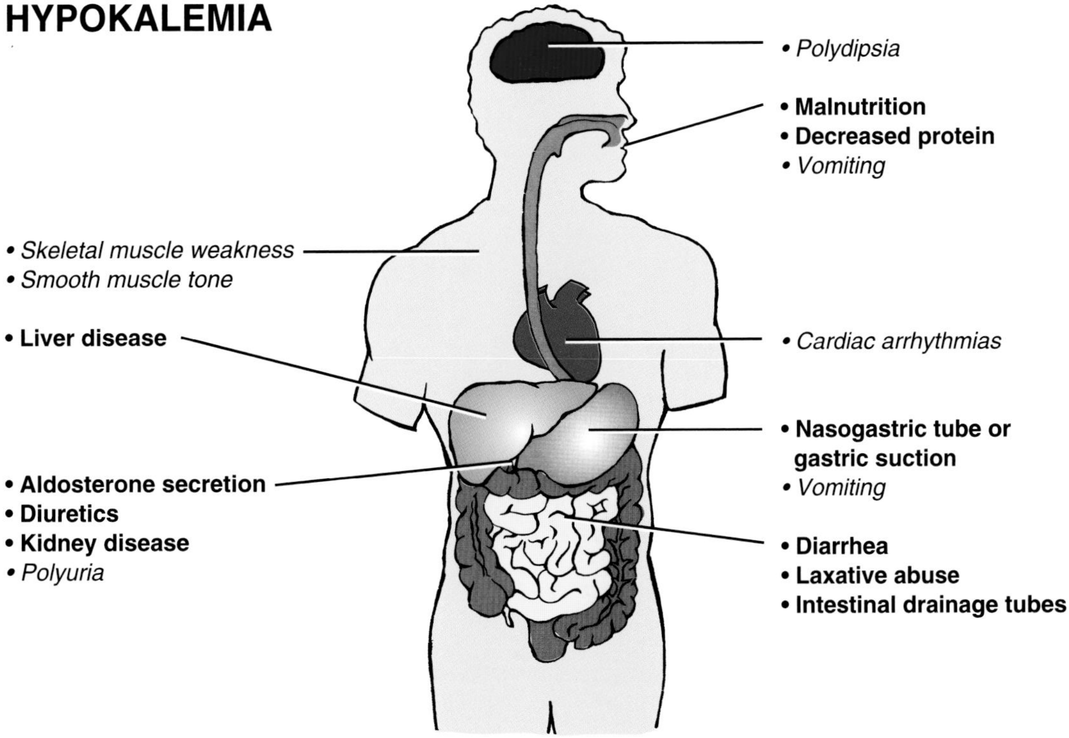

Pathophysiologic Effects

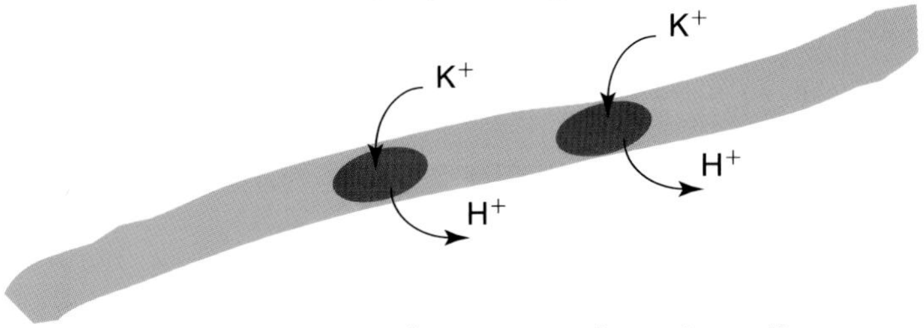

When potassium moves into the cell, it causes hypokalemia. In turn, hydrogen moves out of the cell, making the extracellular fluid more normalized or acidotic.

Associated signs and symptoms *(italics)* and causes of clinical syndromes **(bold)** are shown by organ systems.

HYPERKALEMIA

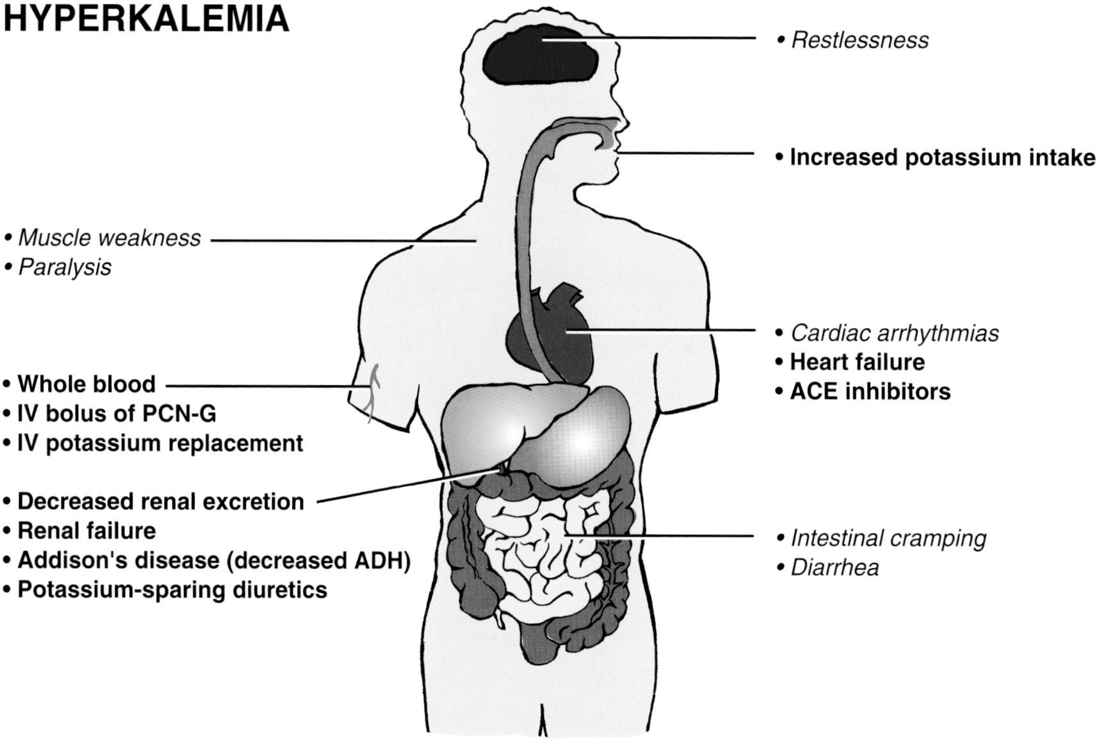

Pathophysiologic Effects

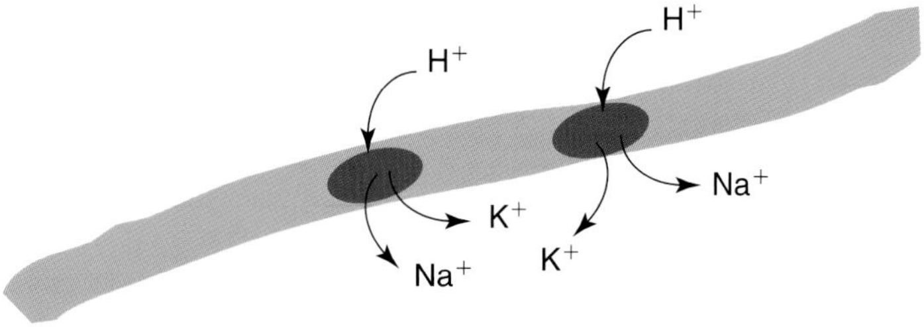

Hydrogen moves into the cell, causing the extracellular fluid to become more normalized or alkalotic. In turn, potassium and sodium move out of the cell, which causes hyperkalemia.

Associated signs and symptoms *(italics)* and causes of clinical syndromes **(bold)** are shown by organ systems.

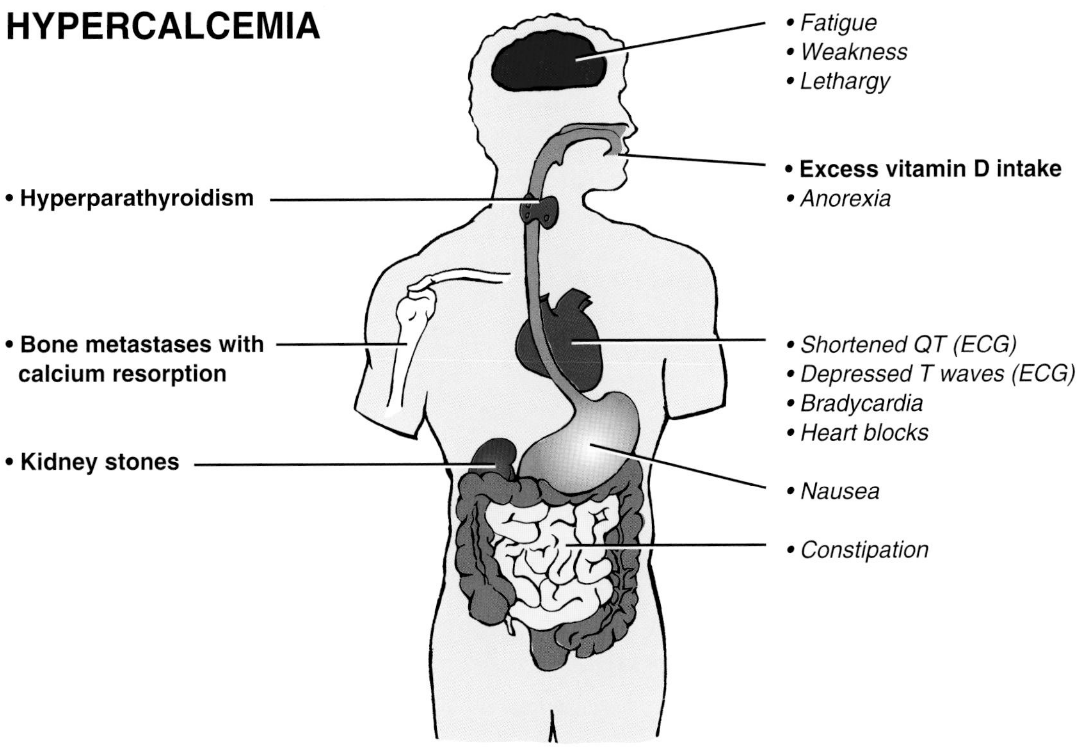

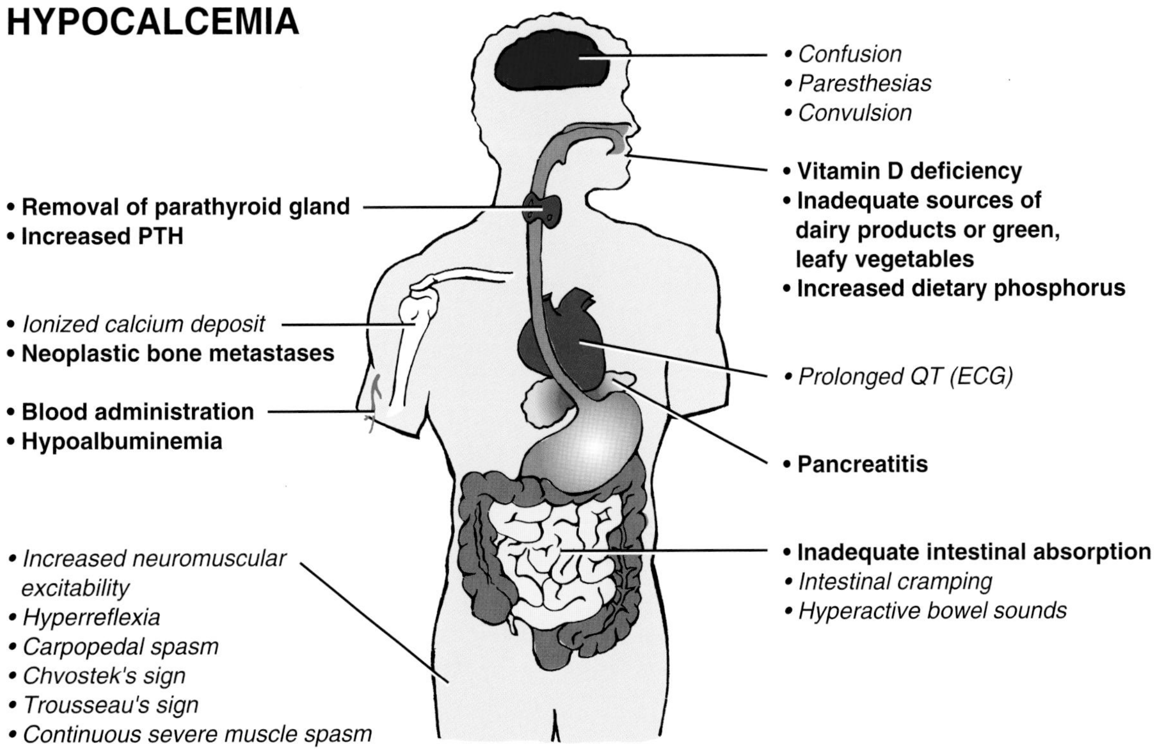

Associated signs and symptoms *(italics)* and causes of clinical syndromes **(bold)** are shown by organ systems.

HYPERPHOSPHATEMIA

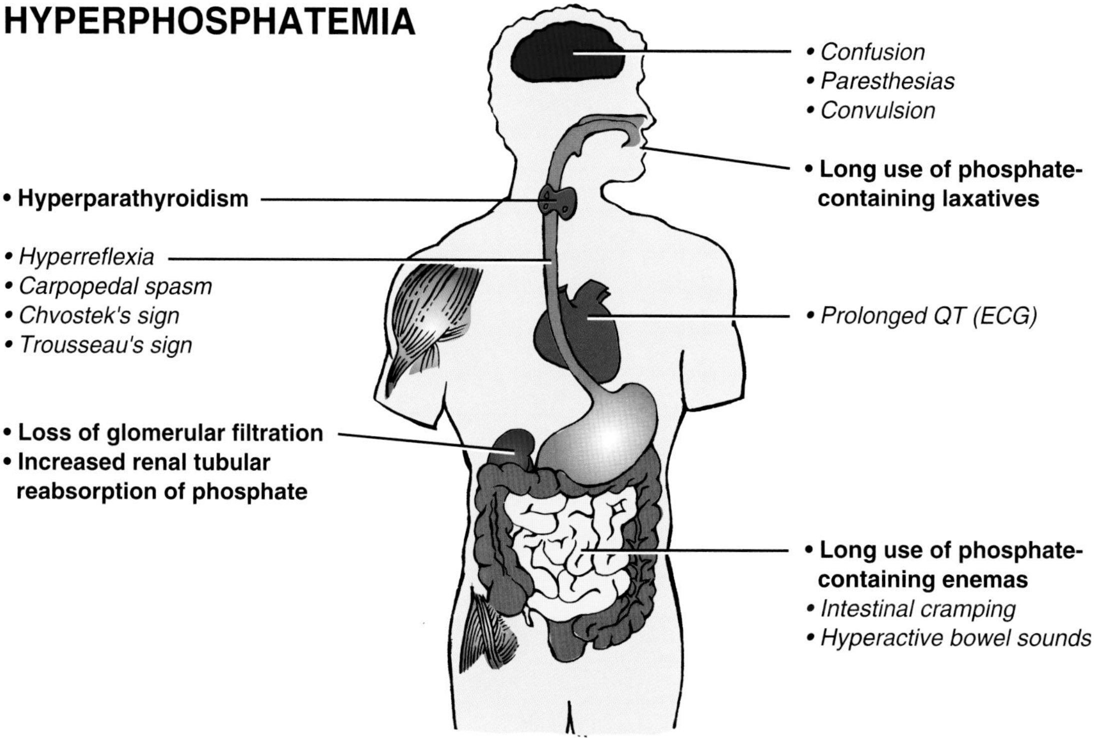

HYPOPHOSPHATEMIA

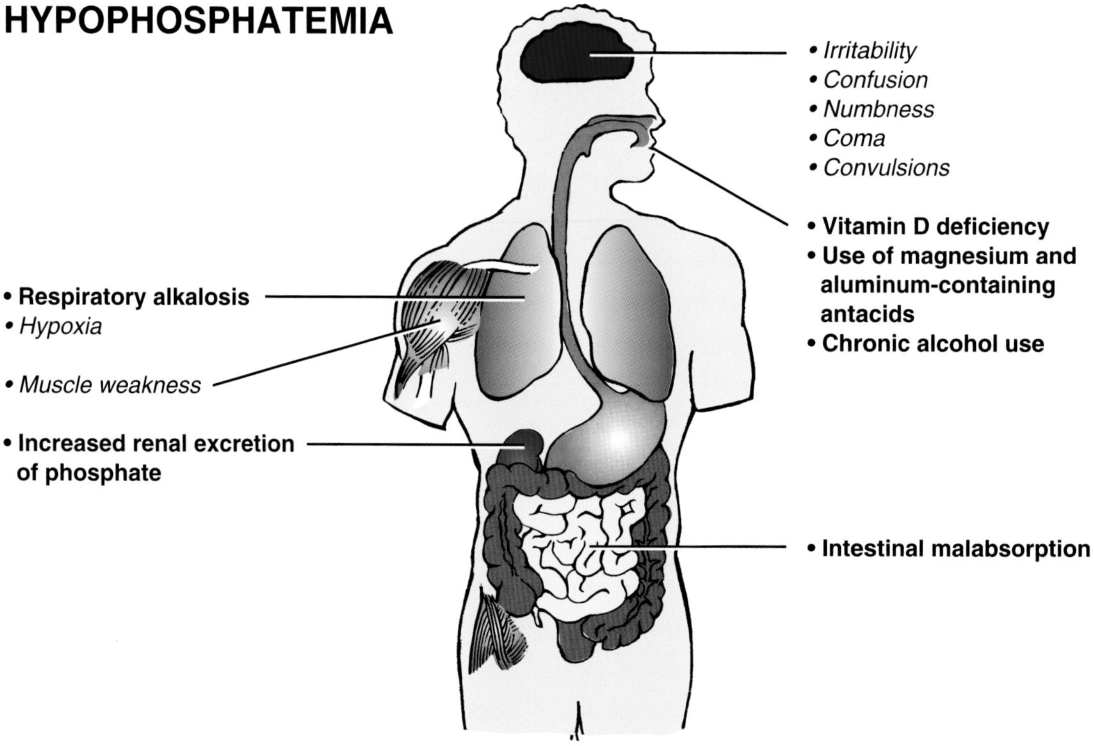

Associated signs and symptoms *(italics)* and causes of clinical syndromes **(bold)** are shown by organ systems.

HYPERMAGNESEMIA

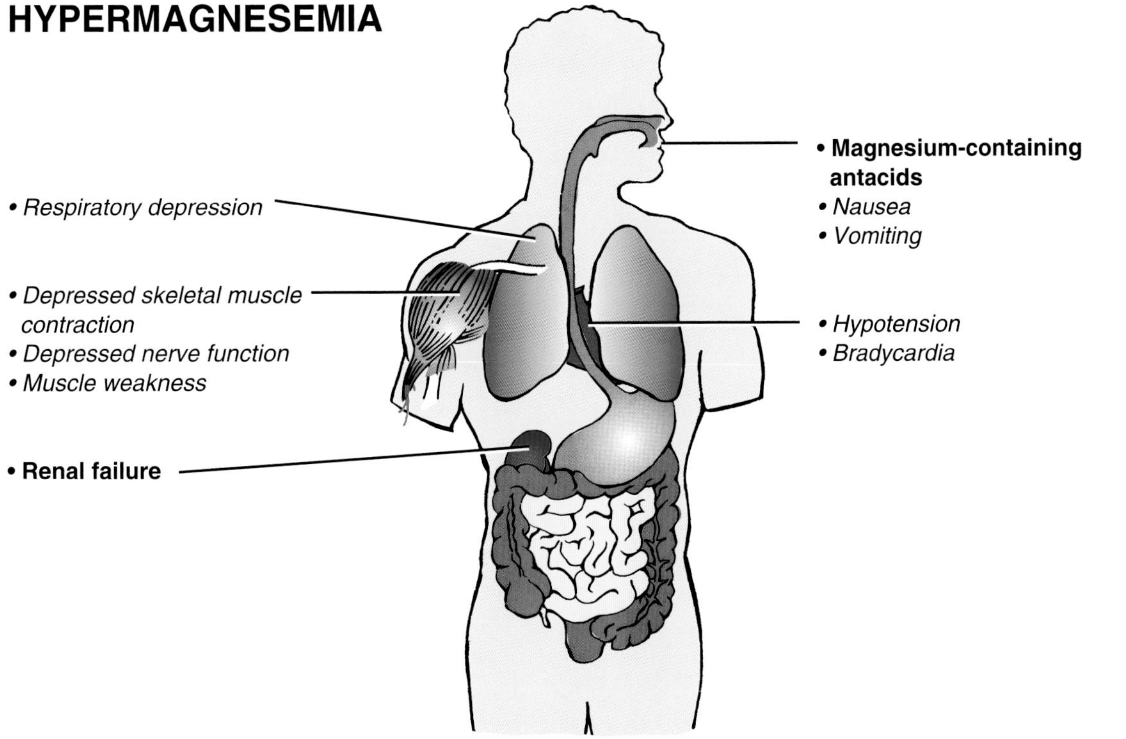

HYPOMAGNESEMIA

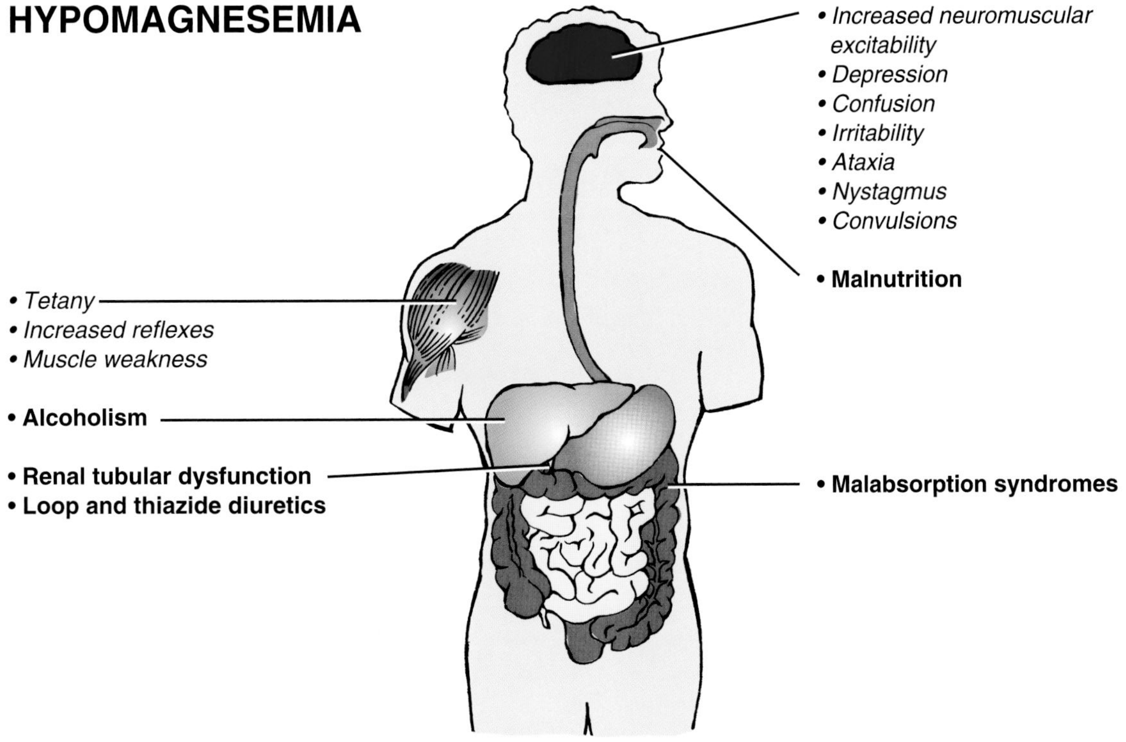

Associated signs and symptoms *(italics)* and causes of clinical syndromes **(bold)** are shown by organ systems.

HYPERCHLOREMIA

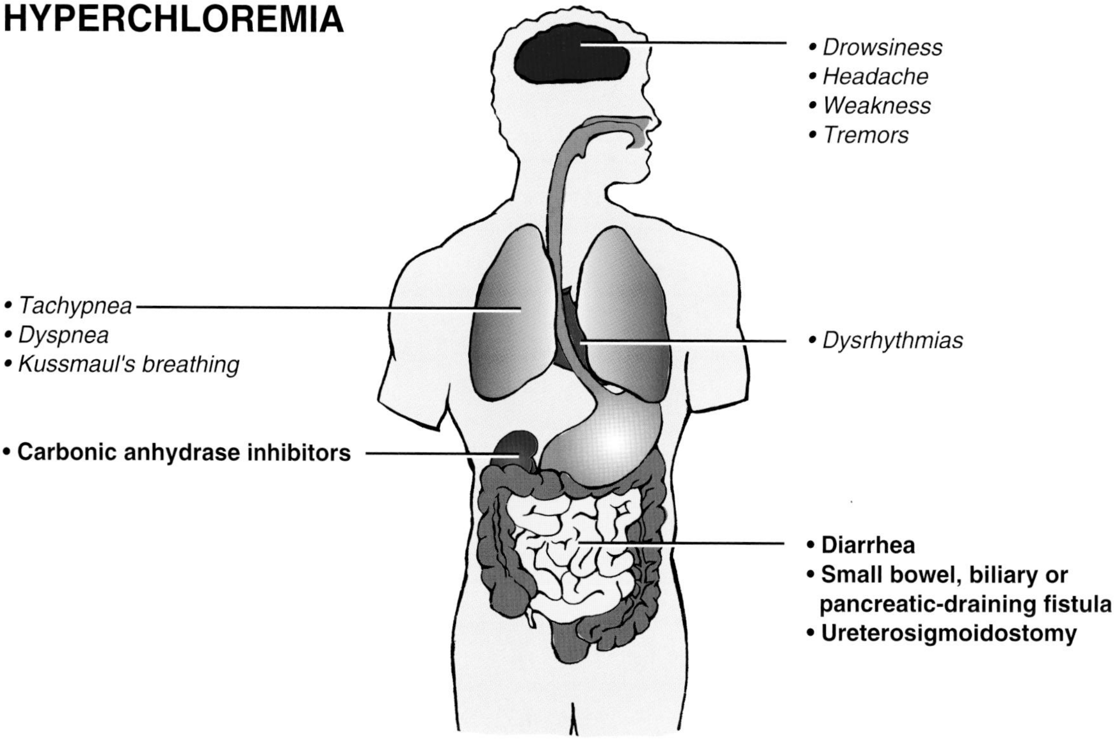

HYPOCHLOREMIA

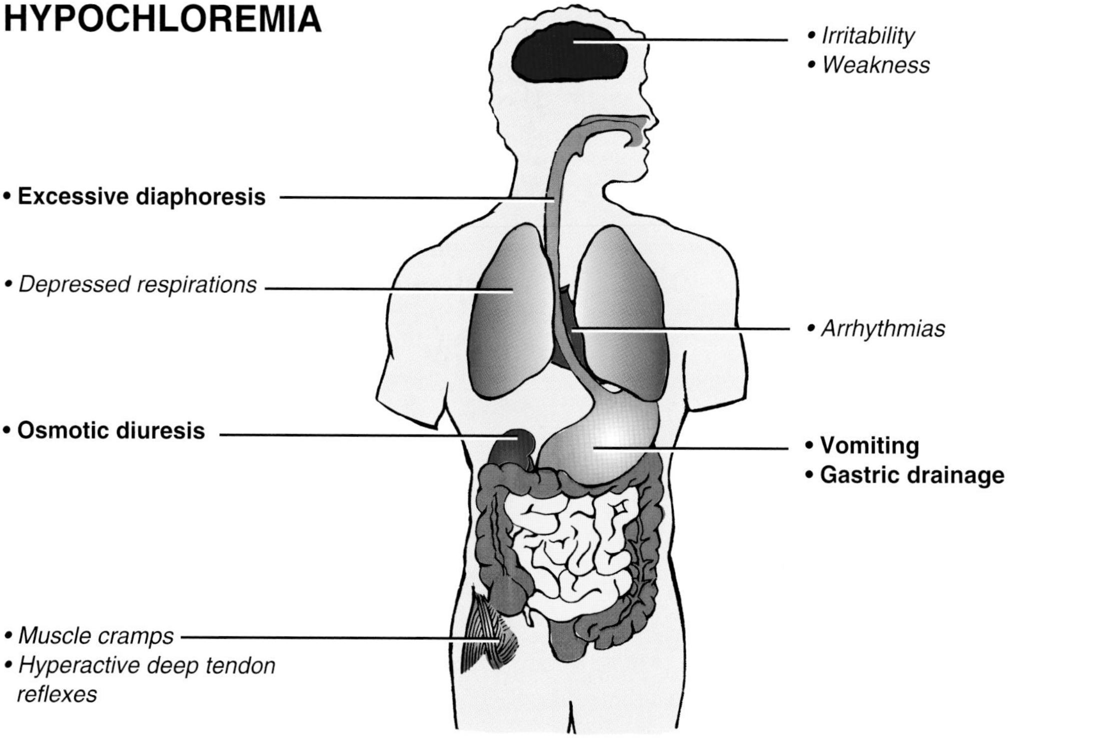

Associated signs and symptoms *(italics)* and causes of clinical syndromes **(bold)** are shown by organ systems.

3. Calcium is necessary for the synaptic release of neurotransmitters for transmission of nerve impulses.
4. Skeletal and cardiac muscle contractions are initiated by release of calcium ions from the intracellular sarcoplasmic reticulum as a result of sodium movement into the cell, causing depolarization.
5. Calcium, in addition to sodium, potassium, and magnesium, helps to maintain muscle tone.
6. Calcium helps regulate the heartbeat and blood pressure.
7. Calcium helps form blood clots by stimulating the release of thromboplastin from platelets and is a co-factor in the conversion of prothrombin to thrombin and in the conversion of fibrinogen to fibrin.

Do You UNDERSTAND?

DIRECTIONS: **Match the definitions in column A with the terms in column B.**

Column A	Column B
1. _____ Requires absorption of calcium	a. Oranges
2. _____ Enhances absorption of calcium	b. Albumin
3. _____ Hormone secreted in response to decreased calcium levels and acts to raise calcium	c. Acid environment
	d. Soybeans
	e. PTH
	f. Vitamin D
4. _____ Hormone secreted in response to an increase in calcium and acts to decrease calcium levels	g. TCT or calcitonin
5. _____ Food item high in calcium	
6. _____ Food item low in calcium	
7. _____ Serum protein, which binds with calcium	

What IS Hypercalcemia?

A serum calcium level above 11 mg/dL is called *hypercalcemia* (serum ionized level of above 5 mEq/L), which can be caused by several processes.

Answers: 1. f; 2. c; 3. e; 4. g; 5. d; 6. a; 7. b.

What You NEED TO KNOW

An excessive intake of calcium can lead to hypercalcemia. Increased amounts of or absorption of vitamin D, or vitamin A excess can raise the calcium level. Endocrine disorders leading to hypercalcemia include hyperparathyroidism, thyrotoxicosis, and adrenal insufficiency, which increases the calcium resorption from bone, reabsorption from the kidneys, and absorption from the intestines.

Malignant causes of hypercalcemia include lymphoproliferative diseases, such as multiple myeloma, lymphoma, or tumors that produce parathyroid-related proteins as part of a paraneoplastic syndrome (ovarian, kidney, and lung cancer) that causes increased bone resorption and a rise in the serum calcium concentration. Bone metastases causes the breakdown of bone and the release of calcium.

Conditions such as osteoporosis, sarcoidosis, benign parathyroid adenoma, Paget's disease, hypophosphatemia, chronic or end stage renal failure, and multiple fractures can increase the serum calcium level. Prolonged immobilization causes bone resorption and decreased bone formation, often with increased serum calcium levels.

Hypercalcemia may be observed with prolonged use of aluminum-containing antacids, which also causes a phosphorus deficit. Lithium and thiazide diuretics can cause hypercalcemia by decreasing the excretion of calcium from the kidneys.

Signs and Symptoms of Hypercalcemia

Excess calcium blocks the effect of sodium in skeletal muscles, reducing the excitation of muscles and nerves (decreasing neuromuscular activity), resulting in the classic symptoms of hypercalcemia listed on p. 145. The signs and symptoms are usually more extreme when the calcium level is 15 mg/dL or higher.

Signs and Symptoms of Hypercalcemia

- Anorexia, nausea, vomiting
- Constipation
- Paralytic ileus
- Confusion
- Muscle weakness
- Lethargy
- Decreased deep tendon reflexes
- Polydipsia, polyuria, dehydration
- Personality changes
- Impaired concentration
- Blurred vision
- Bone pain
- Cardiac symptoms (similar to digitalis effects) include arrhythmias (mostly bradycardia), shortened QT interval, and increased contractility
- Cardiac arrest

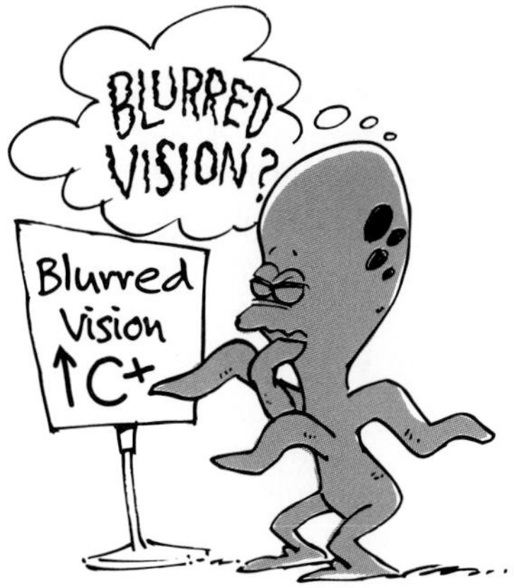

Blurred vision can be a symptom of hypercalcemia.

What You DO

Treatment of hypercalcemia is aimed at identifying and eliminating the cause. The immediate goal of hypercalcemia treatment is to increase urinary excretion of calcium and decrease resorption of calcium from bone. The health care provider should do the following:

- Discontinue medications that may be causing hypercalcemia and treat malignancies.
- Apply emergency treatment: induce natriuresis (excretion of calcium is accompanied by excretion of sodium) by administering intravenous (IV) saline fluids with a loop diuretic such as furosemide. IV phosphate may be used but only in hypercalcemic crisis because of the potential for soft-tissue calcification and renal failure if the calcium decreases too fast.
- Begin aggressive hydration with IV therapy with normal saline to increase renal blood flow and urinary calcium excretion.
- Keep in mind that hypocalcemic drugs are often used.
- IV bisphosphonates, such as pamidronate and etidronate, obstruct calcium release from the bone by inhibiting the action of osteoclasts, ultimately reducing bone resorption. Bisphosphonates lower serum calcium gradually over several days.
- IV calcitonin, which decreases calcium by directly inhibiting bone resorption and promoting renal excretion of calcium, has a rapid onset. The IV site should be continually examined for erythema and pain.

TAKE HOME POINTS

A serum calcium level greater than 12 mg/dL is considered life-threatening and should be treated immediately. Because calcium plays a role in cell permeability, nearly all body organs are affected by hypercalcemia.

TAKE HOME POINTS

It is important that diuretics are administered after rehydration and not for patients who are dehydrated.

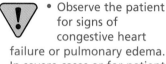

- Observe the patient for signs of congestive heart failure or pulmonary edema. In severe cases or for patients with a history of cardiac instability, cardiac monitoring may be required.
- For patients/families coping with end-stage terminal illnesses, it is important for the registered nurse to explain the rationale for not treating hypercalcemia as the appropriate course, because being in a state of hypercalcemia is not uncomfortable and may offer a mild euphoric/sedative effect.

- In cancer-associated hypercalcemia, corticosteroids and mithramycin may be used.
- In mild cases, remember that oral fluids of 3 to 4 L a day are recommended.
- Monitor vital signs during treatment.
- Check and record the neurologic status every 4 hours, and continue cardiac monitoring for arrhythmias. Reassess for hallmark signs and symptoms of hypercalcemia such as anorexia, confusion, polydipsia, polyuria, and weakness.
- Assess for bone pain, administer analgesics, and assess the effectiveness of pain control. For patients who have pain associated with bone metastasis, standard nursing care includes placing them on analgesics consisting of opioids (long-acting morphine) and nonopioids (nonsteroidal antiinflammatory agents [NSAIDs] or acetaminophen) on a scheduled regimen.
- Treat nausea with antiemetics.
- Because constipation is a common problem, administer laxatives and stool softeners.
- Institute safety measures tailored to the current symptomatology of patients who have the potential for injury related to mental status changes (falls), neurologic irritability (seizures), fatigue, or fractures.
- Explain the rationale for all treatment procedures to the patient and family. When appropriate, review and provide a list of foods and antacids that are high in calcium, and review recommended dietary allowances for gender and age.

Do You UNDERSTAND?

DIRECTIONS: Complete the crossword puzzle using the following hints.

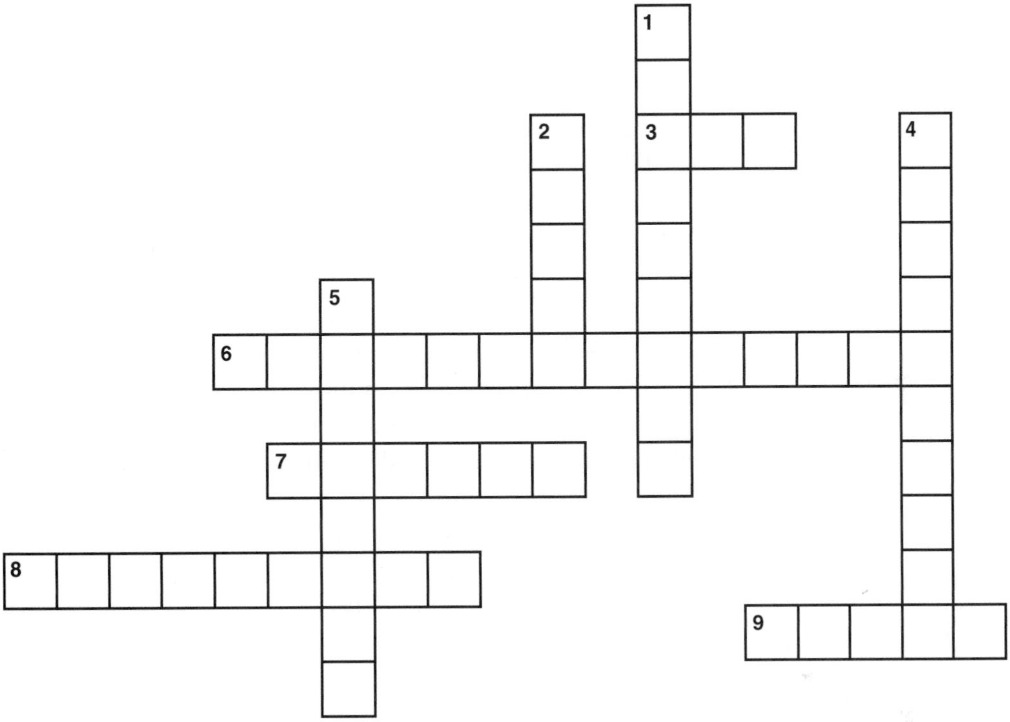

Across

3. The health care provider should assess for signs of heart overload, known as ____________________, when administering IV fluids.
6. Most common malignant-related problem that causes hypercalcemia.
7. GI symptom of hypercalcemia
8. Common neurologic symptom of hypercalcemia
9. Bisphosphonates are medications given to ____________ serum calcium levels slowly.

Down

1. In hypercalcemia, the deep tendon reflexes will become ______.
2. Hypercalcemia can lead to cardiac arrhythmias, and in severe cases, this organ may stop working.
4. The generic name of loop diuretic given to induce excretion of calcium for treatment of severe hypercalcemia
5. A commonly used over-the-counter category of agents for gastritis, which, when taken in excessive amounts, can cause hypercalcemia

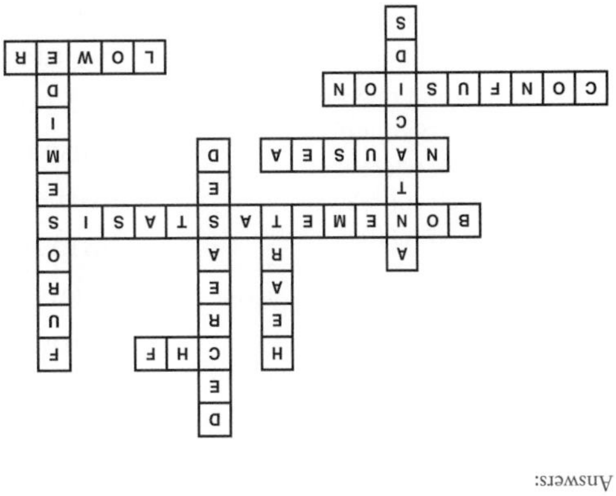

What IS Hypocalcemia?

A serum calcium level of less than 8.5 mg/dL is called *hypocalcemia* (serum ionized level below 4.5 mEq/L).

What You NEED TO KNOW

The most common cause of hypocalcemia is renal failure. Hypocalcemia can be caused by a decreased intake or absorption, as seen in conditions such as malabsorption, small bowel resection, or vitamin D deficiency.

Decreased calcium dietary intake does not usually lead to hypocalcemia because of large stores in the bones. Increased loss of calcium and failure to absorb calcium from alcoholism, pancreatic disease, chronic renal insufficiency, excessive diarrhea, and aggressive diuretic therapy can also lead to hypocalcemia.

Certain endocrine disorders such as acute pancreatitis, hypoparathyroidism, pseudohypoparathyroidism, and thyroid medullary carcinoma may lead to hypocalcemia. Parathyroidectomy can result in life-threatening hypocalcemia if not properly treated. Any surgery or injury to the thyroid can cause acute hypocalcemia if the parathyroid gland is removed or damaged in the process.

A low magnesium level can decrease parathyroid hormone secretion, which causes hypocalcemia. Physiologic causes of hypocalcemia include decreased serum albumin, hyperphosphatemia, multiple blood transfusions, and septicemia. The administration of blood transfusions with citrate added (to prevent clotting) may bind with calcium, decreasing the amount available. Alkalosis causes calcium to bind to albumin, decreasing the amount of available calcium.

Vitamin D deficiency can lead to hypocalcemia. Classic rickets is caused by a lack of sunlight, which prevents the synthesis of vitamin D in the skin, resulting in hypocalcemia and bone malformation. Other forms of rickets include malabsorption (celiac disease, giardiasis, hepatobiliary disease), hereditary tubular renal disease (hypophosphatemia, fibrous dysplasia, neurofibromatosis, Fanconi's syndrome, and distal renal tubular acidosis), and acquired renal disease (chronic glomerular renal failure).

CULTURE

In the past, rickets (a condition of childhood caused by vitamin D deficiency) was a common result of calcium deficiency, with bone decalcification and softening, but because of vitamin D–fortified milk and supplements, this form of rickets is uncommon in the United States.

Medications known to lower calcium levels include bisphosphonates, aminoglycoside antibiotics (gentamicin), anticonvulsants (phenytoin and phenobarbital), calcitonin, loop diuretics (furosemide), edetate sodium (EDTA) (given for lead poisoning), certain antiviral agents (foscarnet), and certain chemotherapy agents (cisplatin). Phosphate given via IV or by mouth binds with calcium and can cause hypocalcemia.

Signs and Symptoms of Hypocalcemia

The classic signs and symptoms of hypocalcemia are from the neural excitability and include the following:

- Spasm of skeletal muscle, causing cramps and tetany
- Laryngospasm with stridor
- Convulsions
- Paresthesias of lips and extremities

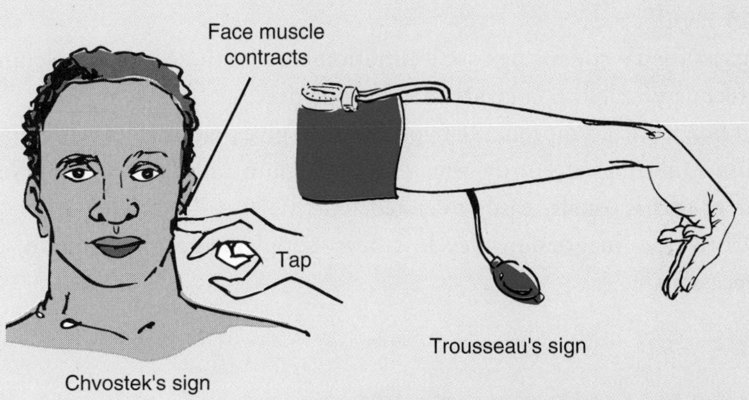

- Chvostek's sign (contraction of the facial muscle in response to tapping the facial nerve against the bone anterior to the ear)
- Trousseau's sign (carpal spasm occurring after occlusion of the brachial artery with a blood pressure cuff for 3 minutes)
- Arrhythmias such as heart block, ventricular fibrillation, and a type of ventricular tachycardia called torsades de pointes (related to QT interval prolongation)
- Brittle nails
- Insomnia
- Periodontal disease
- Seizures
- Increased peristalsis and diarrhea
- Osteoporosis

TAKE HOME POINTS

- Damage to the parathyroid gland can cause life-threatening hypocalcemia. The health care provider should be certain that calcium gluconate and a tracheotomy tray are at the bedside of any patient recovering from thyroid or parathyroid surgery.
- Frequently assess for signs and symptoms of sudden hypocalcemia, such as stridor, dyspnea, cardiac arrhythmias, and a positive Chvostek's or Trousseau's sign.
- If hypocalcemia is associated with hypoalbuminemia (low serum albumin), calcium replacement may not be necessary.

What You DO

The goal of hypocalcemia management is to correct the imbalance by identifying and removing the precipitating cause and treating the underlying disease.

- Initiate emergency care for acute hypocalcemia if tetany (muscle twitching), arrhythmias, or seizures are present. Administer calcium gluconate 10% (10 to 20 mL) IV for 10 to 15 minutes, followed by an infusion of calcium gluconate or calcium chloride in D_5W given for 4 to 6 hours.
- Monitor the serum calcium level every 4 to 6 hours, and adjust IV infusion rate accordingly with the goal of maintaining a level of 7 to 8.5 mg/dL.
- Assess the IV site for signs of infiltration because these agents (calcium gluconate, calcium chloride) cause tissue necrosis.
- In nonacute, asymptomatic hypocalcemia, give oral calcium with vitamin D during or shortly after meals. Calcium carbonate is a supplement that is usually easily tolerated.
- When the magnesium level is low, supplemental magnesium is necessary.

Critical levels: less than 7 mg/dL may cause tetany and less than 6 mg/dL may cause death. Levels greater than 12 mg/dL may lead to coma, and greater than 14 mg/dL may cause death.

Do You UNDERSTAND?

DIRECTIONS: Indicate in the spaces provided whether the following statements are *true* or *false*.

1. _____ The most common cause of hypocalcemia is renal failure.
2. _____ A life-threatening symptom of hypocalcemia is osteoporosis.
3. _____ Trousseau's sign, which is the contraction of the facial muscle in response to tapping the bone anterior to the ear, may be seen in hypocalcemia.

References

Belton NR: Biochemical and physiological tables and reference ranges for laboratory tests. In McIntosh N, Helms P, Smyth R, editors:

Answers: 1. True. Hypocalcemia is not as common as hypercalcemia, but the leading cause of low serum calcium is excessive renal excretion as a result of renal disease; 2. False. Osteoporosis is a serious condition that can be caused by chronic low calcium intake, which can be quite debilitating but is usually not life threatening; 3. False. Trousseau's sign, which occurs in hypocalcemia, is carpal spasm in response to occlusion of the brachial artery. The contraction of facial muscle in response to being tapped is called Chvostek's sign and is also observed in hypocalcemia.

Forfar & Arneil's textbook of pediatrics, New York, 2003, Churchill Livingstone.

Huether SE: The cellular environment: fluids and electrolytes, acids and bases. In McCance KL, Huether SE, editors: *Pathophysiology: the biologic basis for disease in adults and children,* St Louis, 2002, Mosby.

Jamison JR: *Clinical guide to nutrition and dietary supplements in disease,* St Louis, 2003, Mosby.

Kelnar JH, Butler GE: Endocrine gland disorders and disorders of growth and puberty. In Mcintosh N, Helms P, Smyth R, editors: *Forfar & Arneil's textbook of pediatrics,* New York, 2003, Churchill Livingstone.

Kryspin MD, Reeder SJ: Hypercalcemia. In Chernecky C, Berger BJ, editors: *Advanced and critical care oncology nursing: managing primary complications,* Philadelphia, 1998, Saunders.

Lehne RA: *Pharmacology for nursing care,* St Louis, 2004, Saunders.

Notes

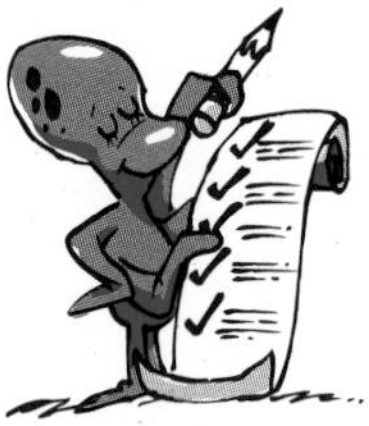

NCLEX® Review

1. Which of the following signs and symptoms would you observe with hypocalcemia?
   1 Nausea and vomiting
   2 Constipation
   3 Muscle spasms
   4 Confusion

2. All of the following are excellent sources of calcium *except:*
   1 Cheese
   2 Broccoli
   3 Yogurt
   4 Carrots

3. Which symptom of hypocalcemia should the nurse report immediately?
   1 Lethargy
   2 Polyuria
   3 Cardiac arrhythmia
   4 Muscle cramps

4. The most common cause of hypocalcemia is:
   1 Rickets
   2 Renal failure
   3 Inadequate diet
   4 Diarrhea

5. A common cause of hypercalcemia is:
   1 Metastatic cancer
   2 Infection
   3 Diarrhea
   4 Hypothyroidism

6. Which fat-soluble vitamin is necessary for the absorption and use of calcium and phosphorus in the body?
   1 Vitamin A
   2 Vitamin D
   3 Vitamin E
   4 Vitamin K

7. Which surgical procedure may cause sudden hypocalcemia?
   1 Nephrectomy
   2 Gastrectomy
   3 Colectomy
   4 Thyroidectomy

8. What is the daily recommended dietary allowance of calcium for a regular (nonpregnant) adult?

9. Chronic hypocalcemia causes bone mass loss that results in brittle bones and is associated primarily with what condition?

10. What vitamin aids in calcium absorption, and how is this vitamin generated?

11. In caring for a malnourished and underweight older patient, it is important to interpret the serum calcium level in relation to what other laboratory value?

NCLEX® Review Answers

1. **3** Hypocalcemia causes increased sensitivity to nerve impulses, which causes muscle spasms and tetany.

2. **4** Carrots are not a source of calcium.

3. **3** Cardiac arrhythmias associated with hypocalcemia are life threatening and need to be treated immediately. Muscle cramps are a sign of hypocalcemia, but they are usually not life threatening. Lethargy and poluria are signs of hypercalcemia.

4. **2** Renal failure causes a decreased production of active vitamin D and causes hyperphosphatemia, both of which contribute to calcium loss. Rickets

is rare in the United States with the advent of vitamin D–fortified milk. The bone mass usually supplies an adequate source of calcium, even in calcium-poor diets. Although acute and prolonged diarrhea can lead to hypocalcemia, this is not the most common cause.

5. 1 Metastatic cancer to the bone causes accelerated bone resorption and bone demineralization, which increases serum calcium. Also, certain tumors produce parathyroid hormone–related proteins that may increase renal tubular reabsorption of calcium.

6. 2 Vitamin D in the active form enhances calcium absorption in the intestines.

7. 4 Thyroidectomy may result in hypocalcemia if the parathyroid glands are inadvertently removed (surgically induced hypoparathyroidism).

8. 800 to 1200 mg

9. Osteoporosis

10. Vitamin D is manufactured by photochemical activation of cholecalciferol in the skin when triggered by ultraviolet light.

11. Serum albumin (protein) is protein bound. In patients with catabolic wasting, less calcium is protein bound. Hypercalcemia is suggested when the calcium level is normal with a low serum albumin.

Notes

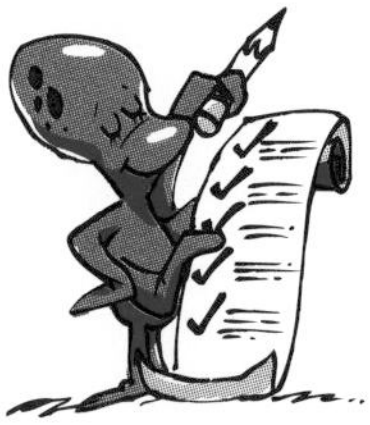

Chapter 9

Elements and Minerals: Fluoride, Iodine, Iron, Selenium, and Zinc

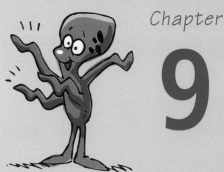

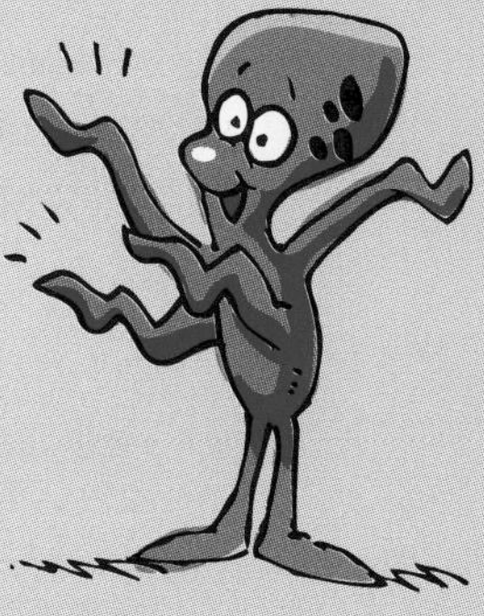

What You WILL LEARN

After reading this chapter, you will know how to do the following:

- ✔ State one function of fluoride in the human body.
- ✔ Differentiate fluoride excess from fluoride deficiency.
- ✔ State one function of iodine in the human body.
- ✔ Identify one disease/condition associated with excess iodine.
- ✔ Describe the signs/symptoms of iodine deficiency.
- ✔ State one function of iron in the human body.
- ✔ Define hematochromatosis.
- ✔ Describe two outcomes of iron deficiency.
- ✔ Identify one role that selenium plays in body function.
- ✔ Define selenosis.
- ✔ State two potential results of selenium deficiency.
- ✔ State one function of zinc in relation to one body system.
- ✔ Differentiate zinc toxicity from zinc deficiency.

Fluoride, iodine, iron, selenium, and zinc are classified as trace minerals because they are present in minute amounts in the body tissue. Despite the relatively small body requirements and content, each mineral plays an essential role in body functions and in growth, health, and development and may cause adverse reactions if not consumed in the proper amounts (Table 1).

What IS Fluoride?

Fluoride is necessary to strengthen bones and teeth. Adequate amounts of fluoride intake can aid in preventing cavities **(dental caries)**; however, it cannot decrease bone loss and therefore supplements do not prevent osteoporosis.

Approximately 2.6 g fluoride are present in the average human body. The greatest concentration of fluoride is found in the bones and tooth enamel. The average skeletal bone structure contains 2.5 mg fluoride.

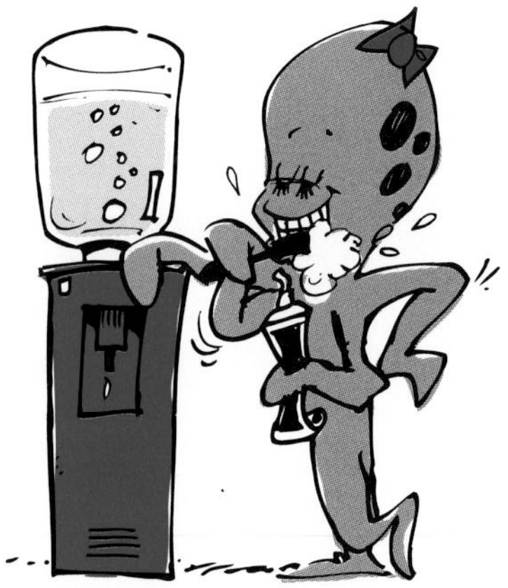

The main source of fluoride is fluoridated water.

What You NEED TO KNOW

Sources of Fluoride

Fluoride is derived from numerous ingested **(exogenous)** sources. Trace amounts are present in soil, water, and plants. A major dietary source of fluoride is fluoridated water.

Dental products are also fluoridated, but add only small amounts with unintentional ingestion. Significant fluoride content is found in tea leaves and seafood, especially salmon and sardines with the bones. Smaller amounts are obtained from soups and stews made with seafood or meat bones.

Control of Fluoride

Ingested fluoride is absorbed in the gastrointestinal (GI) tract by passive diffusion and is inversely related to the blood pH. When gastric acid secretion increases, the rate of fluoride absorption increases. Fluoride absorption is rapid, with approximately 50% absorbed and deposited in teeth and bone within 24 hours of ingestion. The major route of removal of fluoride from the body is renal excretion, with less than 20% excreted in the feces.

Recommended Daily Allowances of Fluoride

Adults: 1.5 to 4.0 mg
Children age 7 years or older: 1.5 to 2.5 mg
Children ages 4 to 6 years: 1.0 to 2.5 mg
Children ages 1 to 3 years: 0.5 to 1.5 mg
Infants: 0.1 to 1.0 mg

Functions of Fluoride

The main function of fluoride is to protect developing and mature teeth from dental caries. Fluoride ions substitute for the hydroxyl group on the calcium phosphate salt structure of the bones and teeth to form fluoridated hydroxylapatite. This increases the stability of the tooth enamel crystals because fluoridated hydroxylapatite is less soluble in organic acids.

1. Fluoride in saliva can decrease the rate of demineralization and facilitate remineralization of early dental caries.
2. High concentrations of fluoride inhibit growth of acidogenic bacteria found in dental plaque. In low concentrations, fluoride inhibits bacterial enzymes and reduces acid production.
3. Fluoride stimulates osteoblastic activity and causes increased bone mass.

Do You UNDERSTAND?

DIRECTIONS: Place a check next to each item that contains fluoride.

1. _____ Seafood	6. _____ Mouthwash
2. _____ Milk	7. _____ Tea
3. _____ Teeth	8. _____ Coffee
4. _____ Liver	9. _____ Toothpaste
5. _____ Bone	10. _____ Chicken

Answers: 1; 3; 5; 7; 9.

What IS Excess of Fluoride?

Fluorosis, or excess fluoride levels, occurs when the daily doses of fluoride exceed two parts per million (ppm) water. Mild fluorosis can occur with as little as 0.1 mg/kg a day.

What You NEED TO KNOW

LIFE SPAN

The most common cause of fluorosis in children is eating toothpaste with fluoride.

The most common cause of fluorosis in children is eating toothpaste with fluoride. Because teeth are forming between birth and 14 years of age, dental fluorosis is limited to this age group.

Fluoride becomes deposited in teeth enamel, resulting in mottling and browning of the teeth. Chronic excess fluoride intake causes the deposit of crystals in the bones (**osteosclerosis**), resulting in decreased elasticity, joint pain, and increased risk of stress fractures.

Signs and Symptoms of Fluorosis

- White or brown stains on teeth
- White opaque flecks on teeth
- Tooth enamel pitting
- Nausea
- Diarrhea
- Chest pain
- Itching
- Vomiting
- Stiffness or pain in joints
- Chronic joint pain
- Osteoporosis of long bones
- Muscle wasting

What You DO

The goal of managing fluorosis is to limit the intake of fluoride. The health care provider should do the following:

- Eliminate fluoride supplements and limit the amount of toothpaste to prevent excess fluoride intake.
- Inform parents of the risk of fluoride excess, including the potential problems from eating or sucking on toothpaste.

Do You UNDERSTAND?

DIRECTIONS: **Fill in the blanks.**

1. Fluorosis occurs primarily in ________________ between ages ____________________________.
2. One sign of fluorosis is ________________ or ________________ on teeth.
3. The most common cause of fluorosis is eating ________________.

What IS a Fluoride Deficit?

The recommended dietary allowance of fluoride depends on the age of the individual.

TAKE HOME POINTS

Fluoride deficits are more critical for individuals under 14 years of age because of the developing dental structures.

What You NEED TO KNOW

Lack of fluoride promotes dental caries. Chronic fluoride deficiency for individuals younger than 50 years of age can increase the severity of osteoporosis.

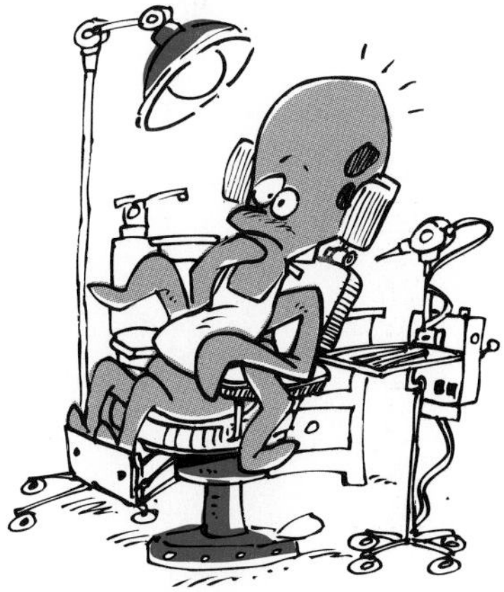

Fluoride deficiency leads to dental caries.

Signs and Symptoms of Fluoride Deficiency

- Dental caries
- Osteoporosis

Answers: 1. children, birth to 14 years; 2. stains, flecks; 3. toothpaste.

What You DO

Prevention is key. The health care provider should do the following:

- Explain the importance of fluoride supplements for communities with well water that does not contain natural fluoride.
- Provide written information on fluoride dose and prescription or the phone number of the public health department that may provide fluoride supplements.
- Explain the importance of not eating fluoride toothpaste to the parent and the child.

Potential Interactions

- Calcium supplements
- Calcium and aluminum-containing antacids

Do You UNDERSTAND?

DIRECTIONS: **Indicate in the spaces provided whether the following statements are *true* or *false*.**

1. _____ Fluoride is necessary for growth and development of the skeletal system.
2. _____ Fluoride is no longer needed after age 50.
3. _____ Excess fluoride can cause brown tooth staining.
4. _____ Fluoride accumulates in new bone formation sites and results in a net gain in bone mass; however, in higher doses, the new bone may be structurally abnormal.

What IS Iodine?

Most *iodine* in the body is found in the thyroid gland and is an essential component of the thyroid hormones throxine and triiodothyronine. Iodine functions as part of the thyroid hormone thyroxine to regulate

Answers: **1. true; 2. false; 3. true; 4. true.**

growth and development, bone turnover, metabolic rate, and body temperature. Iodine levels are only measured in rare cases when iodine toxicity is suspected.

Recommended Daily Allowances of Iodine

Adolescents and adults: 150 μg
Pregnant women: 175 μg
Lactating women: 200 μg
Children ages 7 to 10 years: 120 μg
Children ages 4 to 6 years: 90 μg
Children ages 1 to 3 years: 70 μg
Infants up to 1 year: 50 μg

The body contains approximately 20 to 30 mg of iodine, with approximately 75% concentrated in the thyroid gland. The remainder is distributed in the lactating mammary gland, the gastric mucosa, and the blood. Iodine is stored in the thyroid gland and the liver.

Iodine intake is assessed by measurement of 24-hour urinary excretion.

What You NEED TO KNOW

Sources of Iodine

Iodine is found abundantly in the ocean and in the deeper layers of the soil. Iodine is present in the soil and sea as iodide ions, which are oxidized by the sunlight and escape into the atmosphere. Plants that are grown in older, sun-exposed surfaces that have been iodine depleted will produce iodine-deficient food crops.

Excellent nutritional sources of iodine include fresh saltwater fish, shellfish (e.g., clams, lobster, oysters), iodized salt, and vegetables grown in iodine-rich soil. Milk and milk products may be good sources of iodine, depending on the iodine in the cow feed.

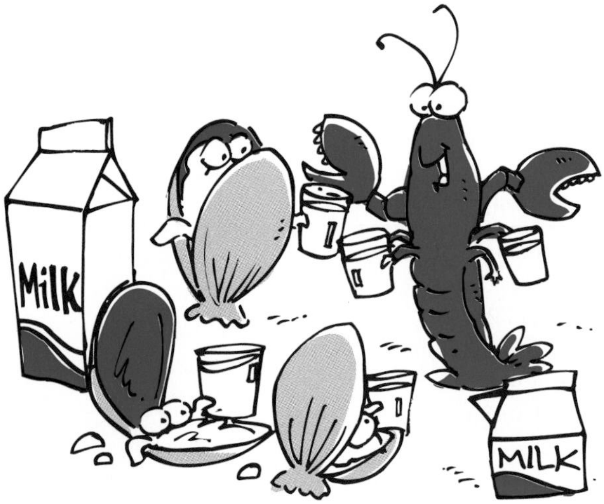

Iodine is found in fresh saltwater fish, shellfish, iodized salt, and vegetables grown in iodine-rich soil.

CULTURE

Milk products in the United States typically contain a fair amount of iodine.

Control of Iodine

Iodine is absorbed in the form of iodide ions. Iodine is stored in the thyroid and used to synthesize two hormones: triiodothyronine (T_3) and thyroxine (T_4). When the hormones are broken down, iodine is stored, if needed, in the liver. Iodine is eliminated primarily in the urine with small amounts excreted in the feces.

Functions of Iodine

1. Iodine is used in the synthesis of the thyroid hormones T_3 and T_4, which are released by the thyroid gland and regulate body temperature, metabolic rate, growth and development, nerve and muscle function, and cellular consumption of oxygen.
2. The thyroid gland takes iodine from the circulation and combines it with tyrosine, which is then converted to T_3 and T_4.
3. The thyroid gland stores T_3 and T_4 until it is released under the stimulation of thyroid-stimulating hormone (TSH).

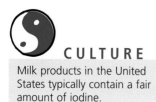

Do You UNDERSTAND?

DIRECTIONS: Unscramble the italicized words after the definitions.

1. Element used in the synthesis of thyroid hormone
   ______________________________ *(iinedo)*
2. Hormone involved in metabolism
   ______________________________ *(ydiorht)*
3. Source of iodine (a category)
   ______________________________ *(shhsiflle)*
4. Source of iodine or where fish live
   ______________________________ *(eanoc)*
5. Vital sign
   ______________________________ *(oybd remtpeurtea)*
6. Crustacean that is a source of iodine
   ______________________________ *(tsblore)*

What IS Excess Iodine?

Iodine excess, or *iodism,* is rare and is usually a result of chronic, long-term excessive iodine intake or acute poisoning by iodine solutions.

What You NEED TO KNOW

Chronic excess iodine intake that exceeds 25 times the recommended dietary intake may produce an enlarged, hyperactive thyroid or goiter.

The overactive thyroid causes disruption in the feedback regulatory mechanisms that control thyroid hormone function. As a result, hyperthyroidism or Graves' disease can occur.

Answers: **1. iodine; 2. thyroid; 3. shellfish; 4. ocean; 5. body temperature; 6. lobster.**

Signs and Symptoms of Iodism

- Anxiety
- Soreness of teeth and gums
- Weight loss
- Increased metabolic rate
- Heat intolerance
- Bulging eyeballs (**exophthalmos**)
- Tachycardia
- Hypertension

With acute poisoning by iodine solutions, severe damage to the tissue of the gastrointestinal (GI) tract occurs from local irritation.

What You DO

The treatment for hyperthyroidism is antithyroid medications or radioiodine. The health care provider should be certain that the excessive intake of iodine is discontinued.

Do You UNDERSTAND?

DIRECTIONS: **Indicate in the spaces provided whether the following statements are *true* or *false*.**

1. ______ Excess iodine may produce an enlarged, hyperactive thyroid.
2. ______ Hyperthyroidism causes a decrease in metabolic rate.

What IS Iodine Deficiency?

Iodine deficiency is associated with simple goiter and hypothyroidism. When there is an iodine deficiency, the thyroid hormones function normally until the iodine stores are exhausted. The pituitary gland, which identifies the deficiency and lack of thyroid function activity, releases hormones that stimulate the thyroid gland to produce thyroid hormones. This overstimulation of the thyroid gland causes goiter (enlarged thyroid gland), which may become multinodular and grow to great size.

Answers: **1. true; 2. false.**

Iodine-deficiency disorders account for stunting and suboptimal mental development in millions of children worldwide and in adults in developing regions with low-iodine water supplies. Worlwide, iodine deficiency is the most common cause of preventable mental deficiency. Selenium deficiency may influence the response to iodine deficiency, especially in regions within China.

TAKE HOME POINTS

Patients with thyroid goiters are usually euthyroid (normal thyroid), but some become hypothyroid or hyperthyroid.

What You NEED TO KNOW

Signs and Symptoms of Iodine Deficiency in Adult Populations

- Weakness and fatigue
- Cold intolerance
- Constipation
- Depression
- Excessive menstrual bleeding (**menorrhagia**)
- Hoarseness
- Dry skin
- Bradycardia
- Delayed deep tendon reflexes
- Anemia
- Hyponatremia
- Low T_4 and elevated TSH
- Hyaluronic acid accumulation in interstitial spaces, causing myxedema changes: puffy appearance, hypoventilation, and carbon dioxide retention from respiratory muscle changes

LIFE SPAN

Iodine deficiency during gestation causes cretinism in infants, which is characterized by extreme and irreversible mental and physical retardation, spasticity, bilateral paralysis **(diplegia)**, or paralysis of all four limbs **(quadriplegia)**, deaf-mutism, shortened stature, shuffling gait, or hypothyroidism.

What You DO

Management of hypothyroidism involves thyroid replacement therapy given orally and adequate consumption of iodine in the diet. Dietary supplementation of iodine is necessary to treat iodine-deficient states, but does not necessarily shrink established goiters. Large multinodular goiters may require thyroidectomy.

The health care provider should do the following:

- Review and provide a list of foods high in iodine and cooking preparation of raw vegetables.

- Instruct patients on the minimum dietary requirement for iodine (50 μg daily).

Potential Interactions

- Decreased absorption
  - Soybeans
  - Selenium excess or deficiency
  - Lithium

Do You UNDERSTAND?

DIRECTIONS: **Identify whether the following symptoms may be seen in *hyperthyroidism* or *hypothyroidism*.**

1. ______________________ Weight loss
2. ______________________ Dry skin
3. ______________________ Tachycardia
4. ______________________ Fatigue
5. ______________________ Bradycardia
6. ______________________ Constipation
7. ______________________ Hypertension
8. ______________________ Anxiety

What IS Iron?

Iron is an essential nutrient and is abundant in numerous food sources. Most iron is found in hemoglobin in red blood cells and is critical for oxygen transfer, normal brain development and function, and synthesis and function of neurotransmitters.

Approximately 70% of iron is found in hemoglobin. The remainder of iron in the body is stored in the liver, spleen, and bone marrow.

Answers: **1. hyperthyroidism; 2. hypothyroidism; 3. hyperthyroidism; 4. hypothyroidism; 5. hypothyroidism; 6. hypothyroidism; 7. hyperthyroidism; 8. hyperthyroidism.**

Normal Serum Iron Values, Hemoglobin, and Hematocrit

Iron (Fe): Adults 50-150 μg/dL; Newborn 110-279 μg/100 mL; Children 6 months to 3 years 60-175 μg/100 mL

Serum ferritin (protein that carries iron): 40 to 160 μg/L

Total iron-binding capacity (TIBC): Adults 300-360 μg/L; Newborns 59-175 μg/100 mL; 6 months to 3 years 250–400 μg/100 mL

Transferrin (plasma protein that transports iron from mucosa of intestines to iron storage sites in the body): 240-480 mg/dL

Transferrin saturation (a calculation using serum iron level and TIBC to determine the cause of abnormal iron levels and abnormal TIBC levels): 20%-50%

Serum iron × 100 = % of transferrin saturation TIBC

Hemoglobin
- Women: 12-15 g/dL
- Men: 13-17 g/dL
- Birth to 2 weeks: 14/9-23.7 g/dL
- 2 weeks: 13/4-19.8 g/dL
- 6 months: 10-13 g/dL
- 2 to 6 years: 11-13.8 g/dL
- 6 to 12 years: 11.1-14.7 g/dL
- 12 to 18 years female: 12/1-15.1 g/dL
- 12 to 18 years male: 12.1-16.6 g/dL

Hematocrit: 37% to 47%
- Women: 36%-45%
- Men: 39%-51%
- Birth: 0.47-0.75
- 2 weeks: 0.41-0.65
- 2 months: 0.28-0.42
- 6 months: 0.3-0.38
- 1 year: 0.3-0.38
- 2 to 12 years: 0.32-0.4
- 12 to 18 years female: 0.35-044
- 12 to 18 years male: 0.35-0.49

Serum iron levels may be increased in toxic and infective liver disease.

Recommended Daily Allowances of Iron

Men: 10 mg
Women: 15 mg
Pregnant: 30 mg
Lactating: 15 mg
Infants: 6 mg
Children ages 1 to 10 years: 10 mg
Women ages 11 to 24 years: 15 mg
Men ages 11 to 24 years: 10-12 mg

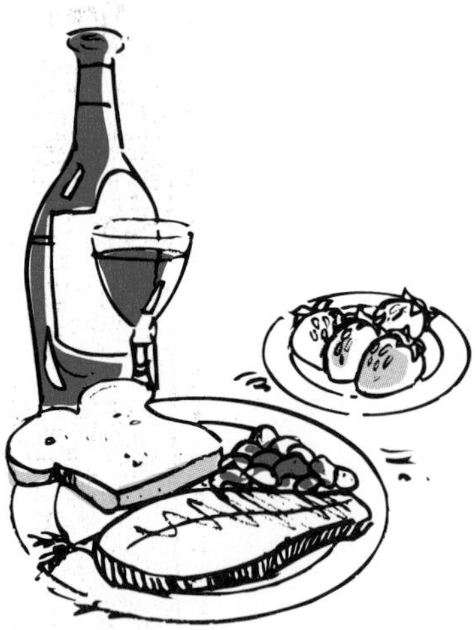

Some foods that contain iron are whole grain breads, egg yolks, dark molasses, wines, green peas, strawberries, tomato juice, Brussels sprouts, winter squash, blackberries, and nuts.

What You NEED TO KNOW

Sources of Iron

Iron sources consist of dietary iron and iron supplements. Excellent sources of dietary iron include liver, oysters, shrimp, kidney, heart, lean meat, poultry, fish, prune juice, dried beans, and dark green vegetables. Other foods that contain iron are whole grain breads and cereals, egg yolks, dark molasses, wines, raisins, green peas, strawberries, tomato juice, Brussels sprouts, winter squash, blackberries, and nuts.

Low-dose iron supplements and iron-fortified foods are poorly absorbed but can contribute slightly to dietary requirements.

Control of Iron

Dietary iron exists in heme iron found in hemoglobin, myoglobin, and some enzymes, and in nonheme iron found predominantly in plant foods. Iron is absorbed in the stomach, duodenum, and upper jejunum. Only approximately 10% of the dietary iron is absorbed.

Gastric secretions and meal consumption have a minimal effect on the absorption of iron. Gastric acid secretion enhances the change of iron into a soluble form, and absorption is enhanced by ingestion of vitamin C. Iron absorption is controlled by the intestinal mucosa depending on the body's requirements.

Transferrin saturation is the percentage of iron bound to transferrin, a protein that carries iron. The total iron–binding capacity (TIBC) is the maximum amount of iron that can be bound to transferrin and is a useful blood test in distinguishing the cause of anemia. If the TIBC is high, then less iron will be absorbed (the iron is utilized because it is bound).

Decreased gastric secretion, increased intestinal motility, and poor fat digestion may cause a decrease in iron absorption. Iron is lost from the body through blood loss and in extremely small amounts through fecal excretion and sweat. Most of the dietary iron that is not absorbed is excreted in the feces.

LIFE SPAN

Under certain conditions, such as pregnancy, growth, and iron deficiency, the body will absorb more iron.

Functions of Iron

1. Iron is the oxygen-binding site of hemoglobin. The hemoglobin molecule carries and releases oxygen to the tissues and then binds to carbon dioxide, carrying it to the lungs, where it is exhaled from the body.
2. Iron, as an oxygen-carrying component, is responsible for delivery of oxygen to muscles, thereby regulating contractions and strength,

enzyme activity, and normal function of many organs such as the brain, heart, liver, and kidneys.

3. Iron is necessary for normal brain development and function.
4. Iron is involved in immune function.
5. Iron is important in the function and synthesis of neurotransmitters.

Do You UNDERSTAND?

DIRECTIONS: **Indicate in the spaces provided whether the following statements are *true* or *false*.**

1. _____ Iron plays a role in transporting oxygen to the cells.
2. _____ An excellent source of dietary iron is milk.

What IS Hemochromatosis?

Under normal conditions, iron excess is rare because iron absorption is regulated by the body's requirements. *Hemochromatosis,* a genetic disorder occurring more predominantly in men, causes excessive iron accumulation in soft tissue and the liver and can result in cirrhosis, heart problems, such as coronary heart disease, and congestive heart failure, stroke, diabetes, arthritis, and blood clots. Acquired hemochromatosis can occur from excessive transfusions.

What You NEED TO KNOW

Signs and Symptoms of Hemochromatosis

- Hyperpigmentation of the skin
- Fatigue
- Cardiac arrhythmias
- Cardiomyopathy
- Cardiac failure
- Arthritis

Answers: **1. true; 2. false.**

What You DO

- Administer phlebotomies to treat hemochromatosis to reach normal hemoglobin and hematocrit levels.
- Educate the patient about hemochromatosis and the purpose of phlebotomies.
- Obtain a family history, and discuss the screening of children.

Keep iron tablets out of the reach of children. Excess intake of iron products can be fatal.

Do You UNDERSTAND?

DIRECTIONS: **Unscramble the italicized words that follow the definitions.**

1. Element that helps carry oxygen
   ______________________________ *(nori)*
2. Condition of iron overload
   ______________________________ *(soifnmachehrtoas)*
3. Carries oxygen
   ______________________________ *(mnbeohlgi)*
4. Protein that carries iron
   ______________________________ *(rernirtrasnf)*

What IS Iron Deficiency?

Decreased dietary intake of iron and increased losses of iron are the primary reasons for the development of *iron deficiency.* Malabsorption states or conditions involving decreased gastric acid secretion may also interfere with iron absorption, causing iron deficiency.

Answers: 1. iron; 2. hemochromatosis; 3. hemoglobin; 4. transferrin.

What You NEED TO KNOW

Iron deficiency anemia is a classic sign and symptom of iron deficiency.

Iron deficiency results in decreased red blood cell production once all the body's iron stores have been depleted.

Clinical symptoms of iron deficiency affect the cardiovascular and neurologic systems, as well as growth and development.

Signs and Symptoms of Iron Deficiency

- Hypochromic, microcytic anemia
- Pallor
- Fatigue
- Cardiac arrhythmias
- Impaired mental status
- Weakness
- Headaches
- Apathy
- Poor resistance to cold temperatures
- Appetite for nonfood substances (**pica**)

CULTURE

Iron deficiency is the leading cause of anemia in the United States from either a lack of dietary iron or GI bleeding.

What You DO

The goals of iron deficiency management are to identify the cause, such as excessive blood loss from menstruation or the GI tract, malabsorption disorders, or poor dietary intake.

Iron replacement, such as ferrous sulfate 325 mg po tid, is the most common treatment and is optimally absorbed when taken on an empty stomach. However, for patients who cannot tolerate this treatment, ferrous sulfate should be taken with food.

Occasionally iron may be ordered intravenously (IV). A 25-mg test dose is given over 5 minutes and the patient is observed for anaphylaxis or allergy symptoms. After 1 hour, the remaining portion is given IV. The intermuscular (IM) route is very irritating to the tissue, and if this is the only route available, the Z-track IM technique must be used in administration.

Blood transfusions are given when the anemia is severe (hemoglobin below 8 g/dL) or if the patient is symptomatic.

The health care provider should do the following:

- Provide a list of foods that are high in iron.
- Suggest measures to prevent constipation, such as a high-fiber diet, increased water intake, and stool softeners, if necessary.

TAKE HOME POINTS

Because iron supplements usually cause constipation, starting at a low dose (one tablet a day) and gradually increasing to three times a day may be helpful in addition to a high-fiber diet.

A test dose of iron to assess for allergic reactions must be given before starting the infusion.

Potential Interactions

- Enhance absorption
  - Calcium
  - Vitamin C–rich foods: orange juice, lemon, tomatoes, peppers
  - Meat, fish, poultry
- Inhibit absorption:
  - Coffee, tea, wine
  - Legumes, grains, rice, tofu
  - Acid-pump inhibitors, H_2 blockers, antacids
  - Tetracyclines, quinolones

Do You UNDERSTAND?

DIRECTIONS: **Indicate whether the following conditions are caused by an iron *excess* or *deficit*.**

1. ____________________ Hemochromatosis
2. ____________________ Anemia
3. ____________________ Skin hyperpigmentation
4. ____________________ Increased risk for stroke
5. ____________________ Pica
6. ____________________ Pallor

What IS Selenium?

Selenium is an essential mineral that is a component of the antioxidant enzyme glutathione peroxidase. This enzyme protects red blood cells and cell membranes from damage caused by free radicals, as well as the toxic effects of mercury and cadmium. Selenium also aids in immunoglobulin synthesis.

Answers: **1. excess; 2. deficit; 3. excess; 4. excess; 5. deficit; 6. deficit.**

The highest concentrations of selenium in the body are in the liver, kidney, heart, and spleen. Smaller amounts of selenium are widely distributed in the body as part of the enzyme glutathione peroxidase structure.

Recommended Daily Allowances of Selenium

Adolescents and adults: 40 to 70 μg
Pregnant women: 65 μg
Lactating women: 70 μg
Children ages 7 to 10 years: 30 μg
Children ages 1 to 6 years: 20 μg
Infants up to 1 year: 10 to 15 μg

What You NEED TO KNOW

Sources of Selenium

Selenium content in food depends on the concentration in soil and water where the food was grown. Food sources high in selenium include Brazil nuts, whole wheat, selenium-rich nutritional yeast, brown rice, oatmeal, poultry, low-fat milk products, extra-lean meat, organ meats, and fish. States that have selenium-rich soil are Montana, Utah, South Dakota, Wyoming, New Mexico, Colorado, and Tennessee.

Control of Selenium

Absorption of selenium occurs in the upper segment of the small intestine. Increased intake results in increased excretion of selenium in the urine. The organic forms are absorbed more efficiently and are less likely to cause toxic symptoms than the inorganic forms. Excess selenium intake of approximately two to three times the recommended daily requirements may cause hair and nail loss, nausea, fatigue, nerve damage, and muscle problems. Children are more susceptible to selenium toxicity, which may result in tooth decay and tooth loss.

LIFE SPAN

Children are more susceptible to selenium toxicity, which may result in tooth decay and tooth loss.

Functions of Selenium

1. Serves as a component of antioxidant enzyme glutathione peroxidase, which protects red blood cells and cell membranes from damage by free radicals.

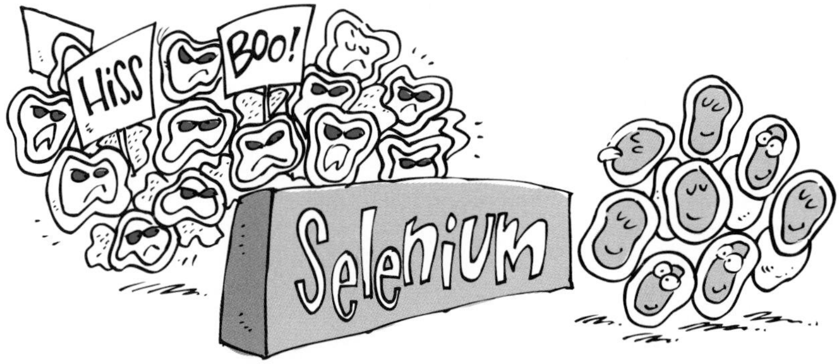

A free radical is an electrically charged atom with an unpaired electron. The unpaired electron (free radical) is unstable, and it attempts to become stable by either giving up an electron to another molecule or stealing an electron from another one. This process (of giving up or stealing an electron) causes an injurious bond formation with proteins, lipids, and carbohydrates, the key molecule in membranes and nucleic acids. Antioxidants such as selenium inactivate or terminate free radicals by attracting and neutralizing the free radicals, preventing them from stealing or shedding electrons.

2. Functions in correlation with the antioxidant vitamin E.
3. May reduce the incidence of leukemia and cancers of the colon, rectum, ovaries, and lung by the antioxidant effect.
4. Facilitates production of prostaglandins, which regulate inflammatory processes.
5. Reduces menopausal hot flashes.
6. Reduces free radical damage to the heart muscle, possibly preventing early-stage heart disease.
7. Enhances the immune system by stimulating activity of macrophages and the release of lymphocytes.
8. Reduces the quantity of damaging compounds such as hydrogen peroxide, which promotes inflammation associated with rheumatoid arthritis.
9. Protects the skin from damaging effects of ultraviolet light.

Do You UNDERSTAND?

DIRECTIONS: **Indicate in the spaces provided whether the following statements are *true* or *false*.**

1. _____ Selenium facilitates oxygenation of tissues.
2. _____ Selenium protects cells from free radical damage.

Answers: **1. false; 2. true.**

3. _____ Selenium-rich soil is found in Florida and Wisconsin.
4. _____ Selenium is found in many sources of dietary grain.

What IS Selenosis?

Selenium toxicity or *selenosis* is rare and involves consuming selenium in excess of three times the recommended daily allowance.

What You NEED TO KNOW

Signs and Symptoms of Selenosis

- Skin and nail changes
- Hair loss
- Swelling of the fingers
- Fatigue
- Nausea
- Vomiting
- Tooth decay

What You DO

The goal of selenosis management is to decrease intake of selenium and to facilitate excretion of excess selenium by the kidneys through the use of diuretics and hydration. The health care provider should provide a review of recommended dietary allowances of selenium.

Answers: 3. false; 4. true.

Do You UNDERSTAND?

DIRECTIONS: **Provide checks next to the signs and symptoms of selenosis.**

1. _____ Dry mouth
2. _____ Heart palpitations
3. _____ Fatigue
4. _____ Sleeplessness
5. _____ Tooth decay
6. _____ Nail changes
7. _____ Depression

What IS Selenium Deficiency?

Selenium deficiency is rare, and manifestations may take years to develop.

What You NEED TO KNOW

LIFE SPAN

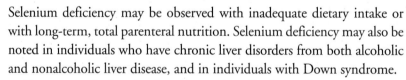

- Keshan disease, a form of cardiomyopathy, affects children.
- One of the signs of selenium deficiency in neonates is jaundice.

Selenium deficiency may be observed with inadequate dietary intake or with long-term, total parenteral nutrition. Selenium deficiency may also be noted in individuals who have chronic liver disorders from both alcoholic and nonalcoholic liver disease, and in individuals with Down syndrome.

Decreased selenium intake affects primarily the cardiovascular system as a result of weakened and damaged heart muscle. Cardiomyopathy can occur and increase the risk for early-stage heart disease and myocardial infarction.

Signs and Symptoms of Selenium Deficiency

- Cardiomyopathy
- Neonatal jaundice
- Seborrheic dermatitis
- Macular degeneration
- Decreased thyroid function

Answers: 3; 5; 6.

What You DO

Management of selenium deficiency involves the replacement of selenium by dietary or supplemental intake.

- Provide a list of foods containing selenium.
- Explain the importance of taking supplements as prescribed.

Potential Interactions

- Inhibit absorption:
  - Vitamin C in high doses
- Synergistic affect:
  - Iodine
  - Vitamin E

Do You UNDERSTAND?

DIRECTIONS: Indicate in the spaces provided whether the following statements are *true* or *false*.

1. _____ Selenium deficiency or excess is rare.
2. _____ Selenium deficiency is often associated with chronic lung disorders.
3. _____ Poultry is an excellent source of selenium.
4. _____ Selenosis can cause nausea and vomiting.

What IS Zinc?

Zinc is a mineral element found abundantly throughout the body. It is second only to iron as a trace element and is the most abundant intracellular trace element. Zinc is involved in numerous catalytic, structural, and regulatory functions and is a component of more than 100 different enzymes.

Answers: **1. true; 2. false; 3. true; 4. true.**

Recommended Daily Allowances of Zinc

Adolescents and adults: 12-15 mg/day Children ages 1 to 10 years: 10 mg/day Infants up to 1 year: 5 mg/day

The highest concentrations of zinc are found in the liver, pancreas, kidney, bone, and muscles. Other tissues with high concentrations include parts of the eye, prostate gland, spermatozoa, skin, hair, fingernails, and toenails. The total body content of zinc is approximately 2 to 3 g.

What You NEED TO KNOW

Sources of Zinc

Zinc intake correlates with protein intake. Approximately 80% of the dietary zinc is obtained from meat, fish, poultry, milk, and milk products. Other good sources of zinc include oysters, shellfish, liver, cheese, whole grain cereals, dry beans, soy products, and nuts.

Control of Zinc

The majority of zinc is absorbed along the small intestine. Small amounts are absorbed in the stomach and the large intestine. The major route of zinc excretion is in the feces, with only 2% to 10% excreted in the urine. The amount of zinc secreted into the gut and, subsequently, the amount of fecal loss depends on dietary intake.

Functions of Zinc

1. Zinc is abundant in the nucleus and stabilizes RNA and DNA structure.
2. Zinc is an essential requirement for the activity of RNA polymerases, which are important in cell division.
3. Zinc maintains normal body cholesterol levels, normal growth and development, and production of prostaglandins.
4. Zinc has a beneficial effect on the immune system by increasing levels of T-lymphocytes and some antibodies and inhibiting the growth of disease-causing bacteria.

CULTURE

The average person in the United States consumes approximately 5 mg of zinc per 1000 calories.

Do You UNDERSTAND?

DIRECTIONS: Indicate in the spaces provided whether the following statements are *true* or *false*.

1. _____ Zinc is found in the extracellular fluid.
2. _____ Foods high in protein are a good source of zinc.

What IS Zinc Toxicity?

Zinc toxicity, caused by excessive zinc ingestion (classified as 100 to 300 mg/day), is rare. Chronic zinc supplementation will interfere with copper absorption.

What You NEED TO KNOW

Zinc toxicity may occur in patients with renal failure who are receiving hemodialysis.

Signs and Symptoms of Zinc Excess

- Anemia
- Fever
- Central nervous system alterations

What You DO

The treatment of zinc toxicity involves decreasing zinc ingestion and zinc supplements.

Answers: 1. false; 2. true.

Do You UNDERSTAND?

DIRECTIONS: Fill in the blanks.

1. Zinc toxicity occurs most often in patients receiving ____________.
2. Zinc excess is classified as greater than ____________ mg/day.

What IS Zinc Deficiency?

Zinc deficiency may occur as a result of a low-protein diet or with a diet high in unrefined cereals or unleavened bread because of the presence of phytates, which bind to zinc and reduce its absorption.

TAKE HOME POINTS

Because zinc is present in numerous cells throughout the body, a wide range of signs and symptoms of zinc deficiency may occur.

What You NEED TO KNOW

Zinc deficiency may also occur as a result of malabsorption syndromes, starvation, or increased loss through urinary, pancreatic, or other exocrine secretions.

Signs and Symptoms of Zinc Deficiency

- Decreased taste acuity (**hypogeusia**)
- Growth retardation
- Delayed sexual maturation
- Decreased semen production (**hypogonadism**) and low count of sperm production (**hypospermia**)
- Baldness (**alopecia**)
- Delayed wound healing
- Skin lesions
- Impaired appetite
- Immune deficiencies
- Behavioral disturbances
- Eye problems, including photophobia and night blindness

Answers: **1. hemodialysis; 2. 100.**

What You DO

Management of zinc deficiency involves increasing dietary intake of zinc or increasing zinc supplements, either orally or parenterally.

- Identify the underlying cause for zinc deficiency.
- Provide a list of foods containing zinc.
- Explain the importance of taking supplements as prescribed.

Potential Interactions

- Enhance absorption:
  - Cysteine-containing proteins
- Decrease absorption:
  - Calcium
  - Iron
  - Caffeine
  - Oxalic acid (spinach, sweet potatoes, rhubarb, beans)

Do You UNDERSTAND?

DIRECTIONS: **Indicate whether the following conditions are related to a zinc *deficit* or *excess.***

1. _____ Growth retardation
2. _____ Alopecia
3. _____ Anemia
4. _____ Photophobia
5. _____ Skin lesions
6. _____ Fever

Answers: **1. deficit; 2. deficit; 3. excess; 4. deficit; 5. deficit; 6. excess.**

Summary of Minerals

Mineral	Body Functions	Sources	Signs/Symptoms: Excess	Signs/Symptoms: Deficiency	Interactions
Fluoride	Strengthen bone and teeth	Fluoridated water	Teeth: stains/flecks Nausea, vomiting, diarrhea Joint pain Chest pain Muscle wasting	Dental caries, osteoporosis	Calcium supplements Calcium- or aluminum-containing antacids
Iodine	Regulate growth and development, metabolic rate, body temperature	Saltwater fish, shellfish, iodized salt	Weight loss Increased metabolic rate Heat intolerance Tachycardia Hypertension Exophthalmos	Weakness Fatigue Cold intolerance Constipation Depression Menorrhagia Hoarseness Dry skin Bradycardia Delayed deep tendon reflex Anemia Hyponatremia Low T_4 and elevated TSH Myxedema changes	Soybeans Selenium excess or deficiency Lithium
Iron	Oxygen transfer Brain development and function Neurotransmitter function	Liver Oysters, shrimp Kidney, heart Poultry Prune juice Dried beans	Skin hyperpigmentation Fatigue Cardiac arrhythmias Cardiomyopathy Cardiac failure	Anemia Pallor Fatigue Cardiac arrhythmias Impaired mental status Weakness	Calcium Vitamin C–rich food Meat, fish, poultry Coffee, tea, wine Legumes, grains Rice, tofu

		Whole grain breads Dark green vegetables Egg yolks Strawberries Tomato juice Blackberries Nuts	Arthritis	Headaches Intolerance to cold Pica	H_2 blockers, antacids Acid pump inhibitors Tetracyclines Quinolones
Selenium	Protects red blood cells and cell membranes Facilitates prostaglandin production Enhances immune system	Brazil nuts Yeast Brown rice Oatmeal Poultry Low-fat milk Lean meat Organ meat Fish	Skin/nail changes Hair loss Fatigue Nausea Vomiting Tooth decay	Cardiomyopathy Neonatal jaundice Seborrheic dermatitis Macular degeneration Decreased thyroid function	Vitamin C in high doses Vitamin E Iodine
Zinc	Maintains normal body cholesterol levels Normal growth and development Prostaglandin production	Meat Fish Poultry Milk Milk products Dry beans Soy Nuts	Anemia Fever Central nervous system alterations	Hypogeusia Growth retardation Delayed sexual maturation Alopecia Impaired appetite Immune deficiencies Visual changes	Cysteine-containing proteins Calcium Iron Caffeine Oxalic acid

References

Burk RF, Levander OA: Selenium. In Shils ME et al, editors: *Modern nutrition in health and disease,* Baltimore, 1999, Williams & Wilkins.

Chernecky C, Berger BJ: *Laboratory tests and diagnostic procedures,* ed 3, Philadelphia, 2000, Saunders.

Decker GM: Commonly used vitamin supplements: implications for clinical practice, *Clin J Oncol Nurs* 2:1-28, 2003.

Herbal medicine handbook, Springhouse, PA, 2001, Springhouse Corporation.

McIntosh N, Helms P, Smyth R: *Forfar & Arneil's textbook of pediatrics,* New York, 2003, Churchill Livingstone.

Mueller D, Burke R: Vitamin and mineral therapy. In Morrison G, Hark L, editors: *Medical nutrition,* Cambridge, 1998, Blackwell Science.

Murray M, Decker GM: Diet, nutrition, and lifestyle changes. In Decker GM, editor: *An introduction to complementary and alternative therapies,* Pittsburgh, 1999, Oncology Nursing Press.

PDR for nutritional supplements, Montvale, NJ, 2001, Medical Economics Company.

Welland D: Eat, 'supp' and be healthy, *Arthritis Today* 17:58-69, 2003.

NCLEX® Review

1. Mr. Gray, age 63, has been recently diagnosed with gastric cancer and has had a partial gastrectomy. It will be important for him to increase which element in his diet because of possible decreased absorption resulting from his recent surgery?
   1 Zinc
   2 Iodine
   3 Selenium
   4 Iron

2. Which foods are considered excellent sources of iron?
   1 Cereals, yellow vegetables, eggs
   2 Green, leafy vegetables; liver; citrus fruits
   3 Pork, fish, milk
   4 Poultry, potatoes, tea

3. Ms. Green, age 19, is a college student at the local community college. Her roommate brings her to the health center because she is concerned that Ms. Green has lost a lot of weight and is looking quite ill. While talking with Ms. Green, she admits to you that she has been starving herself so that she can be thin. She states that she has lost about 30 pounds in 3 months. Her diet consists of carrot sticks and diet coke. Starvation could predispose Ms. Green to which type of deficiency?
   1 Zinc
   2 Selenium
   3 Iron
   4 Fluoride

4. Mrs. White brings her 3-year-old daughter to the well-baby clinic. She is concerned because her daughter's teeth have developed brown spots and pitting of the tooth enamel. She states that she makes sure that her daughter brushes her teeth four times every day using a lot of toothpaste. You are suspicious that her daughter is getting an excess amount of which element?
   1 Zinc
   2 Iodine
   3 Fluoride
   4 Selenium

5. Which one of the following patients is at increased risk for zinc deficiency? The patient who has:
   1 Anorexia
   2 Euthyroid
   3 Osteoporosis
   4 Multiple teeth caries

6. The health care provider is taking care of a family with three small children who live on a farm in Wisconsin. Their water is from a natural well. Which element should be prescribed for the children when the well water test demonstrates that the water does not contain this element?

7. Fluoride is necessary for which body process?
   1 Cardiac contractility
   2 Acid-base balance
   3 Digestion
   4 Bone and teeth formation

8. In addition to calcium, which element is necessary for maintaining bone strength?
   1 Iron
   2 Zinc
   3 Selenium
   4 Fluoride

9. Iodine is stored in which organ?
   1 Thyroid
   2 Bones
   3 Muscle
   4 Gallbladder

10. Iodine is necessary for the synthesis of which hormone?
   1 Estrogen
   2 Testosterone
   3 Parathyroid hormone
   4 Thyroid

11. Mrs. Williams, age 54, has been diagnosed with iron-deficiency anemia. She will be started on oral iron supplements. In an effort to increase absorption of iron, Mrs. Williams should be instructed to increase consumption of:
   1 Coffee
   2 Whole wheat grain breads
   3 Shrimp
   4 Tomatoes

12. Oral iron may cause gastrointestinal distress and constipation. Therefore iron should be taken:
   1 On an empty stomach
   2 With a low-fiber diet
   3 With food or meals
   4 At bedtime

13. Patients taking selenium should be advised not to take high doses of:
   1 Vitamin B_6
   2 Vitamin C
   3 Vitamin D
   4 Vitamin E

14. Which foods are considered excellent sources of selenium?
   1 Whole wheat, brown rice, oatmeal
   2 Green, leafy vegetables; potatoes; tea
   3 Yellow vegetables, whole milk, citrus fruits
   4 Tomatoes, squash, bananas

15. Individuals with hemachromatosis are at increased risk for:
   1 Coronary heart disease
   2 Crohn's disease
   3 Gastric ulcers
   4 Liver cancer

NCLEX® Review Answers

1. 4 Decreased gastric acid secretions will decrease iron absorption.

2. 2 Green, leafy vegetables are high in ascorbic acid, which facilitates iron absorption. Liver is high in iron.

3. 1 Starvation and a low-protein diet are associated with zinc deficiency. She is at risk for developing iron deficiency anemia, but the body will use iron stores over several months before anemia occurs.

4. 3 Excess fluoride from the toothpaste will cause deposits and brown spots on the teeth.

5. 1 Anorexia presents an increased risk for zinc deficiency from starvation. Euthyroid indicates a normal thyroid. Osteoporosis and teeth caries are a result of fluorosis.

6. Fluoride. Fluoride is an important element that helps protect developing teeth from dental caries. Fluoride is usually absent in well water and is rarely found in natural water sources.

7. 4 Bone and teeth formation are dependent on adequate fluoride intake.

8. 4 Fluoride and calcium are necessary to strengthen bones and teeth and to prevent osteoporosis.

9. 1 Thyroid. Iodine is stored mainly in the thyroid and liver.

10. 4 Thyroid. Iodine is used in the synthesis of thyroid hormones T_3 and T_4, which are released by the thyroid gland.

11. 4 Tomatoes. Citrus foods increase absorption of iron.

12. 3 With food or meals. Taking iron with food will decrease gastrointestinal irritation.

13. 2 Vitamin C. The consumption of vitamin C will decrease absorption of selenium.

14. 1 Whole wheat, brown rice, oatmeal. Food sources high in selenium include brazil nuts, whole wheat, brown rice, oatmeal, poultry, low-fat milk products, extra-lean meats, organ meats, and fish.

15. 1 Coronary heart disease. Excessive iron accumulation can cause cirrhosis, heart disease, stroke, diabetes, arthritis, and blood clots.

Notes

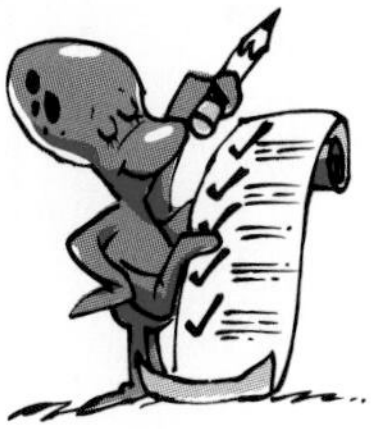

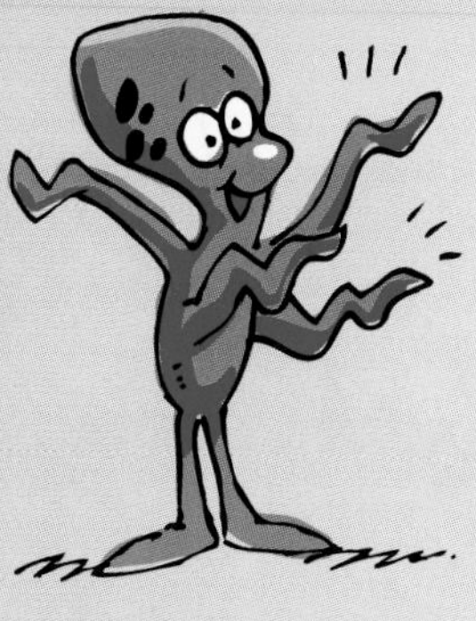

Chapter

10 Health Care Problems of the Neonate

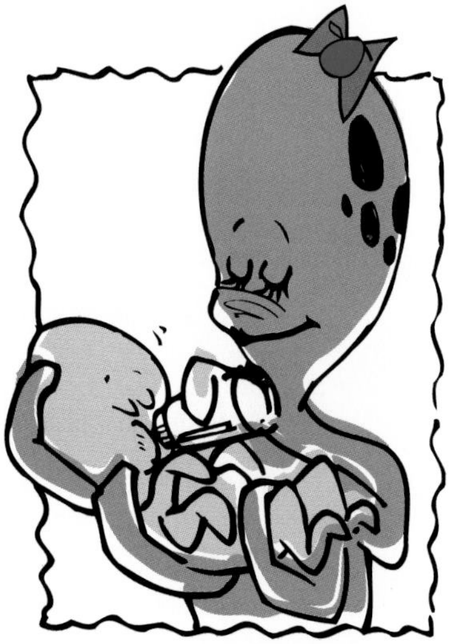

Because of their unique physical proportions and body composition, neonates have fluid and electrolyte requirements that differ from the requirements of adults and older children.

What You WILL LEARN

After reading this chapter, you will know how to do the following:

- ✔ State the maintenance fluid requirement for neonates.
- ✔ Identify two reasons why fluid requirements for neonates are different from fluid requirements for adults.

Now that you understand the basic concepts of fluid and electrolyte metabolism, you are ready to learn the management of patients in various age groups. Newborns can be classified as *full term* (37 or more weeks gestation at birth) or *preterm* (less than 37 weeks gestation at birth). Because of their unique physical proportions and body composition, this group has fluid and electrolyte requirements that differ from the requirements for adults and older children. The ultimate goal of neonatal care is to support normal growth and development. One important aspect of neonatal care is maintaining normal fluid and electrolyte balance.

What IS the Maintenance Fluid Requirement for Neonates?

Total fluid intake refers to liquid taken in as feedings, intravenous (IV) solutions, and medications, and is expressed in milliliters per kilogram per day (mL/kg/day). Measurable fluid output includes urine, stool, and fluid lost via surgical drains and orogastric-nasogastric tubes. Insensible water loss refers to the fluid lost through the skin and respiratory tract. The sum of the fluid needed for growth plus measurable fluid loss plus insensible water loss equals the daily *maintenance fluid requirement.*

What You NEED TO KNOW

You should be able to calculate the infant's total fluid intake and hourly urine output (u/o). Total daily fluid intake (expressed as mL/kg/day) is determined by the following equation:

Total fluid intake = total intake (mL) ÷ weight (kg) ÷ 1 day

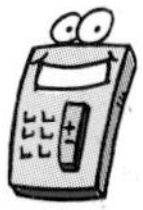

EXAMPLE 1: **The fluid intake including feedings and IV fluid received by a 3.5 kg infant in the past 24 hours was 300 mL.**

Total daily fluid = 300 mL ÷ 3.5 kg ÷ 1 day = 86 mL/kg/day

Daily u/o, expressed as mL/kg/hr, is calculated by the following equation:

u/o = volume of urine in 24 hr (mL) ÷ weight (kg) ÷ 24 hr

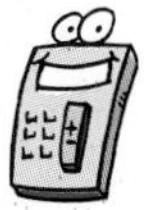

You may be asked to monitor the patient's u/o over a shorter period. You should be able to do so using the equation given to determine whether u/o is below the specified lower limit of normal.

EXAMPLE 2: **The volume of urine produced by the patient in Example 1 was 25 mL in the last 4 hours, or:**

u/o = 25 mL ÷ 3.5 kg ÷ 4 hr = 1.8 mL/kg/hr

Term Infant

The daily neonatal fluid requirement varies with gestational age and maturity at birth.

Neonates contain more total body water per kilogram than older children and adults. Initially, full-term infants require 60 to 100 mL/kg/day of total fluid. This includes fluid needed for replacement of insensible water loss, fluid lost in the urine and stool, and fluid needed for growth.

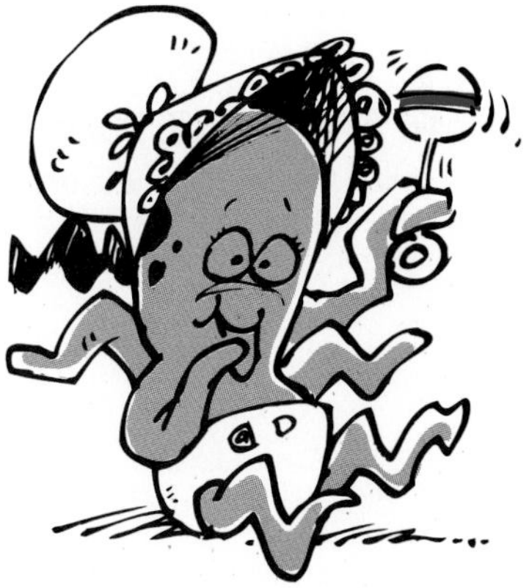

The daily neonatal fluid requirement varies with gestational age and maturity at birth.

Certain conditions alter the normal fluid requirements of neonates. Neonatal jaundice (**hyperbilirubinemia**) is a common problem for both full-term and preterm infants and refers to an excess of bilirubin (a breakdown product of hemoglobin) in the blood. Moderate-to-severe jaundice is often treated in the hospital with phototherapy to avoid the toxic effects of bilirubin on the central nervous system. This treatment can increase insensible water loss.

Sepsis is another condition that may increase a patient's fluid requirements from leakage of fluid out of the blood vessels into the surrounding tissue (**third spacing**). Infants with diarrhea or surgical drains may also have increased fluid loss that requires replacement.

Excessive fluid intake, conversely, can result in fluid overload, edema, and heart failure. Therefore care must be taken to provide adequate but not excessive fluid to the infant. Neonatal fluid balance is best monitored by regular and frequent evaluation of weight, vital signs, total intake and output (I & O), serum electrolyte values, and frequent physical examinations.

The u/o and daily weight are valuable indicators of a newborn's hydration status. Immediately after birth, during the first day of life, the amount of urine produced by infants can be low. However, after this period, most neonates produce at least 1 mL/kg/hr of urine. A u/o of less than this amount could indicate the presence of dehydration or another medical condition warranting investigation. During the first week of life, a physiologic diuresis occurs, resulting in the loss of 7% to 12% of total body weight. Weight loss greater than 15% of the birth weight is considered excessive.

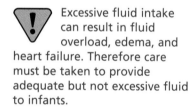

Excessive fluid intake can result in fluid overload, edema, and heart failure. Therefore care must be taken to provide adequate but not excessive fluid to infants.

Serum Electrolyte Values for Term and Preterm Infants

Sodium (Na^+) = 135 to 145 mEq/L
Potassium (K^+) = 3.5 to 5.5 mEq/L
Chloride (Cl^-) = 98 to 108 mEq/L
Bicarbonate (HCO_3^-) = 20 to 24 mEq/L

TAKE HOME POINTS

A sunken anterior fontanelle or decreased skin turgor are signs of moderate dehydration.

Preterm Infant

Basic fluid requirements of premature infants vary tremendously depending on the patient's birth weight and gestational age. In contrast with full-term infants, premature infants have increased total fluid requirements caused by marked insensible water losses through their immature skin and by a larger surface area–to–body weight ratio. For example, an extremely premature infant with a birth weight less than 1000 g may initially require 120 to 220 mL/kg/day to maintain normal fluid and electrolyte balance.

Other factors that increase insensible water loss include an elevated environmental temperature and the use of a radiant warmer or open warmer bed. Factors that decrease insensible water loss are high ambient humidity, plastic shields, closed infant warmers, or topical emollients. The more premature the infant is, the higher the daily fluid requirement will be.

As the degree of prematurity increases, the ability of various organs, such as the kidneys, to perform the normal functions decreases. The premature kidney is less able to concentrate urine effectively or to reabsorb sodium and bicarbonate. Consequently, urine specific gravity is less helpful in determining fluid status. Rather, other indicators, such as daily weight, fluid intake, u/o, blood pressure, and perfusion are used as indicators of hydration status.

Infants born earlier than 34 weeks gestation are prone to developing certain medical conditions as a result of their immaturity. Respiratory distress syndrome (RDS) commonly affects premature infants and is caused by the lack of a substance called surfactant, normally made by the lungs. Surfactant deficiency causes the baby's lungs to inflate inadequately, resulting in low blood oxygen levels.

Some premature infants may develop sepsis or necrotizing enterocolitis (NEC), a bacterial infection of the large and small bowel. Similar to full-term infants with sepsis, these infants have increased fluid requirements caused by third spacing of fluid into the surrounding tissue.

TAKE HOME POINTS

- Electrolytes obtained from the infant during the first day of life reflect the values of the mother before delivery.
- Premature infants have highly variable fluid and electrolyte requirements, depending on their birth weight and gestational age. Physical examination, daily weight, I & O levels, and serum electrolytes are valuable indicators of neonatal fluid balance.

What You DO

The treatment of neonatal jaundice may include hydration and/or administration of special overhead light to the skin **(phototherapy)** to hasten the removal of bilirubin from the blood stream. Phototherapy with overhead lights can increase the patient's insensible water loss and increase the risk for dehydration. Therefore to avoid causing dehydration in a patient being treated with phototherapy, it is often necessary to increase the total fluid intake by 10% to 20% in the form of oral feedings or IV fluid.

TAKE HOME POINTS

Neonates have more total body water per kilogram than adults or older children. Phototherapy with overhead lights and sepsis can increase neonatal fluid requirements.

LIFE SPAN

The potassium level in preterm infants can be elevated to dangerous levels and require extremely close monitoring. Thus, potassium is omitted from IV fluids until the serum potassium is normal and the u/o is greater than 1 mL/kg/hr.

Rapid-volume and bicarbonate infusions are avoided in preterm infants to prevent sudden changes in intravascular volume and/or cerebral blood flow, which increase the risk for the occurrence of brain hemorrhage.

Neonatal fluid balance is best monitored by regular and frequent evaluation of weight, vital signs, total I & O, serum electrolyte values, and frequent physical examinations. To maintain adequate fluid balance and to avoid the problem of inadequate fluid intake, the health care provider must accurately measure and record the newborn's daily weight and all fluid lost into diapers and orogastric or surgical drains. Serial screening of the infant's serum electrolytes is carried out to properly gauge his or her physiologic status and response to fluid therapy.

Extremely premature infants may have inappropriately high u/o (more than 5 mL/kg/hr). Sodium, bicarbonate, and free water intake must be increased, monitored, and adjusted frequently to maintain serum values in the normal range in these patients.

Respiratory distress syndrome is treated with supplemental oxygen, endotracheal intubation, mechanical ventilation, and exogenous surfactant administration. Oxygen is heated and humidified to prevent hypothermia, mucosal drying, and excessive insensible water loss. Patients with RDS are usually kept NPO (nothing by mouth) during their acute illness. In addition, total fluids are restricted during the acute phase of the illness to help improve oxygenation and to decrease the risks for persistent patency of the ductus arteriosus and the subsequent development of chronic lung disease.

Standard neonatal IV fluids vary from institution to institution, but often contain dextrose and sodium chloride. Caregivers may elect to include calcium, bicarbonate, and potassium, as indicated.

Do You UNDERSTAND?

DIRECTIONS: **Indicate in the spaces provided whether the following statements are *true* or *false*.**

1. _____ Total fluid intake refers only to IV fluid.
2. _____ Insensible water loss refers to urine and stool losses.
3. _____ Phototherapy increases insensible water loss.

DIRECTIONS: **Fill in the blanks with the word *increases* or *decreases*.**

4. Total fluid requirement ______________________________ with decreasing birth weight and gestational age.

Answers: 1. false; 2. false; 3. true; 4. increases.

5. Use of plastic shields, closed incubators, and emollients __________ insensible water loss in neonates.
6. Sodium loss ______________ with increasing gestational age.

Answers: 5. **decreases**; 6. **decreases**.

Notes

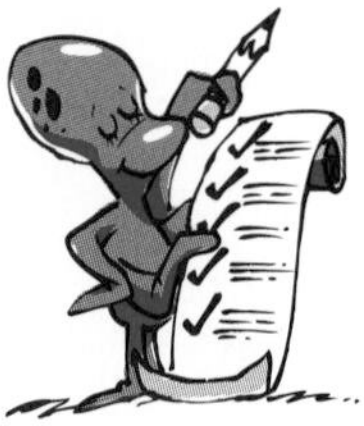

NCLEX® Review

1. What is the total fluid intake per day of a term infant weighing 3.2 kg taking only bottle feedings of 36 mL of formula every 3 hours?
   1 75 mL/kg/day
   2 90 mL/kg/day
   3 100 mL/kg/day
   4 115 mL/kg/day

2. Calculate the urine output during the last 8-hour shift of an infant weighing 2.5 kg with the following output totals:
   0000 to 0800 = 90 mL
   0800 to 1600 = 82 mL
   1600 to 2400 = 66 mL
   1 1.1 mL/kg/hr
   2 2.2 mL/kg/hr
   3 3.3 mL/kg/hr
   4 4.5 mL/kg/hr

3. Total intake of a 3.5-kg full-term infant who received both bottle feeds (320 mL/day) and IV fluids (210 mL/day) was which of the following:
   1 120 mL/kg/day
   2 130 mL/kg/day
   3 140 mL/kg/day
   4 150 mL/kg/day

4. Increased environmental temperature, immature skin, and high ambient humidity __________ the daily fluid requirement, respectively.
   1 Decrease, decrease, and increase
   2 Increase, increase, and increase
   3 Decrease, increase, and decrease
   4 Increase, increase, and decrease

5. What is the total fluid intake in mL/kg/day of a preterm infant weighing 1.2 kg receiving only IV fluid at a rate of 6 mL/hr?
   1 80 mL/kg/day
   2 100 mL/kg/day
   3 120 mL/kg/day
   4 140 mL/kg/day

6. When assessing for fluid imbalance, the most helpful information to collect is:
   1 Total intake and output and daily weight
   2 Food intake
   3 Medication intake
   4 Temperature

7. Premature infants are at risk for fluid imbalance from immature function of which organ?
   1 Lung
   2 Colon
   3 Skin
   4 Brain

8. When caring for an infant admitted with pneumonia, the health care provider should frequently monitor and treat which vital sign?

9. The health care provider is caring for a neonate with a history of prolonged vomiting from a pyloric obstruction. The patient is admitted for a surgical repair and continues to vomit. The patient is at risk for a decrease in which major electrolyte?

10. Jane, 4 years old, had been admitted to the hospital for third-degree burns to her legs. During the first 48 hours after the burn, you notice severe edema of her legs. What electrolyte imbalance is Jane most likely to experience at this time?
    1 Hypomagnesemia
    2 Hyperkalemia
    3 Hypercalcemia
    4 Hypocalcemia

11. True or False: Premature newborns have decreased insensible water loss compared with term newborns.

12. The kidney of a preterm newborn has ________ ability to reabsorb sodium than the kidney of a term newborn.
 1 Greater
 2 Lesser
 3 Equal

13. True or False: Serum electrolytes sampled during the first 24 hours after birth are reflective of the newborn's salt and water balance.

14. A valuable indicator of neonatal fluid balance is:
 1 Temperature
 2 Respiratory rate
 3 Blood glucose
 4 Daily weight

15. Rapid volume and bicarbonate infusions are ________ to preterm infants.
 1 Beneficial
 2 Harmful
 3 Neither harmful or beneficial

NCLEX® Review Answers

1. 2 (36 mL × 8 feeds/day)/3.2 kg = 90 mL/kg/day

2. 3 (66 mL ÷ 8 hr)/2.5 kg = 3.3 mL/kg/hr

3. 4 (320 mL + 210 mL)/3.5 kg = 150 mL/kg/day

4. 4 Increase, increase, and decrease. Immature skin and high environmental temperature increase evaporative water loss; high ambient humidity decreases evaporative water loss.

5. 3 (6 mL/hr x 24 hr)/1.2 kg = 120 mL/kg/day

6. 1 Total intake and output and daily weight are important nursing interventions used to assess fluid balance. Temperature does not usually affect fluid balance unless a fever with excessive perspiration is present.

7. 3 Skin development is immature in the premature infant, causing poor regulation of fluids and electrolytes. Lungs and colon minimally affect fluid imbalance. The brain does not affect it.

8. Temperature, because it is often elevated during infection and can spike rapidly in infants, resulting in dehydration and febrile seizures.

9. Chloride. Prolonged vomiting causes a major loss of chloride from the gastrointestinal tract.

10. 2 Hyperkalemia is common from the massive cellular destruction that occurred as a result of the burn injury.

11. False, preterm infants have increased insensible water loss compared with term infants, owing to their thin skin and increased surface area-to-mass ratio.

12. The preterm kidney has a lesser ability to absorb sodium compared with the term kidney.

13. False. Serum electrolytes measured on the first day are more reflective of maternal salt and water balance.

14. Daily weight is an indicator of neonatal fluid balance. Temperature, respiratory rate, and blood glucose are not indicators of fluid balance.

15. Rapid fluid and bicarbonate infusions are harmful to preterm infants, owing to rapid changes in intravascular volume and/or cerebral blood flow placing these infants at risk for suffering intraventricular hemorrhage.

Notes

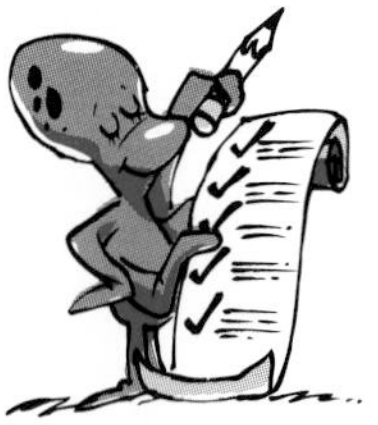

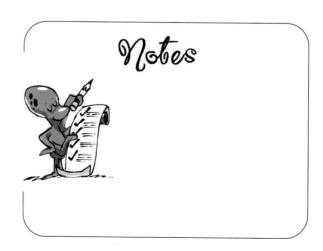

Fluid and Electrolyte Balance in Infants

Chapter 11

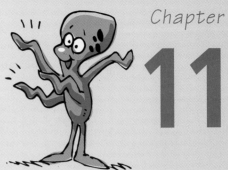

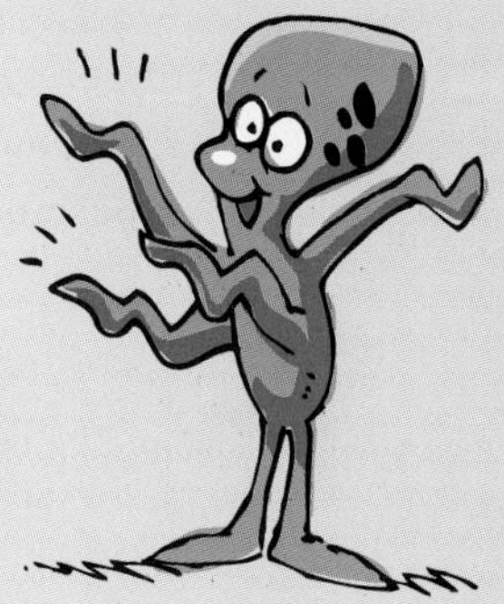

What You WILL LEARN

After reading this chapter, you will know how to do the following:

- ✔ Describe the outcomes of normal fluid and electrolyte status in relation to three body systems.
- ✔ Identify two consequences of fluid imbalance.
- ✔ Identify two electrolyte abnormalities and the disease/condition associated with them.

Infants are highly susceptible to changes in their fluid and electrolyte balance because of a variety of factors. Physiologic differences, which include a higher metabolic rate, larger percentage of extracellular body fluid, greater body surface area compared with older children and adults, and immature kidney function, can place the infant at high risk for developing problems. There is a delicate balance in everyone between intake and output (I & O) that is affected by fluid intake, urine volume, stool volume, sweating, and insensible water loss.

What IS Normal Fluid and Electrolyte Status?

Fluid and electrolyte status in an infant can be assessed by several parameters. The skin of an infant should be warm and pink, indicating good tissue perfusion. Normal capillary refill is less than 2 seconds. Good skin turgor means that when the skin of an infant, including the subcutaneous tissue, is pinched, there is an immediate return to normal appearance.

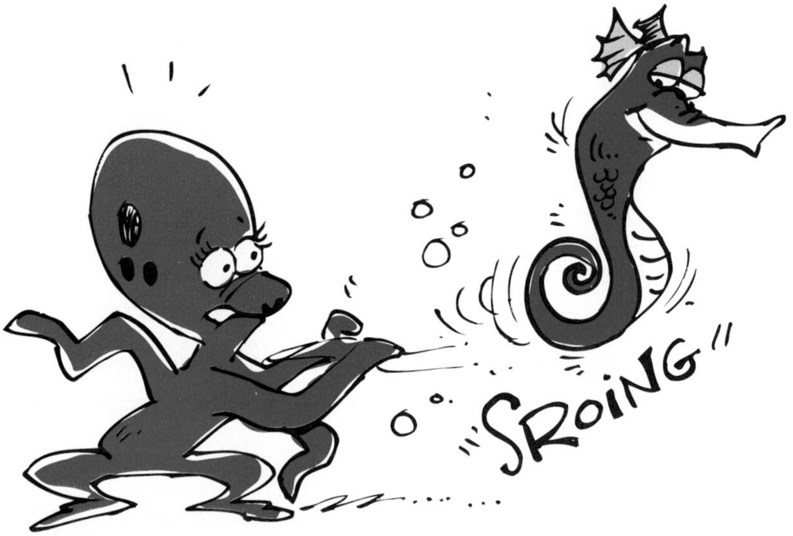

Good skin turgor means that when an infant's skin, including the subcutaneous tissue, is pinched, there is an immediate return to normal appearance.

TAKE HOME POINTS

Pathways of water loss are **F**eces **U**rine **R**espiration **S**weat

TAKE HOME POINTS

- Metabolic or mixed (metabolic and respiratory) acidosis is common in low birth weight infants after delivery.
- Metabolic acidosis in fetal umbilical cord blood at delivery is a sign of cerebral palsy.

An infant's anterior fontanel usually closes by 18 months of age. In a young infant, the fontanel appears flat, often with visible pulsations. The infant's mouth and tongue are moist, indicating good hydration. Tears are usually present by 4 months of age. Blood pressure and heart rate should be within an acceptable range for age. Body weight and length increase incrementally as the infant grows. Plotting an infant's height and weight over time illustrates this concept. The infant urinates at least six times during the day and may have several soft, formed stools. There is no evidence of vomiting, diarrhea, or excessive perspiration.

What You NEED TO KNOW

The body weight of an infant at birth is composed of 75% to 80% water, known as total body water (TBW), which decreases to approximately 67% by the end of the first year of life. Body water is divided between the intracellular fluid (ICF) (fluid within the cells) and extracellular fluid

(ECF) (fluid in the intravascular compartment, which is blood plasma), as well as interstitial fluid, which is between the cells. At birth, the infant's ECF is greater than the ICF. Half of an infant's ECF is exchanged daily.

Normal water losses occur through the kidneys, gastrointestinal (GI) tract, skin, and respiratory tract and must be replaced daily through fluid and dietary means. To remember the pathways of water loss, simply think FURS: *feces, urine, respiration,* and *sweat.*

Infants weighing less than 10 kg require 100 mL of water per kg of body weight every day. Infants above 10 kg require 1000 mL plus 50 mL for each kg over 10 kg. For example, an infant weighing 8.3 kg requires 830 mL of fluid, and an infant weighing 12.5 kg requires 1125 mL. Note the following examples:

EXAMPLE 1: Formula for daily fluid replacement in infants weighing less than 10 kg:

Weight (always stated in kg) × 100 mL = mL of daily fluid replacement

8.3 kg × 100 mL of water = 830 mL of daily fluid replacement

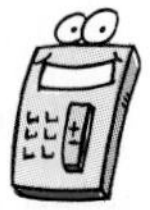

EXAMPLE 2: The formula for daily fluid replacement in infants weighing more than 10 kg:

First, determine how many kilograms more than 10 the patient weighs.

Weight (kg) – 10 kg = A

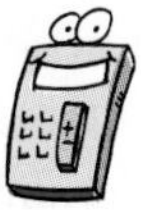

12.5 kg is weight
−10.0
2.5

Then, multiply the result by 50 mL.

2.5
× 50 mL
125.0 mL

Then, add this number to 1000.

125 mL + 1000 mL = 1125 mL of daily fluid replacement

One of the most common causes of fluid and electrolyte imbalance in infants is gastroenteritis, which is an inflammation of the stomach and the gastrointestinal (GI) tract.

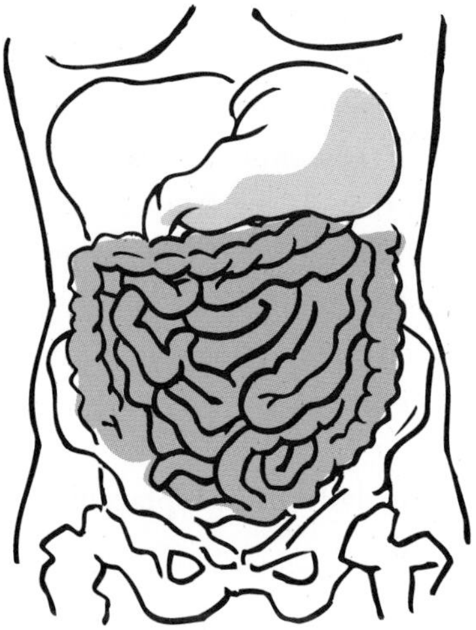

Gastroenteritis

The most common cause of gastroenteritis is a viral infection. For infants, rotavirus is the major cause. Other viruses known to be associated with gastroenteritis include reovirus, coxsackievirus, adenoviruses, echovirus, parvovirus, and polioviruses. In addition, the cause of gastroenteritis may be bacterial or parasitic in origin.

TAKE HOME POINTS

- Frequent and careful hand washing is the best way to prevent transmission of organisms that cause diarrhea in any setting, be it the home, day care facility, hospital, or clinic.
- Infants are at high risk for developing dehydration as a result of gastroenteritis.

The infectious agents involved in gastroenteritis are transmitted via the fecal-oral route. The incubation period is between 24 and 48 hours. Outbreaks may occur in day care centers and schools. Infants may experience vomiting, diarrhea, fever, abdominal pain, and weight loss.

Initial symptoms of gastroenteritis can include vomiting and diarrhea, which predispose the infant to fluid and electrolyte loss. Associated problems with gastroenteritis include metabolic acidosis related to diarrhea and metabolic alkalosis related to prolonged vomiting.

The combination of fluid and electrolyte losses can cause an infant to become dehydrated rapidly and may lead to acid-base imbalance. Sodium, potassium, and chloride are the major electrolytes involved. Sodium is the major extracellular cation, which is accompanied by chloride, the major extracellular anion. Potassium is the major intracellular cation. All three are present in intestinal fluids. Metabolic acidosis occurs with severe diarrhea because bicarbonate is lost in stool. Severe and prolonged vomiting may cause metabolic alkalosis.

! Dehydration from gastroenteritis is a major cause of morbidity in the United States and a major cause of mortality in developing countries.

Signs and Symptoms of Fluid and Electrolyte Loss Based on Causes

Viruses. Vomiting, followed by large watery stools, may be present. Blood is generally not present. Rotavirus generally occurs in the winter.

Bacteria. Stool may be bloody in 50% of cases. Bowel movements are more frequent and smaller in volume. High fever may be present. Shigella and salmonella are examples of bacterial organisms. *Escherichia coli* 0157:H7 has been associated with bloody diarrhea and hemolytic uremic syndrome. *E. coli* has been found in uncooked contaminated beef.

Cryptosporidium, Giardia lamblia, and *Vibrio cholerae* are among the other organisms that cause diarrhea associated with contaminated water supplies.

What You DO

The potential major outcome of vomiting and diarrhea caused by gastroenteritis is dehydration. Dehydration occurs when fluid losses are greater than fluid intake. Nursing care is directed at preventing dehydration while supporting the infant through the illness. Assess the infant for signs and symptoms of dehydration, and document these on the infant's health record.

Assessment of the Severity of Dehydration

Signs and Symptoms	Mild Dehydration	Moderate Dehydration	Severe Dehydration
Infant's appearance and condition	Alert but may be restless	Thirsty, may be restless or lethargic, irritable when touched	Lethargic or comatose; cold, sweaty, or limp; cyanotic with poor peripheral perfusion
Percent of body weight loss	3%-5%	6%-9%	10% or more
Peripheral pulse	Rate and strength within normal	Increased rate and weak	Increased rate, feeble, may be difficult to palpate
Respiratory rate	Within normal limits	Deep but may be rapid	Deep and rapid
Anterior fontanel	Normal, flat	Sunken	Very sunken
Systolic blood pressure	Normotension	Normotensive or low	Hypotensive, may be unable to record

Continued

Assessment of the Severity of Dehydration—cont'd

Signs and Symptoms	Mild Dehydration	Moderate Dehydration	Severe Dehydration
Skin turgor	Immediate return	Slow return	Tenting
Eyes	Normal	Sunken appearance	Very sunken appearance
Tears	Present	Reduced to absent	Absent
Mucous membranes	Moist	Dry	Very dry
Urinary output	May be normal or decreased	Decreased to dry	Absent
Specific gravity	> 1.020	> 1.020	Anuria
Capillary refill	< 2 seconds	± 2 seconds	> 3 seconds
Estimated fluid deficit (mL/kg)	30-50	60-90	100 or more

Adapted from Behrman RE, Kliegman RM, Jenson HB: *Nelson textbook of pediatrics,* ed 16, Philadelphia, 2000, Saunders.

- Assess the infant's vital signs based on the norms for age. The pulse and respiratory rates can increase as dehydration progresses.
- Document the infant's temperature. Fever often accompanies gastroenteritis and causes an increase in evaporative water loss.
- Document the infant's weight. Careful weighing of the infant assists in assessing the severity of dehydration. Weigh the infant unclothed on the same scale each time the weight is measured. Not all scales are calibrated the same. If an infant is to be weighed each day, then he or she must be weighed at the same time of day.
  - Measure total intake and document it. When infants are ill and not taking solid foods, clear liquid diets are indicated. The clear liquids of choice are oral rehydration solutions (ORS), which are available in small volume containers, as ice pops, or as gel cups.
  - Measure all output and document it. Most hospitals and clinics have gram scales on which diapers can be weighed. A dry diaper is weighed, and the amount in grams is noted.

When wet diapers are weighed, the weight of the dry diaper is subtracted to obtain an estimation of urinary output (1 g = 1 mL = 1 cc).

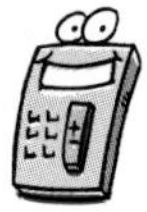

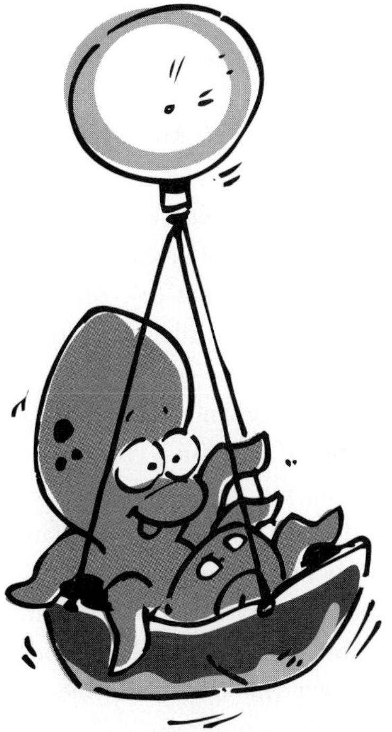

When wet diapers are weighed, the weight of the dry diaper is subtracted to obtain an estimation of urinary output (1 g = 1 mL = 1 cc).

When stools are diarrheal (loose and watery), an estimation of the fluid loss can be made in the same manner. You need to note the color, number, and characteristics of stool. Be aware that some stools may contain blood or mucus.

- Obtain a detailed history of the illness. Ask these questions:
    1. When did the infant first become ill? Are there others in the family with the same type of illness?
    2. Is the infant eating and drinking? How much? What kind and what amount of fluid has the infant taken in the last 24 hours? Is the infant keeping it down?
    3. Is the infant voiding? Infants produce urine at the minimum rate of 1 to 2 mL/kg/hr.
    4. Is diarrhea present? Sodium, potassium, and chloride are lost from the body in excessive amounts when an infant has diarrhea. The infant is likely to experience metabolic acidosis.
    5. Does the infant have tears?
    6. Is the inside of the mouth moist?
    7. Does the family drink water from a well?

TAKE HOME POINTS

- When caring for an infant with gastroenteritis, note that your most important nursing intervention is maintaining fluid and electrolyte balance to restore the infant to the former state of wellness.
- Occasionally, it is difficult for a mother to tell whether her baby's diaper is wet because disposable diapers have super-absorbing capabilities and tend to feel dry even when wet. To determine whether a baby is urinating, disposable paper tissues or cotton balls can be placed in the diaper. The tissue or cotton will absorb the urine and make urine output easier to access and assess.

LIFE SPAN

Frequently, infants are fussy and irritable when experiencing gastroenteritis and may refuse to eat or drink. Some infants may experience intestinal cramping caused by the increased motility of the GI tract.

8. Have the infant and family traveled outside of the country?
9. Does the infant have any health problem that makes him or her immunocompromised?
10. Is the infant in day care? Are other infants in the day care center ill?

- Frequent diarrheal stools may cause redness and excoriation of the perianal area. Change diapers after each stool. Wash the area with a mild soap in warm water and pat dry. An infant's perianal area can remain undiapered, especially while asleep, to allow thorough drying and to prevent rash.
- Monitor infants who are receiving intravenous (IV) infusions for rehydration closely. The site of infusion is checked for patency and signs of infection. Fluid volume and rate of infusion are monitored to prevent the overload or underload of fluids. The infant must urinate before potassium is added to any IV infusion.
- Offer oral feedings, as tolerated, such as infant rice cereal, mashed bananas, and vegetable juice, during the period of rehydration. It has been demonstrated that the small intestine absorbs up to 60% of nutrients even during the acute stage.

Infant formula and milk may be added, when tolerated. Infants who are receiving solid foods may tolerate smaller, more frequent meals. Foods should be easily digestible and rich in energy.

The type of dehydration is based on the value of the serum sodium. Sodium controls fluid between the fluid compartments in the body. Normal serum sodium levels for infants are 139 to 146 μmol/L. There are three types of dehydration based on the serum sodium concentration and the osmotic gradient:

TAKE HOME POINTS

Parents need to receive anticipatory guidance regarding the possibility of diarrhea and the potential for dehydration during well-baby visits so that they can initiate oral rehydration therapy before the infant becomes dehydrated.

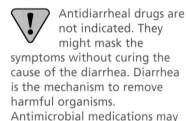

Antidiarrheal drugs are not indicated. They might mask the symptoms without curing the cause of the diarrhea. Diarrhea is the mechanism to remove harmful organisms. Antimicrobial medications may be indicated in certain cases.

- Withholding fluids and giving the bowel a rest is contraindicated and might prolong diarrhea.
- Home remedies, such as flavored gelatins, sports drinks, soft drinks, apple juice, and broth, are not recommended because they do not have the correct carbohydrate-to-sodium ratios. Fluids with a high sugar content, such as apple juice or colas, may cause osmotic diarrhea. Diet drinks should never be used in treating dehydration.

Three Types of Dehydration Based on Serum Sodium Concentration and Osmotic Gradient

Type	Serum Sodium	Physiologic Mechanism
Hypotonic	< 130 mEq/L	Shift of ECF to the ICF with a decrease in ECF can lead to circulatory collapse
Isotonic	130-150 mEq/L	No osmotic gradient across cell walls
Hypertonic	> 150 mEq/L	Shift of ICF to ECF with decrease in ICF

ECF, Extracellular fluid; *ICF*, intracellular fluid.

Treatment of Dehydration

MILD DEHYDRATION
For a 3% to 5% loss of body weight, give ORS at the rate of 50 mL/kg over 4 hours; can usually be treated at home. Offer an additional 60 to 120 mL of ORS for each diarrheal stool.
MODERATE DEHYDRATION
For a 6% to 9% loss of body weight, give ORS at the rate of 100 mL/kg over 4 hours; may be hospitalized, depending on infant's condition; if infant does not want to drink from a bottle, offer ORS by spoon or dropper at frequent intervals.
SEVERE DEHYDRATION
For a 10% or greater loss of body weight, prepare to administer IV fluids as prescribed. Isotonic solutions (e.g., NS, LR solution) are used in the initial treatment. Infant is usually hospitalized.

IV, Intravenous; *LR,* lactated Ringer's; *NS,* normal saline; *ORS,* oral rehydration solutions.

TAKE HOME POINTS

Breast-feeding should continue during acute gastroenteritis.

It is important to monitor laboratory values. However, treatment should not be delayed while awaiting the results of the blood tests. Hemoglobin and hematocrit may be elevated by fluid loss, a condition known as hemoconcentration. Serum potassium levels for infants range from 3.5 to 6.0 fmol/L but may be normal or elevated from dehydration caused by diarrhea. Normal serum bicarbonate levels vary between 21 and 28 mEq/L and may decrease as dehydration progresses. The specific gravity of urine will become more concentrated with dehydration (increased specific gravity).

Mild dehydration usually can be treated with oral fluids that have a physiologic carbohydrate-to-sodium ratio plus other electrolytes. These fluids are known as oral rehydration therapy (ORT).

Commercial ORS include Pedialyte, Lytren, Rehydralyte, and Ricelyte. Electrolyte solutions are sold under a variety of brand names. They may be packaged as liquids, gelatins, or popsicles for freezing. Parents should be encouraged to keep a form of ORS on hand to use as needed. These solutions can be purchased at most drug stores and supermarkets, and are available in hospitals and clinics.

Do You UNDERSTAND?

1. Scott Miller, 4 months old, weighed 6.6 kilograms last week at his regular checkup. Calculate his required fluid intake per day in milliliters.
2. Yesterday, Scott began to experience diarrhea and had five loose, watery stools before he is brought to the clinic. He is refusing to drink any fluids. You weigh him today and note that he weighs 6.23 kilograms. What is his percentage body loss in his weight?

Answers: **1. 100 mL × 6.6 = 660 mL; 2. 6.60 − 6.23 = 0.37 kg in weight loss, 0.37 ÷ 6.6 = 5% weight loss.**

TAKE HOME POINTS

- The health care provider will prescribe replacement fluids and electrolytes depending on the type and severity of dehydration. IV fluid replacement is administered in cases of severe dehydration or when the infant refuses oral intake or has persistent vomiting.
- Most infants with mild-to-moderate dehydration can be treated at home. Infants with severe dehydration should be hospitalized.

3. What is Scott's degree of dehydration?
4. What is the best way of rehydrating Scott?

DIRECTIONS: **Unscramble the words to indicate the three major electrolyte imbalances found in an infant with gastroenteritis:**

5. _____ *(moduis)*
6. _____ *(sumistpoa)*
7. _____ *(delroihc)*

DIRECTIONS: **Fill in the blanks.**

8. What classification of medications is not indicated for an infant with diarrhea?

   ____

9. The incubation period for infectious agents involved in gastroenteritis is _____ to _____ hours.
10. What symptom that often accompanies gastroenteritis causes an increase in evaporative water loss?

   ____

References

Chernecky CC, Berger BJ: *Laboratory tests and diagnostic procedures,* ed 4, Philadelphia, 2004, Saunders.

Hankins GD, Speer M: Defining the pathogenesis and pathophysiology of neonatal encephalopathy and cerebral palsy, *Obstet Gynecol* 102(3):628-36, 2003.

Kecskes ZB, Davies MW: Rapid correlation of early metabolic acidaemia in comparison with placebo, no intervention or slow correction in LBW infants, *The Cochrane Library* (Oxford), ID #CD002976, 2004.

Eliason BC, Lewan RB: Gastroenteritis in children: principles of diagnosis and treatment, *Am Family Phys* 58:1769, 1998.

Kleinman RE, editor: *Pediatric nutrition handbook,* ed 4, Elk Grove Village, Ill, 1998, American Academy of Pediatrics.

Kleinman RE, Sack D, Riikonen CB: Infant diarrhea: management and comfort, *Pediatr Basics* 91(Spring):16, 2000.

Answers: **3. mild dehydration, 3% to 5% of body weight; 4. offering small amounts (5 to 10 mL) of ORS frequently, either by nipple, syringe, dropper, or spoon, and calculating his fluid requirement and monitoring his intake of the solution; 5. sodium; 6. potassium; 7. chloride; 8. antidiarrheals; 9. 24, 48; 10. fever.**

NCLEX® Review

1. An infant has experienced a 7% fluid loss because of rotavirus infection. Which of the following signs and symptoms would you least expect to find?
   1 Increased pulse rate
   2 Flat anterior fontanel
   3 Decreased urinary output
   4 Capillary refill of less than 2 seconds

2. Which of the following fluids is acceptable for an infant with diarrhea?
   1 Chicken broth
   2 Decarbonated ginger ale
   3 Infalyte
   4 Apple juice

3. To assess an infant for a change in hydration status, the most reliable method is which of the following?
   1 Assess skin turgor.
   2 Measure intake and output.
   3 Weigh the infant.
   4 Obtain blood for serum sodium levels.

4. Which of the following is the correct amount of Pedialyte to give an infant weighing 8.5 kg who is mildly dehydrated?
   1 250 mL over 4 hours
   2 500 mL over 4 hours
   3 625 mL over 4 hours
   4 425 mL over 4 hours

5. A mother reports that her infant son has been having loose, watery stools. Your first response to her should be what?
   1 "When did it begin, and how many stools has he had?"
   2 "Give him some diluted cola to keep him hydrated."
   3 "Diarrhea has been going around. Don't worry. He should be better in a few days."
   4 "What have you been feeding him?"

6. Water loss occurs during fever by which mechanism?
   1 Perspiration or sweat
   2 Renal damage
   3 Hypotension
   4 Hypertension

7. Which route transmits infectious agents that cause gastroenteritis in infants?
   1 Intramuscular
   2 Pulmonary inhalation
   3 Fecal
   4 Cerebrospinal fluid

8. Severe diarrhea in an infant causes bicarbonate loss in the stool, leading to which acid-base imbalance?
   1 Hyperchloremia
   2 Metabolic acidosis
   3 Respiratory alkalosis
   4 Hypermagnesemia

9. An infant is admitted in the emergency room with vomiting followed by large, watery stools and no bloody diarrhea. Based on these signs and symptoms, which is the most likely cause?
   1 Bacteria
   2 Virus
   3 Protozoa
   4 Allergic reaction to medication

10. Dehydration in an infant will cause what type of change in cardiac pulse?

11. True or False: The total body weight of an infant at birth is approximately 75% to 80% water.

12. True or False: Use of antidiarrheal mediations is common health care practice in treating diarrhea caused by infections in infants.

13. What condition is a major cause of dehydration in infants?

14. Clear liquids of choice for infants who are ill and not taking solid food are called ORS. What does ORS stand for?

15. If 1 gram of net diaper equals 1 mL of urine output, then how much urine output has the infant had whose net diaper weight is 42 grams?

NCLEX® Review Answers

1. **2** A flat anterior fontanel is a normal finding in an infant. An infant with a rotavirus infection is expected to be dehydrated. Symptoms of dehydration include increased pulse rate, decreased urinary output, and capillary refill time greater than 2 seconds.

2. **3** An infant with diarrhea should receive a solution such as Infalyte to address electrolyte and fluid loss. Chicken broth is high in sodium and does not replenish electrolytes (i.e., is not physiologic). Ginger ale and apple juice are high in glucose, low in sodium, and do not replenish electrolytes (i.e., are not physiologic).

3. **3** The most reliable method to assess an infant's hydration status is to weigh the infant regularly because water loss can be measured from changes in weight. Assessing skin turgor and measuring input and output are assessment parameters but are not the most reliable. Blood tests for serum levels are assessment parameters but they require laboratory analysis. The health care practitioner cannot wait for lab findings to begin treatment for dehydration.

4. **4** The required amount of Pedialyte is 50 mL/kg ($8.5 \times 50 = 425$); 250 mL over 4 hours is a volume of 29.4 mL/kg; 500 mL over 4 hours is a volume of 58.8 mL/kg; and 625 mL over 4 hours is a volume of 75.5 mL/kg.

5. **2** First, you should determine the history of the illness. Instructing the mother to keep her son hydrated does not explore all the circumstances of the illness but provides a response. "Don't worry" provides false reassurance without exploring all the circumstances of the illness. "What have you been feeding him?" is an adversarial question, which may make the mother feel that she is at fault and not explore all the circumstances of the illness.

6. **1** Fever is associated with high temperature and perspiration. Hypotension and hypertension are indicators of blood pressure. Renal damage is not a result of fever.

7. **3** Infants frequently acquire gastroenteritis from transmission from the fecal-oral route. Gastroenteritis is neither an airborne pathogen nor a muscle or cerebrospinal fluid infection.

8. **2** Metabolic acidosis occurs in the infant caused by a loss of bicarbonate in the stool from diarrhea. Hyperchloremia is the result of a high chloride intake. Hypermagnesemia is the result of high magnesium intake. Respiratory alkalosis results from hyperventilation.

9. **2** Typically, viruses are associated with vomiting followed by large, watery stools. Bacteria cause bloody bowel movements and frequent, small stools. High fever may be present. Protozoa cause formed but soft stools. Allergic reactions to medication may cause hives.

10. Pulse will increase.

11. True.

12. False. Diarrhea is the body's way of ridding the infection from the body, and, therefore, no medication to stop diarrhea should be taken. The health care practitioner may prescribe an antimicrobial agent, if indicated.

13. Viruses, especially gastroenteritis.

14. Oral rehydration solutions.

15. 42 mL.

Health Care Problems of the Toddler

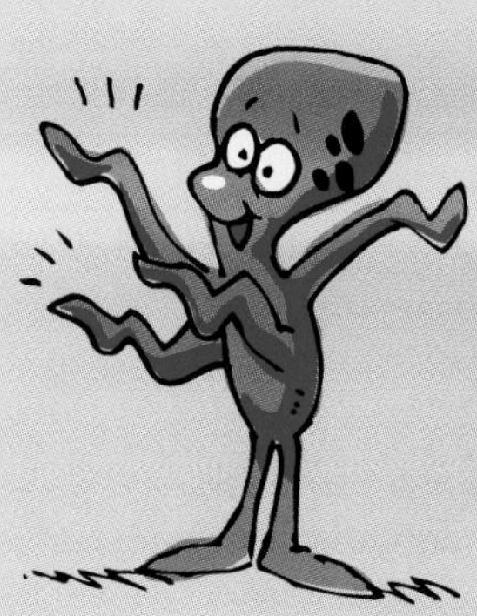

Chapter 12

What You WILL LEARN

After reading this chapter, you will know how to do the following:

- ✔ Define burns in relation to body surface area.
- ✔ Describe one fluid and two electrolyte imbalances associated with full-thickness burns.

The ages between 12 and 36 months are referred to as the *toddler years.* Children in this age group are often curious and may be prone to injury when not closely supervised.

The major cause of death in toddlers is injury. Young children love to explore their environment, without concern for their own safety. Injuries are often a result of motor vehicle accidents, falls, or burns sustained when the toddler reaches for pots on the stove. The toddler is at a risk for fluid and electrolyte imbalances for the following reasons:

1. Fever with insensible fluid loss
2. Respiratory problems with fast breathing **(tachypnea)**
3. Kidney disease
4. Burns
5. Vomiting and diarrhea (gastroenteritis)

A brief summary of the risk factors for fluid and electrolyte imbalances in the toddler can be found in the table on p. 210.

TAKE HOME POINTS

Toddlers/children with allergic diseases who are treated with elimination diets may develop ketotic hypoglycemia.

Summary of Injury Risk Factors in Toddlers

Risk Factors	Causes	Signs and Symptoms	Treatments
Fever	Infection (viral or bacterial)	Fever, thirst, decreased urine output	Reduce fever with acetaminophen, tepid bath; treat infection as prescribed by health care provider
Vomiting and diarrhea	Gastroenteritis, dehydration, infection	Persistent vomiting and large amounts of diarrhea; thirst and decreased urine output	Replace fluids orally (may need to use intravenous hydration if unable to take fluids by mouth; antiemetics as prescribed
Kidney disease	Trauma, kidney infection, congenital disease of the kidney	Symptoms may vary, depending on the underlying disease; in some cases, decreased or increased urine output may be observed; protein and blood may be observed in the urine	Treat underlying cause; replace fluids and electrolytes as prescribed by the health care provider
Respiratory problems	Infections, pulmonary disease (e.g., cystic fibrosis)	Increased respiratory rate may lead to insensible fluid loss	Treat underlying cause

The major cause of death in toddlers is injury.

The goal of this chapter is to discuss fluid and electrolyte imbalances related to burn injuries in the toddler. Although burns are not the most common cause of fluid and electrolyte imbalances, they reveal some of the more dramatic symptoms and complications.

What ARE Burns?

Burns rank second among girls and third among boys as a cause of death. The causes of burns in this age group are numerous and include the following:

- Accidental scalding when they reach for pots and pans on a stove or when they are placed in bath water that is too hot.
- Flame injuries when they play with matches or candles and accidentally set themselves on fire.
- Electrical burns when they play with cords and electric appliances.
- Chemical burns when they play with caustic agents such as cleaning products or batteries.

TAKE HOME POINTS

Mustard gas, such as that used in a weapon, produces chronic blepharitis and corneal scarring.

What You NEED TO KNOW

TAKE HOME POINTS

The most common type of burn injury in this age group is related to scalding, although fires cause 33% of all burns.

Prevention of Burn Injury

Type of Burn Injury	Prevention
Scalds from pulling pots with hot liquids off of the stove	Do not leave children unattended. Turn pot handles toward the back of the stove. Keep cords and appliances (coffee maker) out of reach. Do not leave the oven door open.
Scalds from submersion in hot water	Do not leave children unattended. Regulate water temperature to less than 120° F. Monitor water temperature with a meat thermometer before placing the toddler in the tub. Test water temperature with your elbow.
Flame injuries from candles and matches	Do not leave the toddlers unattended. Keep matches and candles out of reach. Do not leave lit candles or fires unattended. Remember that all homes should be equipped with a smoke detector and fire alarm.
Electrical burns	Place protective guards in all electrical outlets when not in use. Do not let child play with electrical cords or batteries.
Burns related to child abuse (e.g., scalding, cigarette burns)	Identify high-risk patients. Parent education and support. Remove child from home if in immediate danger.

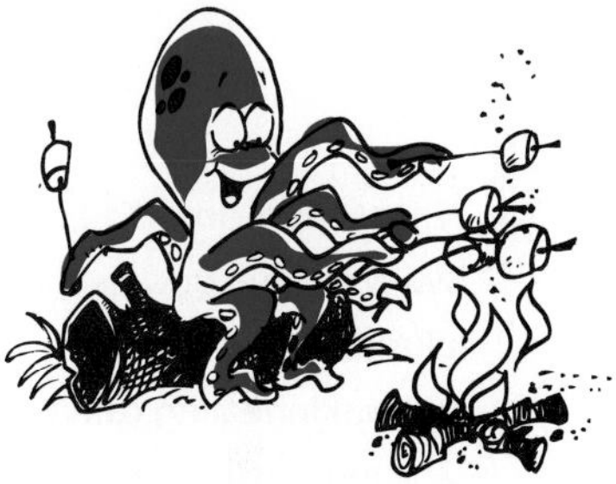

Burns rank second among girls and third among boys as a cause of death.

Burns are typically classified in two ways, the first of which is related to the depth of the injury and includes *first-degree, second-degree, third-degree,* and *fourth-degree* burns. The second is based on the extent of the burn and includes *superficial, partial-thickness,* and *full-thickness* burns.

Types of Burns

Degree	Prevention	Signs and Symptoms
FIRST		
Superficial	Sunburn	Red surface blanches to touch Burn is dry without any open lesions
SECOND		
Partial thickness	Scalds and flames	Red surface had blisters and areas of clear (serous) drainage Blanches to touch
THIRD		
Full thickness	Fire	Involves the epidermis (outer layer of skin) and subcutaneous tissue (below the skin) Does not blanch
FOURTH		
Full thickness	Fire and prolonged contact with a hot object	Involves underlying structures such as muscle, fat, and bone Very serious

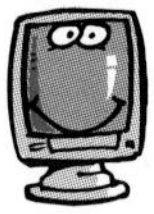

Chest Medicine On-Line
www.nlm.nih.gov/medlineplus/burns.html
www.skinhealing.com/2_2_skinburnsscars.shtml

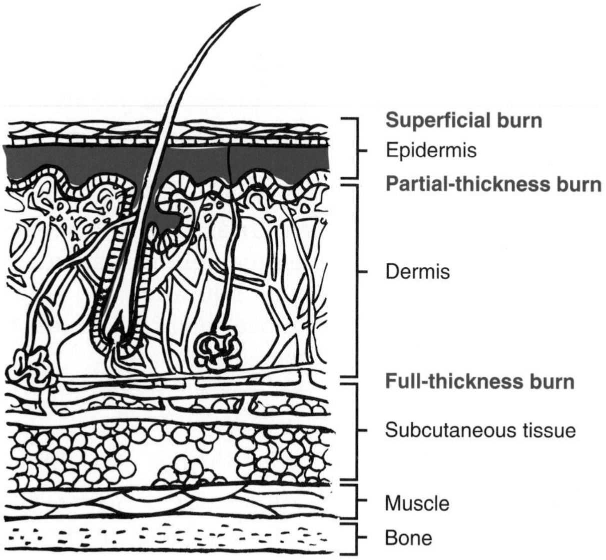

Layers of the skin.

All burns can be painful. Typically, full-thickness burns (third- and fourth-degree) destroy nerve endings, but there are often superficial first- and second-degree burns around the full-thickness burn that can be quite painful. Also, patients with third-degree burns lose their sweat glands, which creates a problem with temperature regulation. After resolution of the burn, there can be the sequellae of life-long itching as an irritant. This usually occurs in 60% of burn patients and can be helped by the use of the medication gabapentin.

TAKE HOME POINTS

Young children under 2 years of age are at risk for developing toxic shock syndrome (TSS) after a burn.

What You DO

Emergency Treatment of Burns

Most burn injuries will occur outside the hospital or medical setting. All burns need immediate attention.

- Stop the burning process.

  Flames:
  - Place the child in a horizontal position (on the floor), and wrap the child in a blanket or rug. Roll the child on the floor until the flames are extinguished.
  - Apply cool (not cold) water to the burned area.
  - Remove burned clothing or jewelry to prevent further burning of the skin.

  Chemical:
  - Wash the burn with copious amounts of water to remove the chemical from the skin.
  - Do not place water on a powder, but brush the powder off. Adding water may cause increased burning as the powder becomes a liquid.
- Make certain that the child is breathing and has a heartbeat and good circulation. Apply the basics of cardiopulmonary resuscitation (CPR) if the patient is not breathing or does not have a heartbeat.
- Cover the burn with a clean cloth or dressing if there is risk for contamination or for full-thickness burns that may be painful when exposed to air.
- Seek immediate medical attention if needed (especially for partial- and full-thickness burns). A combination cream of hyaluronic acid and silver sulfadiazine significantly reduces the healing time of second-degree burns.

- Burned clothing or jewelry should be removed to prevent further burning of the skin.
- Do not place water on a powder. This may cause increased burning as the powder becomes a liquid.
- Do not attempt to "pop" or drain blisters. This process may cause infection to the burned area.

Do You UNDERSTAND?

DIRECTIONS: **Match the types of burns in column A with the degree(s) of burn in column B.**

Column A	Column B
1. _____ Superficial burns	a. First-degree
2. _____ Partial-thickness	b. Second-degree burns
3. _____ Full-thickness	c. Third-degree burns
	d. Fourth-degree
	e. Third- and fourth-degree

DIRECTIONS: **Indicate in the spaces provided whether the following statements are *true* or *false*.**

4. _____ All burns can be painful.
5. _____ Burns are the most common cause of fluid and electrolyte loss in toddlers.

What You NEED TO KNOW

There are several potential complications related to burn injury:

- ***Swelling.*** As related to tissue damage.
- ***Fluid and electrolyte losses.*** Burned patients can lose tremendous amounts of fluids and electrolytes when the protective layer of the skin is damaged. Hypomagnesemia, hypokalemia, and hypocalcemia are common.
- ***Kidney damage.*** If the fluids and electrolytes are not replaced, damage may occur. The kidneys' normal defense mechanism is to constrict the blood vessels when fluids and electrolytes are reduced. Prolonged constriction of these vessels can cause damage to the kidneys.

Answers: **1. a. Superficial burns are also called first-degree; 2. b. Partial-thickness burns are also called second-degree; 3. e. Full-thickness burns are also called third- and fourth-degree; 4. True. Full-thickness burns (third- and fourth-degree) often destroy nerve endings that are responsible for pain. Most of these burns, however, typically cause pain (sometimes severe) because they have first- and second-degree burns on the periphery; 5. False.**

- ***Pulmonary (lung) damage.*** Smoke inhalation or tissue damage from swallowing caustic agents, such as drain cleaner or battery acid, can damage the lungs.
- ***Infection.*** The skin is the first line of defense in the prevention of infection. Damage caused by burns can lead to infection.
- ***Pain.*** The tissue damage related to the burn can cause severe pain.
- ***Mobility problems.*** As related to contractures (shortening of the muscle) caused by damaged tissue.
- ***Circulation problems.*** As related to damaged tissue and blood vessels.

What You DO

Toddlers who receive minor burns (superficial and some partial-thickness burns) may be treated on an outpatient basis. Major burns (some partial-thickness and full-thickness burns) may require an inpatient hospitalization. Some of these children will be hospitalized for extended periods.

The treatment of burns is based on the extent of the injury. The major goals of treatment are as follows:

1. Cleaning the wound
2. Removing dead tissue **(débriding)**
3. Closing the wound or burn
4. Preventing infection
5. Managing pain
6. Preventing contractures and scars
   - Topical medications are often applied directly to the burn (as prescribed by the health care provider).
   - Skin grafts are occasionally required to close major burn wounds.
   - Physical and occupational therapy is often required to prevent contractures and scars. Many children will be required to wear splints or elasticized garments to prevent scarring and contractures.
   - Intravenous fluids and electrolytes will be needed for major burns.

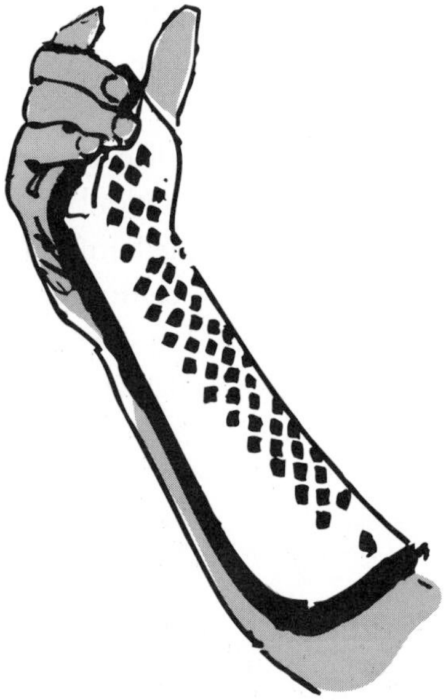

Splint.

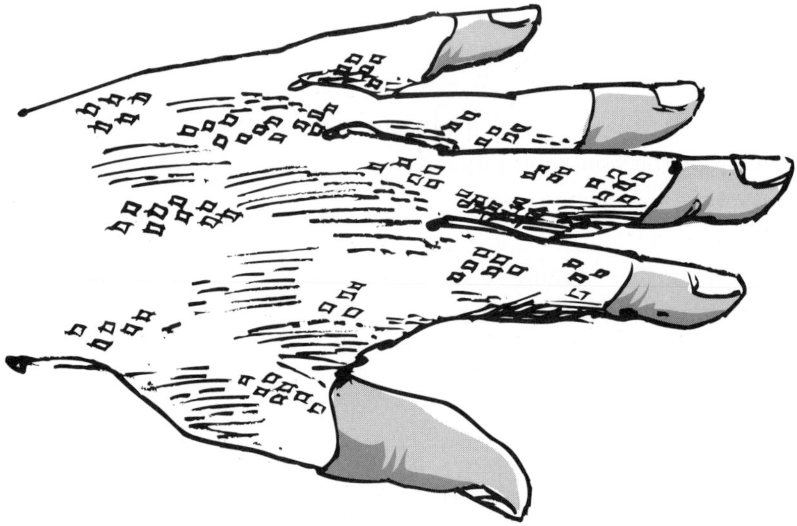

Pressure dressing.

The major long-term complication after moderate-to-severe burns is scarring. Scar tissue can cause contractures and deformity, with loss in flexibility and mobility.

Scarring should be minimized:

- Apply uniform pressure to the scarred area, which should be done under the supervision of a health care provider or therapist who is experienced in burns and wound healing. Pressure is usually applied by elastic bandages or customized bandages, based on the severity and location of the burn.
- Splints and other adaptive devices are often used to minimize contractures and to promote mobility.
- Scar tissue is often "itchy" as it heals. Medications and creams should be applied as prescribed by the health care provider to minimize scratching and further damage to the skin.

Major burns can cause a great deal of permanent scarring. Discharge planning for the burned child should include a plan for dealing with disturbances in body image. This plan will need to be modified as the child grows and reaches different levels of maturity.

TAKE HOME POINTS

Burn dressings need to be changed on a regular basis (as prescribed by the health care provider) to remove dead tissue and prevent infection. The removal of these dressings can be painful. The child should be premedicated for pain as needed.

Scarred tissue does not contain sweat glands. Care should be taken during hot weather to make sure that the child with major burns (and scarred tissue) does not get overheated (**hyperthermia**). Avoid prolonged exposure to sun and other heat sources.

Do You UNDERSTAND?

DIRECTIONS: List three of the complications that may occur in the burned patient.

1. ____

____

____

DIRECTIONS: Match the correct answer from column B in the space provided in column A.

	Column A	Column B
2.	_____ The first step in caring for the burned patient is what?	a. False
		b. True
3.	_____ When should medical care be sought?	c. Stop the burning process.

Answer: 1. swelling, pain, infection, contractures, circulation problems, kidney and lung damage, fluid and electrolyte losses; 2. c. This action prevents further damage to the skin and underlying tissues; 3. d. Medical care is especially needed if the child is having difficulty breathing or if he or she has suffered partial- or full-thickness burns.

4. _____ The second step in caring for the burned patient is what?
5. _____ All chemical burns should be washed with water. (*true* or *false*)
6. _____ All burns should be covered. (*true* or *false*)
7. _____ All blisters should be "popped" to allow the fluid to drain. (*true* or *false*)

d. As needed, especially for partial- or full-thickness burns.
e. Assess the child to make sure that he or she is breathing and has a heartbeat. Start CPR if needed.

DIRECTIONS: Indicate in the spaces provided whether the following statements are *true* or *false*.

8. _____ A long-term side effect of burns is infection.
9. _____ A long-term side effect of burns includes scarring.
10. _____ Casting is frequently applied to minimize scarring related to burns.
11. _____ Children with extensive areas of scarred tissue are at risk for hypothermia (body temperature below normal).

Answer: 4. e; 5. a. Liquid chemicals should be washed off with water. Powder chemicals should not be washed off because washing may cause further burning and damage; 6. a. Burns should be covered when there is a risk for contamination or when air movement is painful to the patient. Cover with a clean cloth when necessary; 7. a. Do not "pop" or manipulate blisters. This may increase the risk of infection; 8. False. Infection is a complication that is typically observed in the acute phase of burns; 9. True. Scarring (often permanent) is the major long-term complication related to burn injuries; 10. False. Scarring is minimized by the use of elastic bandages or garments. Casting is not used; 11. False. Hyperthermia (body temperature that is above normal) is a risk for children with major areas of scarring because scarred areas do not contain sweat glands.

DIRECTIONS: Find and circle the common causes of burns of toddlers.

C	X	V	R	S	E	M	A	L	F	B	X	C	N	E
M	H	S	X	E	Y	R	Q	Y	D	U	T	S	Y	L
L	S	E	E	V	L	N	M	A	E	L	H	X	I	E
D	J	G	M	I	Q	D	N	A	D	D	O	E	U	C
R	P	M	L	I	R	V	D	X	D	S	T	L	Q	T
K	O	K	K	S	C	E	Q	O	O	L	W	C	S	R
A	T	S	P	G	F	A	T	A	T	U	A	N	X	I
G	R	G	O	O	D	L	L	T	K	R	T	W	Q	C
N	U	M	U	U	E	S	W	Z	A	O	E	M	X	A
S	O	N	B	V	C	X	Z	A	S	B	R	D	E	L
D	X	C	I	G	A	R	E	T	T	E	B	U	R	N
L	I	E	R	T	Y	U	I	O	P	L	K	J	H	G
A	P	O	I	S	E	H	C	T	A	M	U	Y	T	R
C	Z	N	M	L	K	C	A	N	D	L	E	S	A	Q
S	X	C	B	E	S	U	B	A	D	L	I	H	C	E

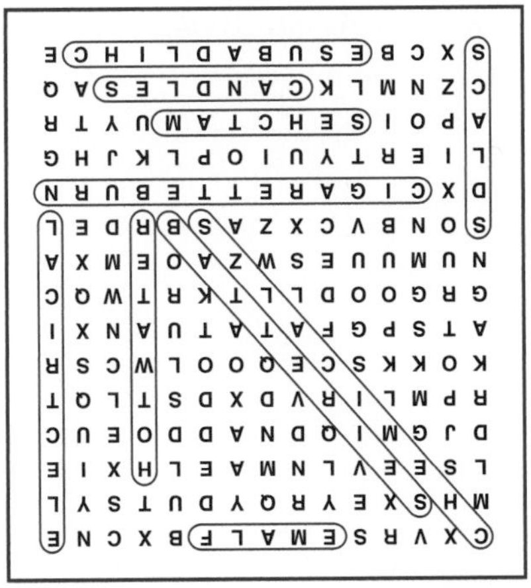

Answers: hot water; chemical; flame; electrical; candles; child abuse; cigarette burn; scalds; batteries; matches.

References

Barret JP et al: Biobrane versus 1% silver sulfadiazine in second-degree pediatric burns, *Plast Reconstr Surg* 105(1):62, 2000.

Engum SA et al: Prehospital triage in the injured pediatric patient, *J Pediatr Surg* 35(1):82, 2000.

Koller J: Topical treatment of partial thickness burns by silver sulfadiazine plus hyaluronic acid compared to silver sulfadiazine alone: a double-blind, clinical study, *Drugs Under Experimental & Clinical Research* 30(5-6):183-190, 2004.

Matsubara T et al: Ketotic hypoglycemia in patients with allergic diseases, *Pediatrics International* 45(16):653, 2003.

Mendham JE: Gabapentin for the treatment of itching produced by burns and wound healing in children: a pilot study, *Burns* 30(8):851-853, 2004.

Meyers-Paal R et al: Physical and psychologic rehabilitation outcomes for pediatric patients who suffer 80% or more TBSA, 70% or more third degree burns, *J Burn Care Rehabil* 21:43, 2000.

Rayatt SS, Grew P, Powell BW: A custom-made thermoplastic boot splint for the treatment of burns, contractures of the feet in children, *Burns* 26(1):106, 2000.

Tyack ZF, Ziviani J, Pegg S: The functional outcome of children after a burn injury: a pilot study, *J Burn Care Rehabil* 20(5):367, 1999.

Willebrand M et al: Pruritis, personality traits and coping in long-term follow-up of burn-injured patients, *Acta Dermato-Venereologica* 84(5):375-380, 2004.

NCLEX® Review

1. What cause of a fluid and electrolyte imbalance in the toddler is associated with the risk factors of vomiting and diarrhea?
   1 Gastroenteritis
   2 Kidney infection
   3 Cystic fibrosis
   4 Pulmonary disease

2. A sunburn is a common cause of which degree of burn?
   1 First degree
   2 Second degree
   3 Third degree
   4 Fourth degree

3. Which type of burn typically destroys nerve endings, thereby making the patient feel less pain?
   1 First degree
   2 Superficial
   3 Second degree
   4 Third and fourth degree

4. The first intervention of emergency treatment of a child who is burning is to:
   1 Wrap the child in a blanket or rug.
   2 Spray the child with water bursts.
   3 Remove any jewelry or metal objects from the child.
   4 Fan child to extinguish the flames.

5. Blisters on the skin of a burned patient should not be "popped" or drained because this can lead to which of the following:
   1 Kidney failure
   2 Gastroenteritis
   3 Infection
   4 Severe hypotension

6. Which vital organ is damaged when the patient swallows battery acid?
   1 Lungs
   2 Skin
   3 Heart
   4 Brain

7. Contractures and deformities after a burn are most likely a result of what?
   1 Dead tissue
   2 Scarring
   3 Loss of fluids
   4 Fever

8. To avoid hyperthermia, a child who has had burns with multiple areas of scarring should avoid which of the following?
   1 Sunbathing
   2 Bowling
   3 Video games
   4 Talking on the telephone

9. What terminology is used to identify a superficial burn?

10. What is the most common type of burn injury to the toddler in the 12- to 36-month age group?
    1 Flame
    2 Electrical
    3 Chemical
    4 Accidental scalding

11. Potential complications of burn injuries include which of the following?
    1 Swelling
    2 Fluid and electrolyte imbalance
    3 Infection
    4 All of the above

12. What is the major long-term complication after a moderate-to-severe burn?
    1 Pain
    2 Infection
    3 Scarring
    4 Bleeding

13. Signs and symptoms of first-degree (superficial) burns include:
    1 Red surface that blanches to the touch
    2 Red surface with blisters
    3 Muscle damage
    4 Serous (clear) drainage

14. Which of the following is not a cause of pain in third-degree burns?
    1 Superficial burns surrounding a third-degree burn
    2 Destruction of nerve endings
    3 Contractures
    4 Fluid and electrolyte imbalance

15. True or False: The major cause of death for toddlers is injury.

16. True or False: Urine output will increase during fever in a toddler.

17. What type of burn can occur when a toddler reaches for a pot/pan on an active stove?
    A ________ burn

18. Why should you remove burnt clothing and jewelry from a burned child?

19. What is débriding?

20. Because scarred tissue does not contain sweat glands, children with major burns need to be assessed for _____thermia.

NCLEX® Review Answers

1. 1 Gastroenteritis is associated with vomiting and diarrhea in the toddler. Kidney infection would cause pain. Cystic fibrosis has pulmonary symptoms. Pulmonary disease would cause difficulty breathing.

2. 1 Sunburn is a common cause of first-degree burns with red surfaces that blanche to the touch. Second-degree burns would have blisters. Third- and fourth-degree burns would involve deep tissue damage.

3. 4 Both third- and fourth-degree burns (full-thickness burns) destroy nerve endings. First- and second-degree burns are superficial.

4. 1 Wrapping the child in a blanket or rug will extinguish the flames and stop the burning process. After the burning process has been stopped, any metal objects should be removed. The child should not be sprayed with water because this would actually increase the burning process of chemical burns (if water is placed on a powder). Fanning a child may actually spread the fire.

5. 3 Blisters that are "popped" or drained may cause infection to the burned area. Kidney failure, gastroenteritis, and severe hypotension are not associated with blisters.

6. 1 The lungs are damaged from swallowing caustic agents such as drain cleaner or battery acid. Skin is not affected by swallowing. The heart is not directly affected. Caustic agents do not affect the brain unless they are inhaled.

7. 2 Scarring causes contractures and deformities with loss of flexibility and mobility. Dead tissue is pliable and usually débrided, adding to flexibility. Loss of fluids does not affect contractures. Fever is a symptom of infection and not related to mobility or flexibility.

8. 1 Sunbathing or any activity that would cause the child to overheat should be avoided because scar tissue contains no sweat glands. Bowling, playing video games, and talking on the telephone would be acceptable diversions for burn patients who can tolerate such activities.

9. A first-degree burn.

10. 4 Accidental scalding is the most common cause of burn injury in the toddler age group. Toddlers are curious about their surroundings and will reach for pots and other hot items on the stove.

Flame injury, electrical burns, and chemical burns are not common among toddlers but are more common in older children.

11. 4 All of the choices are potential complications of burn injuries. Swelling is caused by tissue damage. Infection occurs because the skin is the first line of defense in the prevention of infection.

12. 3 A major long-term complication following moderate-to-severe burns is scarring. Scar tissue can cause contractures and deformity, with losses in flexibility and mobility. Pain, infection, and bleeding are acute complications of burns.

13. 1 Superficial burns cause a red surface that blanches to the touch. A first-degree burn is dry without any open lesions or drainage. Blisters are common in second-degree burns. Muscle damage is common in fourth-degree burns.

14. 4 All burns can be painful. Typically, full-thickness burns (third- or fourth-degree) destroy nerve endings that sense pain. Frequently however, there are superficial (first- and second-degree) burns around the full-thickness burn that can be quite painful. Any contractures that occur from the tightening of skin around the burn are also painful.

15. True.

16. False. Urine output decreases as sweating uses up some fluid that would have otherwise been output.

17. Scalding.

18. Removal prevents further burning of the skin and underlying muscle and tissues.

19. Débriding is the surgical removal of dead tissue.

20. "Hyper" as in "hyperthermia".

Notes

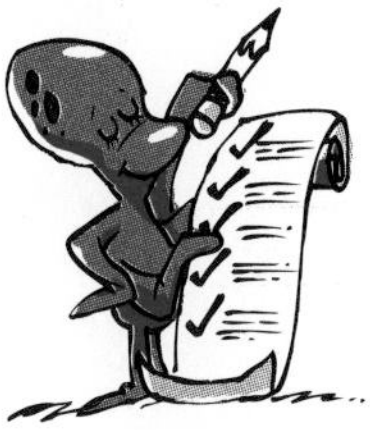

Chapter

13

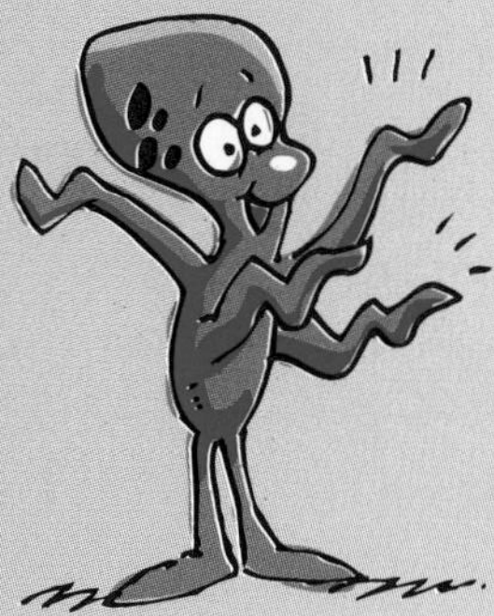

Health Care Problems of the Adolescent

What You WILL LEARN

After reading this chapter, you will know how to do the following:

- ✔ Name two potential health care conditions of adolescence.
- ✔ Define anorexia nervosa.
- ✔ Identify one fluid and two potential electrolyte imbalances in persons with anorexia nervosa.

Adolescence is the time when individuals try to achieve identity and emotional independence and prepare for the future. This can be a turbulent time of physical, emotional, and social changes, yet these changes are necessary to help the transition from childhood to young adulthood. Conditions such as scoliosis, acne, sexually transmitted diseases **(STDs)**, substance abuse, obesity, and eating disorders occur during adolescence and influence this transition.

Scoliosis, a lateral S-shaped curvature of the spine, is a common skeletal deformity. Adolescent scoliosis (the cause of which remains unknown) is the most common. Girls often develop more severe curves than boys, and therefore more girls than boys present for treatment.

During adolescence, the sebaceous glands increase their production of sebum in response to a rise in circulating androgen. It is estimated that nearly 80% of all adolescents suffer from acne. Although acne cannot be cured, it can be controlled. Aggressive intervention is necessary to quell the physical and emotional concerns the adolescent may have concerning this problem.

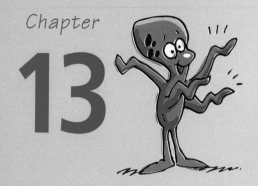

Adolescents become sexually active for various reasons. An Internet resource to recommend for patients seeking more information on becoming sexually active is called "The Safer Sex Page." Unfortunately, many adolescents do not consider the consequences of unprotected intercourse. Approximately 86% of infections and reproductive dysfunction is related to STDs in individuals between the ages of 15 and 29. STDs are responsible for complications later in life, such as pelvic inflammatory disease (PID).

Although substance abuse does not begin abruptly during adolescence, it is a daily pressure in teenage lives. Adolescents experiment with drugs and alcohol for different reasons. These reasons include, but are not limited to, depression, low self-esteem, peer pressure, and anger. Society has a significant influence on the adolescent's decisions. Health care providers must help adolescents with rational decisions about tobacco, alcohol, and other substances and provide them with information necessary to help them avoid or stop using these substances.

Adolescence is a time of accelerated growth and sexual maturation requiring additional nutrients for growth. The need for peer acceptance and concerns with bodily appearance during this time may affect food choices and intake. Approximately 15% of adolescents are obese. Obesity affects the adolescent's self-esteem and social development, which can lead to greater obesity, adult obesity, or eating disorders such as anorexia nervosa, as well as to comorbid diseases, such as hypertension and diabetes mellitus.

The goal of this chapter is to discuss fluid and electrolyte imbalances related to anorexia nervosa. Although anorexia nervosa is not the only health care concern with regard to adolescents, in its advanced stages, anorexia nervosa provides one of the most common causes of fluid and electrolyte imbalance in this age group.

Early diagnosis and intervention is important because untreated scoliosis can lead to disfigurement, impaired mobility, cardiopulmonary complications, and cerebral atrophy.

TAKE HOME POINTS

Diabetic ketoacidosis is the leading cause of morbidity and mortality in children with type 1 diabetes mellitus.

American Diabetes Association
www.diabetes.org

What IS Anorexia Nervosa?

Anorexia nervosa is a complex eating disorder defined as a preoccupation with eating, weight, and body image, during which persistent dieting to lose weight may lead to severe malnutrition. The lifetime prevalence is 0.7%. Anorexia is particularly interesting because it occurs primarily in male and female adolescents. The American Psychiatric Association (APA) characterizes anorexia nervosa as the inability to maintain a

TAKE HOME POINTS

- Individuals with anorexia nervosa use various methods to lose weight, including excessive exercise, diet pills, laxatives, and vomiting, as well as possible binging and purging.
- In bulimia nervosa, hypochloremia and hypokalemia are common electrolyte abnormalities.

CULTURE

- Anorexia nervosa affects approximately 0.6% of white female adolescents from middle and upper classes of Western culture but can also affect male adolescents (0.1% from the same type of culture).
- Debate continues over the idea that sociocultural pressure to diet is a crucial factor in the causation of anorexia nervosa occurring only in Western societies. The emphasis Western culture places on physical attractiveness leaves the impression that beauty is thin, which leads to dieting and the development of eating disorders.

minimally normal body weight and severe weight loss in the absence of physical causes. Diagnosis is based on clinical manifestations and established criteria. Anorexia nervosa has a mortality rate of 3.3% to 6% with a major risk factor being an admission body mass index (BMI) below 15 kg/m^2. There is a 22% suicide attempt rate in persons with anorexia nervosa. Persons who report previous suicide attempts have significantly lower serum cholesterol levels.

Diagnostic Criteria for Anorexia Nervosa

- Refuses to maintain body weight at or above a minimum normal weight for age and height.
- Experiences intense fear of gaining weight or becoming fat, although underweight.
- Is disturbed by the way in which body weight or shape is experienced, overvalues shape or weight, or denies the seriousness of the current low body weight.
- Postmenarcheal girls or women: Experiences an absence of at least three consecutive menstrual cycles.
- Restricting type: During an episode of anorexia nervosa, does not engage in recurrent episodes of binge eating or purging.
- Binge eating and purging type: During an episode of anorexia nervosa, engages in recurrent episodes of binge eating and then purging (bulimia nervosa).

Reprinted with permission from the American Psychiatric Association: *Diagnostic and statistical manual of mental disorders,* ed 4 (DSM-IV), text revision, Washington, DC, 2000, American Psychiatric Association.

What You NEED TO KNOW

Approximately 90% of reported cases occur in young women. Family studies have suggested a biologic vulnerability and also a family environment component that includes rigid, emotional restraint and the avoidance of conflict. Only about 50% of persons will overcome anorexia nervosa.

Young women affected with this disorder usually perform well academically, are considered to be "good children," and are perfectionists. However, they also have difficulty expressing themselves. Affected individuals will have high energy levels and be exercise dependent, despite obvious bodily emaciation. Adolescents with anorexia usually sustain only superficial relationships, and they tend to isolate themselves socially. Their families are usually achievement-oriented but may be over-controlling, rigid, lacking in communication skills, and unable to resolve conflicts.

Dieting and weight loss are usually triggered by a personal emotional event (e.g., parents' divorce, change in schools, insensitive remarks, peer pressure) or adolescent crisis (e.g., the onset of menses). The individual struggles to find his or her identity and feels ineffective, helpless, and out of control, but his or her appearance may say otherwise. Controlling food becomes a way of controlling life. The fear of fatness leads to relentless dieting and exercising, and for reasons unknown, the vital function of eating becomes diminished.

Accelerated growth during adolescence requires proper nutrition and additional calories. In general, adolescent diets are deficient in vitamins and minerals. Poor nutrition can retard growth and delay sexual maturation. In the wake of severe weight loss, physical signs of nutritional compromise appear. Those with anorexia have low serum leptin levels and develop bradycardia, low blood pressure (**hypotension**), hypothermia, and lack menstruation cycles (**amenorrhea**). They have dry skin and brittle nails and develop fine hair covering the body (**lanugo**). These changes are usually reversible with improved nutritional status and adequate weight gain. Left untreated, anorexia can progress to serious fluid and electrolyte imbalances (especially hypophosphatemia), which lead to hypotension and cardiac dysrhythmias. Bone loss, osteoporosis, and renal disease are particular comorbidities that can occur.

Laboratory Data

Urinalysis	Ketones—small, secondary to metabolic demands Protein—small, caused by renal (glomerular) damage Specific gravity—low, caused by renal concentrating defect
Vitamin deficiencies	Rare, because diet usually contains leafy vegetables and fruits
Hemoglobin level, platelet count, albumin, total protein, minerals	Usually within normal limits
White blood cell count	Normal in less malnourished individuals

Continued

TAKE HOME POINTS

High-risk factors in anorexia include having the AA genotype, being a female adolescent of Western culture, having low self-esteem, communicating difficulties, having a family history of affective or eating disorders, having anxiety or obsessive-compulsive disorder, being an older adolescent who chooses a career that requires a lower body weight, and possible sexual or substance abuse. Anorexia nervosa is prevalent across all age groups; it is not uncommon in men and women in their late 20s and 30s.

Anorexia can usually be treated on an outpatient basis with nonspecific supportive therapy shown to be superior to interpersonal psychotherapy. However, in severe cases of malnutrition, cardiac dysrhythmias, or fluid and electrolyte abnormalities, hospitalization is often necessary to prevent physical deterioration. Psychiatric disturbances (suicidal ideation) are also an indication requiring hospitalization.

TAKE HOME POINTS

Anorexia nervosa is multifactorial and psychologic in origin. Depression and suicide can be associated with anorexia. Anorexic individuals may develop bizarre food rituals and may weigh themselves several times a day.

Laboratory Data—cont'd

Hematocrit	Low in severely emaciated individuals, indicating starvation's effect on immunity and anemia
Electrolytes	Abnormal, with dehydration, vomiting, and laxative abuse
Blood urea nitrogen	Can be elevated, secondary to dehydration
Creatinine levels	Usually normal; high in renal failure
LH, FSH, estrogen, testosterone, thyroid hormone	Low, secondary to hypothalamic suppression
Serum hepatic	Mild elevation, caused by fatty degeneration transaminase levels of the liver

FSH, Follicle-stimulating hormone; *LH*, luteinizing hormone.

What You DO

Once all medical crises have resolved, the patient can begin therapeutic management. The damaged self-image and low self-esteem are underlying problems to address in addition to proper nutritional requirements. Management of anorexia nervosa is geared toward the following:

- Increasing body weight
- Correcting malnutrition
- Establishing appropriate eating behaviors
- Increasing self-esteem
- Correcting family disturbances

Eating disorders require long-term, multidisciplinary treatment. The prognosis is best when anorexia is diagnosed early. Approximately 25% of affected individuals will fully recover; 50% will improve but will have a relapse that usually occurs during a time of stress.

The remaining 25% will do poorly despite treatment. Up to 20% of patients have died from complications associated with anorexia nervosa. Research shows that laboratory findings of low serum albumin and high serum creatinine levels are predictors of a chronic or fatal course. Women with past or current eating disorders also deliver infants with low birth weight.

Early recognition of symptoms and restoration of nutritional compromise are crucial for a successful outcome.

Early and Late Symptoms of Anorexia Nervosa

Early Symptoms	Late Symptoms
Significant weight loss	Amenorrhea, muscle wasting
Compulsive activity, exercise, and dieting	Electrolyte imbalances
Low self-esteem	Cardiac dysrhythmias
Preoccupation with food	Hypotension, bradycardia
Rigid calorie counting	Hypothermia, lanugo
Persistent body weight dissatisfaction	Brittle nails, dry skin
Wears loose-fitting clothes to hide weight loss	Loss of hair, facial puffiness

- Discuss the problem with the patient and prepare for referral.
- Determine which family members or friends are part of the support system for the patient.
- Refer all patients suspected of having anorexia nervosa to a specialist familiar with the disorder.
- Obtain health history, laboratory testing, and a physical examination.
- Determine the onset of dieting and what prompted it.
- Ask the individual how he or she perceives appearance.
- Obtain daily vital signs and daily weights and document hourly intake and output.
- Administer treatment: bed rest, hospitalization for intravenous infusion (fluids, electrolytes, vitamins, total parenteral nutrition, and hyperalimentation), oral or tube feedings, psychotherapy, behavior modification, family therapy, and pharmacotherapy.
- Monitor for potential complications, such as electrolyte imbalances (especially hypokalemia; see Chapter 5), kidney failure, heart failure, or coma. For electrolyte imbalances, monitor serum sodium, potassium, and calcium levels. (See Chapters 3, 5, and 8 to review how to treat imbalances of these electrolytes.)
- Monitor the following for possible kidney and heart failure: signs of fluid overload (congestive heart failure, pulmonary edema, hypertension, peripheral edema, and distended neck veins), respirations, low specific gravity of urine, urine output below 400 mL/24 hours or less than 30 mL/hr, level of consciousness, hyperkalemia, hyponatremia, elevated creatinine and blood urea nitrogen, and metabolic acidosis.

TAKE HOME POINTS

Individuals who improve usually nevertheless retain an altered body image. Many continue to see themselves as fat.

Monitor these serum lab tests in anorexia:

- Potassium for hypokalemia/hyperkalemia
- Creatinine for kidney failure
- Sodium for hyponatremia
- Calcium for hypocalcemia

Healthy Weight
www.healthyweight.com

- Monitor for coma or unconsciousness, including the following: level of consciousness, pupils, ocular movements, respirations, motor responses, and reflexes.
- Do not allow manipulative behavior. Formulate a treatment plan on which the hospital staff and patient can agree. Rules must be consistent from one staff member to another.
- Remain with the patient when he or she is eating and at least 30 minutes afterwards to monitor for vomiting. Also, monitor when the patient eats with others.
- Do not accept excuses by the patient to leave the eating area (patient may vomit).
- Set limits on the amount the patient must eat. Reward the patient when he or she adheres to the plan.

Do You UNDERSTAND?

DIRECTIONS: **Indicate in the spaces provided whether the following statements are *true* or *false*.**

1. _____ Risk behaviors for anorexia are high self-esteem and healthy family communication.
2. _____ Anorexia occurs primarily among female adolescents in Western societies.
3. _____ A characteristic of anorexic individuals is low academic achievement.
4. _____ Complications of anorexia include cardiac dysrhythmias and hypotension.
5. _____ The best prognosis for a person with anorexia includes early diagnosis and referral to a professional who deals with the problem of anorexia nervosa.

Answers: 1. False. Individuals usually have low self-esteem, their families lack communication skills, and they are unable to resolve conflicts; 2. False. Although anorexia nervosa affects men, it occurs primarily among women; 3. False. Anorexic individuals usually have high academic grades and are often labeled as perfectionists; 4. True. Cardiac dysrhythmias and hypotension are secondary to fluid and electrolyte imbalances and dehydration; 5. True. Similar to all health care problems, early diagnosis is the key. Early diagnosis leads to early intervention and helps to prevent complications.

DIRECTIONS: Unscramble the italicized words.

6. A risk behavior for anorexia is __________ ______________ *(owl lsfe-etemse)*
7. An early sign of anorexia is __________ __________ __________. *(revees itehwg slos)*
8. Electrolyte disturbances can lead to __________ __________. *(ricadca tsayirdmysh)*
9. A long-term result of inadequate calcium is __________________. *(retosiosopo)*
10. An eating disorder characterized by an extreme loss of weight is __________________ __________________. *(xroainae raesnov)*

TAKE HOME POINTS

Remember, the patient is not the only one affected by his or her disorder. Recovery is a long process that includes the patient's family and close friends.

References

Favaro A et al: Total serum cholesterol and suicidality in anorexia nervosa, *Psychosom Med* 66(4):548-552, 2004.

Franko DL et al: What predicts suicide attempts in women with eating disorders? *Psychol Med* 34(5):843-853, 2004.

Haas V et al: Leptin and body weight regulation in patients with anorexia nervosa before and during weight recovery, *Am J Clin Nutr* 81(4):889-896, 2005.

Kjelsas E, Bjornstrom C, Gotestam KG: Prevalence of eating disorders in female and male adolescents (14-15 years), *Eat Behav* 5(1):13-25, 2004.

Kouba S et al: Pregnancy and neonatal outcomes in women with eating disorders, *Obstet Gynecol* 105(2):255-260, 2005.

McIntosh VV et al: Three psychotherapies for anorexia nervosa: a randomized, controlled trial, *Am J Psychiatry* 162(4):74-77, 2005.

Pinter O et al: The predictive value of body mass index for the weight evolution in anorexia nervosa, *Eat Weight Disord* 9(3):232-235, 2004.

Answers: **6. low self-esteem; 7. severe weight loss; 8. cardiac dysrhythmias; 9. osteoporosis; 10. anorexia nervosa.**

Notes

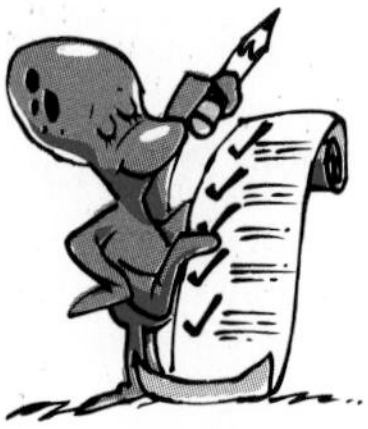

NCLEX® Review

Susan, 15 years of age, is admitted with anorexia nervosa. She is 5'6" in height, weighs 90 pounds, and appears cachectic (malnourished and wasting). Her mother reports that Susan is obsessed with her weight, exercises several hours each day, and eats little. Her mother also states that Susan is a model child and earns As in school. On several occasions, Susan has induced vomiting after having been pressured to eat. Her lab reports indicate serious electrolyte imbalances.

1. Which inference about the patient can the nurse make based on this profile?
1 She is overanxious.
2 She is catatonic.
3 She has an eating disorder.
4 She is health conscious.

2. The health care provider recognizes that the primary benefit the patient achieves from anorexia nervosa is what?
1 Separation from parent via hospitalization
2 Reduction of anxiety via control over food
3 Release from doing homework during her illness
4 Loss of weight

3. Initial treatment of this individual would most likely be which of the following?
1 Family psychotherapy sessions
2 Correcting electrolyte imbalances
3 Medication to treat depression
4 Setting limits on the amount of food she must eat

4. At this time, decisions about her treatment are best made by whom?
1 Patient
2 Patient and family
3 Patient and the dietitian
4 Staff

5. A nursing assessment of a female adolescent with anorexia nervosa would be positive for which physical characteristic?
1 Secondary amenorrhea
2 Moist, supple skin
3 Tachycardia
4 Heat intolerance

6. Untreated scoliosis can lead to complications of which vital organ(s)?
1 Heart
2 Brain
3 Kidneys
4 Adrenal glands

7. During adolescence, the sebaceous glands increase their production of sebum in response to a rise in circulatory androgens. The result of this is what?
1 Scoliosis
2 Substance abuse
3 Acne
4 Pregnancy

8. Research indicates that two laboratory findings are predictors of a chronic or fatal course for individuals with anorexia. What are these two laboratory findings?
1 Low hemoglobin and low white blood cells
2 Low albumin and high creatinine
3 High sodium and low potassium
4 High red blood cells and low BUN level

9. Which of the following is a "late" symptom of a person with anorexia nervosa?
1 Low self-esteem
2 Rigid calorie counting
3 Compulsive exercising
4 Hypotension

10. Pelvic inflammatory disease in a 30-year-old woman may be a result of which past disease?

11. Obesity is a factor that can lead to the development of _________ nervosa, _________ tension, and _________ mellitus.

12. True or False: One sign/symptom of anorexia nervosa is amenorrhea.

13. Name two laboratory tests (one blood test and one urine test) that would indicate renal failure and state if you would expect their values to be increased or decreased in patient's with anorexia nervosa.

14. True or False: Cardiac dysrhythmias are an early sign of anorexia nervosa.

15. Signs of fluid overload from heart or kidney failure due to anorexia nervosa include pulmonary _________, _________ tension, peripheral _________, and _________ neck veins.

NCLEX® Review Answers

1. 3 Patients with eating disorders usually present as female overachievers or "good" children who are obsessed with their weight. An overanxious patient would worry excessively about life events. A catatonic patient is characterized by a lack of movement or activity. A health-conscious person would neither starve himself or herself nor lose such excessive weight.

2. 2 The adolescent demonstrates a mastery over her food intake. Families are usually fused (unable to separate emotionally); separation from parents would not be a desirable gain. Those with anorexia generally excel in academic areas and receive attention and praise; they would not benefit from having this source of attention removed. Severe weight loss and nutritional compromise would not be a benefit.

3. 2 Electrolyte imbalances can be life threatening. Family psychotherapy sessions would be a later therapy. It is more important to treat electrolyte imbalances than to use medication to treat depression. Limits on the amount of food she must consume will be set at a later time. It is most important to treat electrolyte imbalances.

4. 4 At this point, only the staff members have the knowledge to make sound decisions about the patient's treatment. The patient will be involved later. In this late stage of anorexia, the patient is incapable of making sound decisions about treatment, but in the future should be given choices and be involved in the plan of care. The patient with serious electrolyte imbalances requires medical treatment to correct imbalances. The patient does not have the knowledge base to make sound decisions.

5. 1 Secondary amenorrhea is a result of endocrine imbalance, which is possibly a result of damage of the hypothalamus. Someone with anorexia has dry, cracked skin, bradycardia, and cold intolerance.

6. 1 Cardiopulmonary complications can result from untreated scoliosis. The brain, kidneys, and adrenal glands are not affected by curvature of the spine.

7. 3 Acne results from an increase in sebum production. Pregnancy is the result of sexual activity. Scoliosis is a function of heredity. Substance abuse is caused by many factors, both environmental and hereditary, but not by any bodily function.

8. 2 Low protein and high creatinine levels related to renal failure are predictors of death from anorexia. Low albumin and high creatinine are associated with hematology problems and not renal problems. High sodium and low potassium are electrolyte problems that are easily corrected. A high red blood cell count is associated with recent blood transfusion. Low BUN is associated with a low-protein diet.

9. 4 Amenorrhea, cardiac arrhythmias, hypotension, and brittle nails are late symptoms of anorexia nervosa. Low self-esteem, rigid calorie counting, and compulsive exercising are behaviors of an anorexic.

10. She had contracted a sexually transmitted disease as an adolescent.

11. anorexia, hyper (hypertension), diabetes.

12. True.

13. Increased serum blood urea nitrogen or serum creatinine and a decrease in urine specific gravity.

14. False, cardiac dysrhythmias are a late sign.

15. edema, hyper (hypertension), edema, distended.

Health Care Problems of the Young Adult

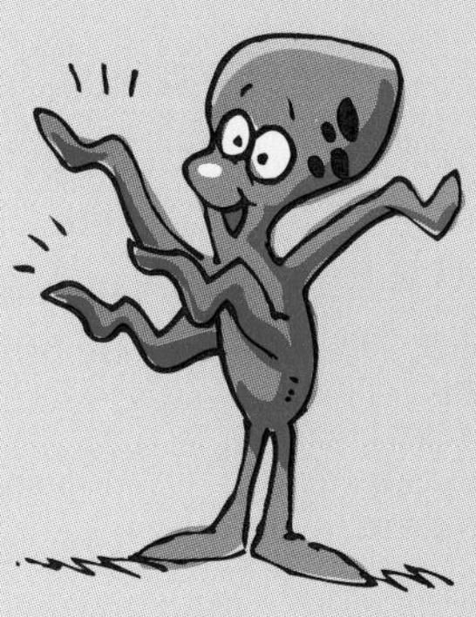

Chapter 14

What You WILL LEARN

After reading this chapter, you will know how to do the following:

- ✔ Define diabetes mellitus.
- ✔ Differentiate the signs and symptoms of hyperglycemia from hypoglycemia.
- ✔ Relate the signs/symptoms of hyperglycemia/hypoglycemia to potential fluid and/or electrolyte imbalances.

In this chapter, three representative disorders affecting fluid and electrolyte balance in the young adult are examined:

- Diabetes mellitus
- Acute renal failure (ARF)
- Crohn's disease

Although these conditions can occur in all age groups, they are common in young adults (18 to 30 years of age). Here are some important facts:

- Type 1, insulin-dependent diabetes mellitus (IDDM) is more common in the young patient than the older patient.
- Type 2, non–insulin-dependent diabetes mellitus (NIDDM) occurs in approximately 90% to 95% of all patients with diabetes but is commonly associated with advancing age. However, with the increase of obesity coupled with inactivity, NIDDM occurrence is rapidly increasing in the young adult.
- Two thirds of patients presenting with hyperglycemic, hyperosmolar, nonketotic syndrome (HHNKS) have not been diagnosed with NIDDM.

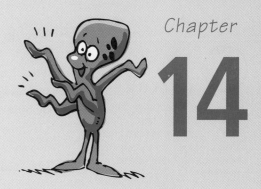

CULTURE

Blacks and American Indians develop diabetes, nephropathy, and renal failure at rates higher than average. Scientists have not been able to explain these higher rates.

- Between 1990 and 1998, diabetes in people aged 30 to 39 increased 70%.
- The chances of suffering from the major complications of diabetes, such as kidney disease, blindness, and nerve damage, can be decreased by 50% to 80% if the disease is controlled early.
- Of those admitted to a general medical-surgical ward in the hospital, 4% to 5% will develop ARF.
- One quarter to one third of patients with Crohn's disease are diagnosed before the age of 20.

What IS Diabetes Mellitus?

American Diabetes Association
www.diabetes.org
CDC—Diabetes Home Page
www.cdc.gov/diabetes

There are two types of *diabetes mellitus.* Type 1, IDDM, is a complex disorder that results from the autoimmune destruction of pancreatic beta cells, causing a partial to an absolute lack of insulin production. Type 2, NIDDM, is generally characterized by peripheral insulin resistance and relative insulin deficiency that may range from predominant insulin secretory defect to insulin resistance. Resistance to the action of insulin takes the form of a decrease in the ability of skeletal muscle to store and use (**oxidize**) glucose, which leads to an increased amount of glucose in the blood (**hyperglycemia**).

What You NEED TO KNOW

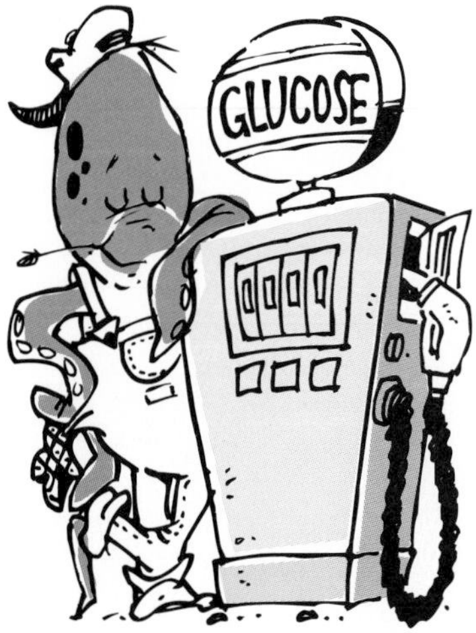

Glucose is the only fuel that the central nervous system can use for energy.

The lack of the necessary amount of insulin causes an elevation of glucose in the blood (hyperglycemia). Without insulin, glucose is unable to enter the cell. Although glucose is present in the blood stream, glucose cannot enter the cell and be used, causing the cells to be "starving for glucose." Glucose is the only fuel that the central nervous system can use for energy. The body responds to starvation by increasing production of glucose from fats and proteins in the liver. This process leads to an accumulation of acids (**ketones**) in the blood, causing metabolic acidosis. The presence of ketoacidosis decreases the brain's ability to oxidize glucose. Blood levels of glucose and ketones continue to rise. With the rise of glucose blood levels, water shifts into the extracellular fluid (ECF). This increase of water and glucose in the plasma causes urine output to increase dramatically in both volume and frequency (**polyuria**). Eventually, polyuria leads to a fluid volume deficit (FVD). With the dehydration, the blood pressure drops, and urine output eventually stops (**anuria**).

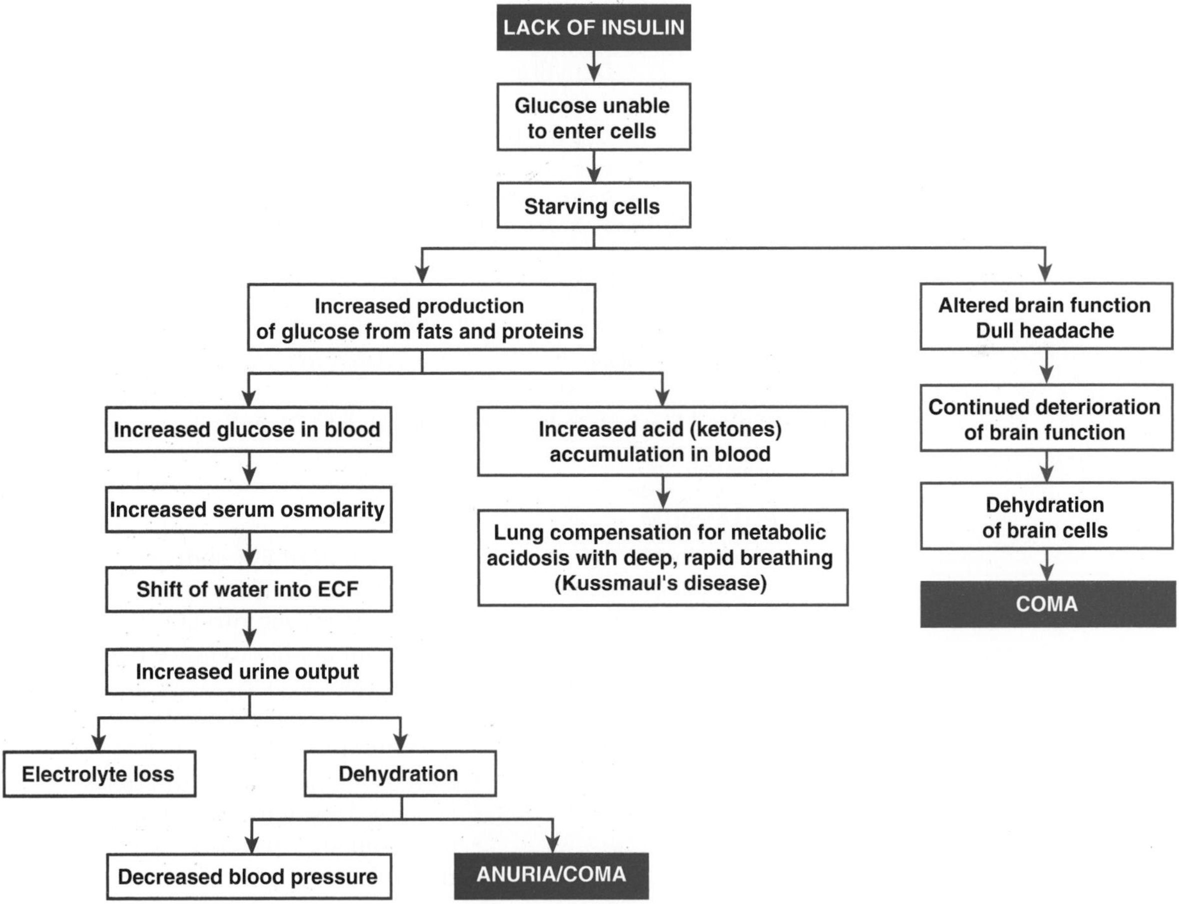

Physiologic responses to lack of insulin

Diabetic ketoacidosis (DKA) is caused by a profound insulin deficiency. DKA is a metabolic disorder consisting of severe hyperglycemia, elevated ketone bodies, metabolic acidosis, profound dehydration, and electrolyte imbalance (see box on page 238). DKA accounts for 14% of all hospital admissions of patients with diabetes and 16% of all diabetes-related fatalities. In children younger than 10 years of age, DKA causes 70% of diabetes-related fatalities. In pregnant patients the fetal mortality rate is as high as 30% and as high as 60% when coma is present.

Precipitating Factors of Diabetic Ketoacidosis in Types 1 and 2 Diabetes

Type	Precipitating Factors
Type 1	• Acute infection (50%-60%) • Failure to take prescribed insulin (20%-30%) • Emotional stress • Trauma • Excessive carbohydrate
Type 2	• Dehydration • Infection • Use of steroids and diuretics • Calcium channel blockers • Pancreatitis

The ketoacidosis and hyperglycemia associated with DKA lead to numerous fluids and electrolyte imbalances. The most serious electrolyte imbalance associated with DKA is related to potassium.

Fluid and Electrolyte Imbalances Related to Diabetic Ketoacidosis

Imbalance	Probable Causes
POTASSIUM Serum levels: low, normal, or elevated Total body stores: lower level	Early: • Osmotic pull of ECF shifts out of ICF • Acidosis moves hydrogen into ICF; potassium moves into ECF • Potassium unable to move back into cell without insulin • Loss in urine caused by osmotic pull of glucosuria • Lack of intake because of anorexia • Increased loss with vomiting • Increased aldosterone secretion with the FVD
HYPERKALEMIA	Late: • FVD • Low or absent output • Continued shift of potassium into ECF • Continued release of potassium from tissue breakdown
HYPONATREMIA Total body store: normal early Total body store: low late	• Osmotic pull of ECF shifts water into plasma for dilution • Shift from ECF into the ICF secondary to loss of potassium • Loss in urine during the polyuria • Loss with vomiting

Continued

Fluid and Electrolyte Imbalances Related to Diabetic Ketoacidosis—cont'd

Imbalance	Probable Causes
HYPOPHOSPHATEMIA	• Loss in urine with attempts to buffer acid • When insulin is administered during treatment, it moves from the ECF to the ICF with insulin, glucose, and potassium
HYPERGLYCEMIA	• Glucose cannot enter cells
GLUCOSURIA	• Glucose level exceeds renal threshold; it spills into the urine

ECF, Extracellular fluid; *FVD*, fluid volume deficit; *ICF*, intracellular fluid.

HHNKS consists of severe hyperglycemia, absence of ketosis, profound dehydration, and neurologic changes. With HHNKS, there is enough insulin produced to prevent ketosis but not enough to prevent hyperglycemia.

This condition causes more severe hyperosmolality, which leads to more profound osmotic diuresing (15% to 25% of body fluid), profound dehydration, and low renal perfusion, which causes increased hyperosmolality.

1. Although DKA can occur with either type of diabetes, HHNKS occurs primarily with Type 2.
2. With HHNKS, the blood sugar tends to be higher than with DKA.
3. Electrolyte loss in HHNKS is similar to the loss in DKA.
4. With DKA, serum potassium levels can be low, normal, or elevated, although the total body store is depleted.
5. Hyperglycemia + ketosis = DKA
6. Hyperglycemia without significant ketosis = HHNKS
7. Hyperglycemia, dehydration, and hyperosmolality are more severe with HHNKS than with DKA.
8. Altered central nervous system function is common with HHNKS.
9. Cerebral edema primarily affects children and is the leading cause of DKA mortality in children (1% of children with DKA, with a mortality rate of 21%).

Signs and Symptoms of Hyperglycemia and Hypoglycemia

Hyperglycemia	Hypoglycemia
Dull headache	Dull headache
Hot skin	Cold, pale, clammy skin
Dry skin	Sweating
Reduced responsiveness or unresponsive	Nervousness, trembling, mental confusion
Fast, weak, thready pulse	Pounding pulse
Postural hypotension	Normal blood pressure

Hyperglycemia: Signs and Symptoms and Probable Causes

Signs and Symptoms	Probable Causes
Glucosuria—classic early sign	Serum glucose elevated about kidney's threshold and is spilled into the urine
Polyuria	Osmotic diuretic effect of hyperglycemia
Large volume and increased frequency	
Excessive thirst **(polydipsia)** classic early sign	Dehydration
Excessive hunger **(polyphagia)** classic sign	Cells are not able to use glucose, which stimulates starvation response

Diabetic Ketoacidosis: Signs and Symptoms and Probable Causes

Signs and Symptoms	Probable Causes
Ketonuria	Ketones buffered by serum bicarbonate and excreted in urine
Rapid deep respiration (Kussmaul's sign), classic symptom	Increase elimination of serum carbon dioxide to raise blood oxygen
Dull headache, early sign	Metabolic acidosis
Fatigue, muscle weakness	Inability to use glucose, loss of potassium
Dry, hot skin and/or dry mucous membranes	Dehydration
Nausea and vomiting with abdominal pain	Electrolyte imbalance and metabolic acidosis Nausea and vomiting occur first (with other diseases, abdominal pain occurs first, followed by nausea and vomiting)

Continued

Diabetic Ketoacidosis: Signs and Symptoms and Probable Causes—cont'd

Signs and Symptoms	Probable Causes
	Symptoms subside 6-8 hr after treatment
Fruity smelling breath classic symptom	Lungs blowing off acetone
Cherry red skin	Vasodilation secondary to ketosis
Mucous membranes	
Sunken soft eye balls	Dehydration
Fast, weak, thready pulse rate	FVD
BP < 10 mm Hg when sitting versus lying position **(postural hypotension)**	FVD
Low urine output **(oliguria)**	FVD
No urine output **(anuria)** late symptom	
Coma	Dehydration of brain cells

BP, Blood pressure; *FVD*, fluid volume deficit.

- Diabetic complications from hyperglycemia can be life threatening with both types of diabetes.
- DKA is the most serious diabetic emergency.

TAKE HOME POINTS

- Although DKA can occur with either type of diabetes, HHNKS occurs primarily with Type 2.
- If Type 2 diabetes remains uncontrolled for a long period of time, more serious symptoms may result. These include severe hyperglycemia (blood sugar over 600 mg), lethargy, confusion, shock, and, ultimately, what doctors call "hyperosmolar hyperglycemic nonketotic coma"

Signs and Symptoms of Diabetes Mellitus

DKA occurs with the passage of time—hours, even days. HHNKS occurs over several days—even weeks. Approximately 80% of DKA occurs with patients who are not newly diagnosed.

Hyperglycemia, dehydration, and hyperosmolality are more severe with HHNKS than with DKA.

Laboratory Values of DKA and HHNKS Compared with Normal Values

	DKA	HHNKS	Normal
Serum	> 250 glucose	High > 800	Fasting 70-100 mg/dL
Osmolality	Variable	> 350 mOsm/L	280-295 mOsm/L
Bicarbonate	< 15 mEq/L	> 20 mEq/L	222-226 mEq/L
pH	< 7.30-7.35	> 7.4	7.35-7.45
Anion gap	Elevated	Normal	12-15 mEq/L
BUN	> 20 mg/dL	60-90 mg/dL	5-20 mg/dL
Creatinine	> 1.5	Elevated	0.7-1.5 mg/dL
Serum sodium	< 137 mEq/L	Usually elevated	136-145 mEq/L
Serum potassium	Low, normal or elevated	Normal or low	3.5-5.0 mEq/L
Urine ketones	Positive	Negative	Negative

DKA, Diabetic ketoacidosis; *HHNKS*, hyperglycemic, hyperosmolar, nonketotic syndrome.

TAKE HOME POINTS

With patients who do not know they have diabetes mellitus, it is extremely important for the health care provider to be able to differentiate between signs of hyperglycemia and hypoglycemia (too little insulin).

TAKE HOME POINTS

- Frequent urination (**polyuria**), excessive thirst (polydipsia), and excessive hunger (polyphagia) are the classic symptoms of hyperglycemia.
- Nausea and vomiting followed by abdominal pain and Kussmaul's respirations are symptoms associated with DKA.
- The classic HHNKS symptom is dehydration.
- Seizures and even reversible hemiparesis can occur with HHNKS.

TAKE HOME POINTS

With HHNKS, the primary treatment is hydration. The fluid of choice in the absence of hypovolemic shock is 0.45% NaCl. Other treatments are similar to the one for DKA.

The classic symptoms of HHNKS are associated with dehydration. It is impossible to develop HHNKS when adequate hydration is maintained. Unlike in DKA, with HHNKS, altered central nervous system function can include generalized focal seizures and even reversible hemiparesis resulting from the severe dehydration and hyperosmolality. Unlike in DKA, nausea, vomiting, and Kussmaul's respirations are absent with HHNKS.

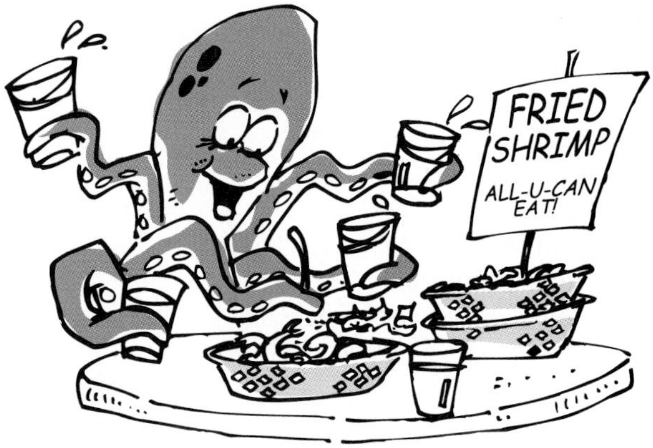

Frequent urination, excessive thirst, and excessive hunger are classic symptoms of hyperglycemia.

What You DO

Treatment is dependent on the response of the patient with DKA. DKA is commonly reversed in 10 to 16 hours. The goals of treatment are to improve hypovolemia and tissue perfusion, decrease serum glucose, correct electrolyte imbalances, and steadily reverse metabolic acidosis.

Improving Hypovolemia and Tissue Perfusion

- **Phase 1: Short phase of rapid rehydration (over 0-2 hours).** Intravenous (IV) solution (0.9% saline) is administered to replenish ECF and ICF, improve blood pressure, stabilize the pulse, and improve urinary output.
- **Phase 2: Slow rehydration.** As hydration improves, blood glucose levels are lowered (below 250 mg/dL), the blood pressure is stabilized and urine output is restored, the IV solution is changed to 0.45% saline, and infusion should continue until 48 hours after admission.

Decreasing Serum Glucose

Insulin is needed to improve the movement of glucose into cells and eliminate the production of glucose from fat. Current research has found that hourly or semi-hourly subcutaneous administration of ultrashort acting insulins (insulin aspart [NovoLog], insulin lispro [Humalog]) have the same effect in treating DKA as administering regular insulin intravenously (the only insulin that may be administered IV). They start to work about 15 minutes after being injected, peak after 1 hour, and last for 3 to 5 hours.

Correcting Electrolyte Imbalances

The serum potassium level needs to be checked every 1 to 2 hours during initial treatment. Glucose and other electrolyte levels should be checked every 2 hours during initial rapid rehydration. If the initial phosphorus level is low, it should be monitored every 4 hours during therapy. Potassium is added (20-40 mEq) to each liter of fluid once serum potassium is below 5.5 mEq/L.

TAKE HOME POINTS

Children: Be alert to headache and altered mental status (e.g., decreased alertness) since these are signs of impending cerebral edema.

Nursing Responsibilities

Nursing responsibilities in the treatment of hyperglycemia include the following:

- **Administer insulin as prescribed.**

Types of Insulin

Type	Route of Administration	Onset	Peak	Duration
lispro (Humalog)	SC	< 15 min	30-60 min	3-4 hr
aspart (NovoLog)	SC	< 15 min	30-60 min	3-4 hr
regular	SC	30-60 min	2-4 hr	5-7 hr
	IV	10-30 min	15-30 min	30-60 min
NPH	SC	1-4 hr	6-12 hr	18-24 hr
Lente	SC	1-2 hr	8-12 hr	18-28 hr
Ultra Lente	SC	4-6 hr	16-24 hr	36 hr
Lantus	SC	1.5 hr	Maintains consistent level	Up to 24 hr
NPH 70/regular 30	SC	30 min	4-8 hr	Up to 24 hr

SC, Subcutaneous; *IV,* intravenous.

- **Maintain patent IV access.**
- **Assess the patient's response to treatment.**
  1. Vital signs: apical pulse, blood pressure (BP) (lying and standing), and respirations (depth and rate)
  2. Skin color and degree of moisture
  3. Intake and output (patient may require a Foley catheter)
  4. Weight (compare with normal weight before admission)

TAKE HOME POINTS

- Rehydration is critical in reversing DKA.
- BP and urine output are key indicators of fluid volume assessment.
- Insulin replacement is necessary for glucose to enter cells.
- Frequent physical assessments and monitoring of laboratory values are important throughout the treatment of DKA.
- Teaching the patient helps prevent DKA.
- More deaths occur from hypokalemia (result of rapid movement of potassium into the ICF with insulin and glucose) than from hyperkalemia.

5. Laboratory results and electrocardiogram (ECG)
6. Deep tendon reflexes
7. Level of consciousness

- **Promote patient safety (e.g., all bed side rails in up position).**
- **Know drug interactions.**
  1. Concurrent ACE inhibitors may elevate serum potassium concentrations.
  2. Potassium-sparing diuretics and potassium-containing salt substitutes can produce severe hyperkalemia.
  3. In patients taking digoxin, hypokalemia may result in digoxin toxicity.
  4. Use caution if discontinuing potassium administration in patients maintained on digoxin.
- **Instruct the patient and family on the following:**
  1. The signs and symptoms of DKA and HHNKS
  2. Activities that alter insulin requirements
  3. The importance of seeking medical attention early when symptoms begin to appear
  4. The importance of proper hydration

Do You UNDERSTAND?

DIRECTIONS: **Match the symptom in column A with the probable cause in column B. Although some of the symptoms have more than one cause, choose the most appropriate.**

Column A	Column B
1. _____ Polyuria	a. Dehydration
2. _____ Polydipsia	b. Osmotic diuretic effect of hyperglycemia
3. _____ Ketonuria	c. Fat metabolism
4. _____ Polyphagia	d. Serum level elevated above renal threshold followed by abdominal pain
5. _____ Glucosuria	e. Brain cells lack glucose
6. _____ Nausea and vomiting	f. Cells starving for glucose
7. _____ Reduced responsiveness	g. Metabolic acidosis

Answers: 1. b; 2. a; 3. c; 4. f; 5. d; 6. g; 7. e.

DIRECTIONS: Fill in the squares to form a word that is the missing link to connect the given words.

8.

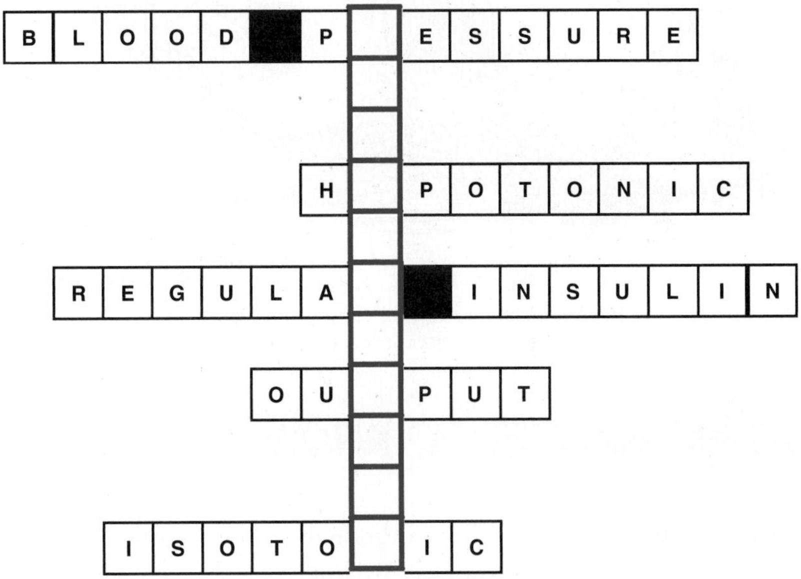

DIRECTIONS: Unscramble the following nursing measures and symptoms indicated for patients with DKA.

9. ______________________ *(niure toutup)*
10. ______________________ *(dolob srepruse)*
11. ______________________ *(cipala spule)*
12. ______________________ *(peed denton flreesex)*

What IS Acute Renal Failure?

Acute renal failure (ARF) is a generic term used to define the abrupt onset of decreased renal function and the retention of nitrogen waste products in the body (**uremia** or **azotemia**). Many forms of ARF are reversible when the cause is identified and treated. If it is not reversible, kidney function fails to return, resulting in chronic renal failure. The mortality rate with ARF is 50% and higher in patients who require hemodialysis.

Answers: **8. rehydration; 9. urine output; 10. blood pressure; 11. apical pulse; 12. deep tendon reflexes.**

National Kidney Foundation
www.kidney.org

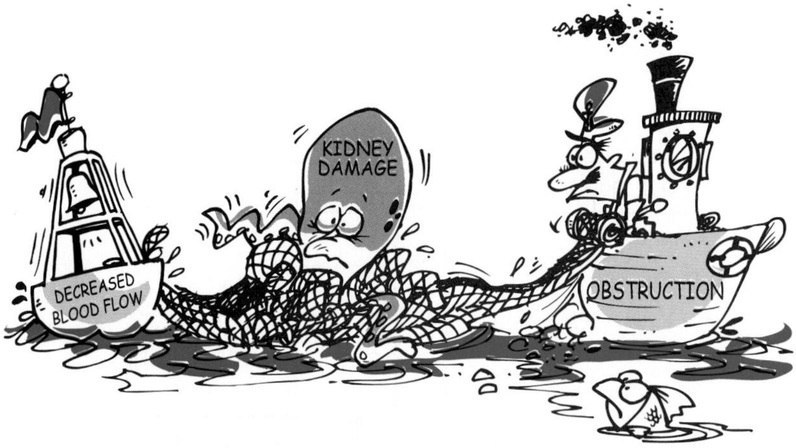

The two main culprits that cause kidney damage are a decreased blood flow and obstruction.

What You NEED TO KNOW

ARF is grouped into three main categories based on the cause: prerenal ARF, intrarenal ARF, and postrenal ARF.

Prerenal ARF occurs when there is a decreased flow of blood to the kidneys such as with the following:

1. Volume depletion, as in the case of hemorrhage, burns, severe FVD, and severe trauma
2. Heart failure

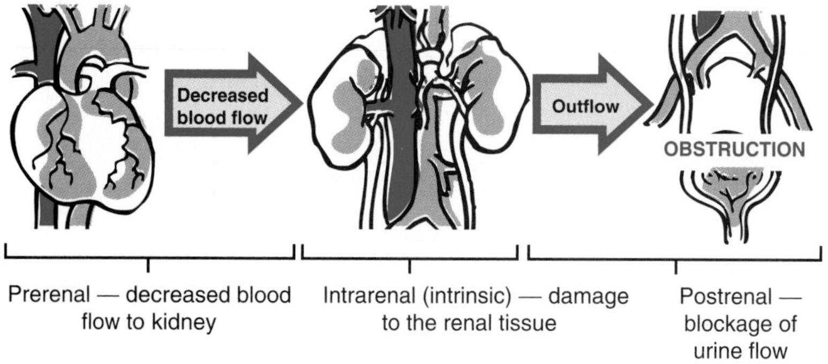

Acute renal failure

3. Sepsis
4. Pulmonary embolism
5. Hemolytic blood transfusion reaction
6. Shock

Intrarenal ARF (**acute tubular necrosis**) can occur when the kidney is damaged. The pathogenesis of "acute tubular necrosis" is unclear, but currently, tubular obstruction, leakage of tubular fluid through damaged tubular epithelium, arteriolar vasoconstriction, and decreased glomerular permeability are all believed to play a role.

The kidney can be damaged by the following:

1. Drugs that are toxic to the kidney, such as the following:
   - Antibiotics, antiinfectives, antivirals (aminoglycosides [gentamycin, kanamycin, tobramycin], amphotericin B, vancomycin, rifampin, methicillin, sulfonamides, tetracycline, pentamidine, acyclovir)
   - Antineoplastics (cisplatin, methotrexate, and cyclophosphamide).
   - Nonsteroidal antiinflammatory drugs (indomethacin)
   - Acetaminophen
   - Cyclosporin
   - Captopril
2. Chemicals that are toxic to the kidney, such as the following:
   - Heavy metals (mercury, lead, arsenic)
   - Radiographic contrast
   - Pesticides
   - Fungicides
3. Lymphoma, leukemia
4. Kidney inflammation (**glomerulonephritis**)
5. Kidney infection (**pyelonephritis**)
6. Renal artery or vein stenosis, thrombosis

Postrenal ARF can occur when there is an obstruction of the urinary tract below the kidney, as with the following:

1. Bladder cancer
2. Prostate cancer
3. Cervical cancer
4. Kidney stones
5. Urethral stricture

Sufficient urine output is necessary for maintaining normal fluid and electrolyte balance. A wide range of fluid and electrolyte imbalances occur, depending on the severity and duration of the renal failure. ARF has two phases: Phase 1—low or no urine output (**oliguric**) and Phase 2—return of urine output (**polyuric**).

TAKE HOME POINTS
Volume depletion is the most common cause of ARF.

Phase 1 Imbalances

1. Hyperkalemia (main cause of death) (see Chapter 5)
2. Fluid volume excess

3. Metabolic acidosis
4. Hypocalcemia (lack of a hormone produced by the kidney, required to create active vitamin D) (see Chapter 8)
5. Hyperphosphatemia (phosphates shift from ICF to ECF as hydrogen moves into the cell) (see Chapter 6)
6. Hyponatremia (result of hemodilution related to fluid volume excess and shift into ICF). Total body store normal (see Chapter 3)
7. Hypermagnesemia (administer magnesium-containing medications such as Milk of Magnesia, Maalox, Gelusil, Riopan, Rulox) (see Chapter 7)
8. Anemia (lack of renal enzyme that stimulates erythropoietin, hyperkalemia, azotemia, and acidosis cause shortened red-cell life spans)

Hyperkalemia is the main cause of death related to ARF.

TAKE HOME POINTS

- Continuous flow of fluid is necessary for proper renal function.
- Many forms of ARF are reversible with early identification.
- Renal failure can occur because of decreased flow to the kidney, damage to the kidney itself, or obstruction of the urinary tract below the kidney.

Phase 2 Imbalances

Usually within 10 to 21 days after the onset of ARF, Phase 2 begins, and urine output begins to increase. Initially, the kidney is unable to concentrate urine. Therefore urine output is increased without conservation of water and electrolytes. All electrolytes excreted by the kidneys (sodium, potassium, phosphate, and magnesium), as well as fluid, are lost. As the nitrogen wastes are excreted, the blood urea nitrogen (BUN) level decreases to the normal range.

Signs and Symptoms of ARF

Symptoms include oliguria or anuria and a variety of signs related to hyperkalemia, hyponatremia, fluid volume excess, metabolic acidosis, uremia, hypocalcemia, hypermagnesemia, hyperphosphatemia, and anemia. They include the following:

- Heart failure
- Hypertension (hypotension with prerenal ARF)
- Shortness of breath, moist wheezes heard in lungs (rales)
- Distended neck veins, elevated central venous pressure
- Weight gain
- Anorexia, nausea
- Lethargy, seizures
- Inflammation of the sac around the heart (**pericarditis**) can occur, which can lead to fluid in the pericardial sac (**pericardial effusion**) and compression of the heart by the fluid in the sac (**cardiac tamponade**).

TAKE HOME POINTS

- Symptoms are related to imbalances that occur with diminished or absent urine output.
- Fluid volume overload is a major cause of symptoms.
- Fluid and electrolyte imbalances continue to occur when urine output returns.

Laboratory studies will show the creatinine level increasing from 1 to 2 mg/dL every 24 to 48 hours (not with prerenal ARF) and BUN level increasing from 10 to 20 mg/dL every 24 to 48 hours. Electrolyte and arterial blood gas (ABG) levels relate to specific imbalance.

What You DO

Overhydration with resultant pulmonary edema is usually a result of attempts to restore urine output before the cause of the renal failure has been established. While the patient is being hydrated and metabolic or electrolyte imbalances are being managed, the cause of the ARF must be established to begin the required interventions.

Prerenal ARF treatment focuses on restoration of the normal circulating blood volume. The major question that must be addressed is the rate at which the fluid should be given. This rate usually depends on the clinical status of the patient. The patient must be constantly reassessed to prevent overhydration. The adequacy of fluid repletion can be assessed from physical examination and by monitoring renal function and urine output.

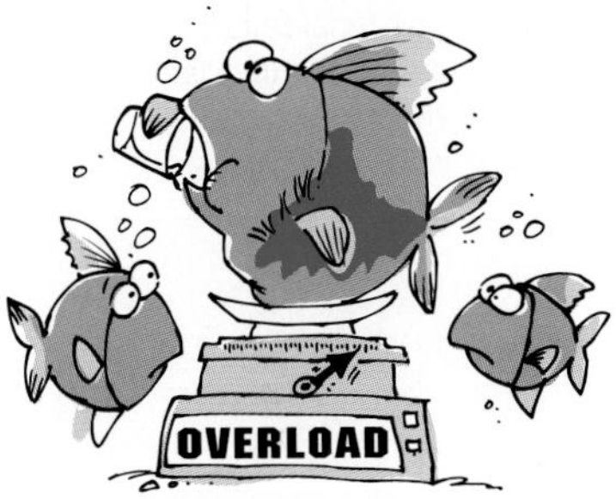

One indication of the need for dialysis is marked fluid overload.

Intrarenal ARF treatment involves correcting electrolyte imbalances by dietary restrictions, medication administration, or dialysis (in severe cases). Fluid volume overload is problematic. Fluid intake should equal fluid output, including urine, emesis, diarrhea, sweating, and respiration. (Review appropriate electrolyte chapters for common treatments.) Diuretics may be used to correct oliguria. Furosemide can be used in high doses alone or with dopamine to increase urine output.

Despite management, some patients require dialysis. Indications for dialysis include the following:

- Marked fluid overload
- Severe hyperkalemia
- The presence of uremic signs or symptoms (pericarditis, nausea and vomiting, confusion, bleeding with coagulopathy)
- BUN level greater than 100

With postrenal ARF, a passage for the drainage of urine must be created. The exact method that is used depends entirely on the level of the obstruction and may be as simple as a urinary catheter or as complex as a percutaneous nephrostomy tube.

The health care provider should do the following:

- Assess the patient for the possibility of ARF. If you can identify patients at risk, then you can frequently prevent ARF from occurring or iden-

The two most common causes of death early in the acute oliguric phase of ARF are hyperkalemia and pulmonary edema.

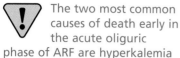

TAKE HOME POINTS

1. Treatment of ARF depends on the type of the failure.
2. With prerenal failure, treatment focuses on restoration of the normal circulating blood.
3. With intrarenal ARF, treatment focuses on correcting electrolyte imbalances by dietary restrictions, medication administration, or, in severe cases, dialysis.
4. With postrenal failure, a passage for the drainage of urine must be created.

- Minimize the potential for infection (major cause of death in ARF) by thoroughly assessing the skin.
- Use tepid water and avoid heating pads for pain, tingling, or numbness because the patient has a limited ability to sense heat.

tify it early, when it is easier to correct and permanent damage to the kidney can be prevented. When assessing patients, it is important to identify conditions in which not enough blood reaches the kidney, the kidney is inflamed or damaged, or there is a potential obstruction below the kidney to identify patients who may be at risk for ARF. Patients at risk for renal failure include the following:

1. Obstetric patients (potential for hemorrhage prepartum and postpartum)
2. Postoperative patients, such as those who have undergone open heart and gastrointestinal surgeries
3. Patients with bowel preps and held nothing by mouth (NPO)
4. Patients having radiograph procedures requiring a contrast medium
5. Critical care patients
6. Any patient on a nephrotoxic drug
7. Patients with decreased cardiac output

- Monitor vital signs, such as the following:
  1. Apical pulse rate and quality
  2. Blood pressure in each arm
  3. Rate and quality of respirations, shortness of breath on exertion, presence of rales, and pleural friction rub (dry, grating sound)
- Monitor laboratory values. Monitoring is important because early changes in the BUN and creatinine levels can signal the onset of ARF (especially when both are increased).
- Assess fluid volume status.
  1. Inspect neck veins for distention. If the veins are distended from the top of the sternum to the angle of the jaw, the patient is fluid overloaded.
  2. Elevate hands in circulatory overload. Hand veins will be clearly visible and will not empty, even with elevation.
  3. Perform daily weights with the same scale at the same time (usually in the morning) and with the same clothing (1 L water = 2.2 lb or 1 kg)
     - Mild-to-rapid loss or 2% total body water (TBW)
     - Moderate-to-rapid loss or 5% TBW
     - Severe-to-rapid loss or 8% TBW
- Perform a thorough skin care assessment. Because of decreased platelet action and uric crystal deposits, patients are highly susceptible to loss of skin integrity, leading to potential infection.
- Assess neurologic alterations, and institute safety measures as indicated. Institute seizure precautions. Assess for pain and tingling, especially in the glove area of the hands and the stocking area of the legs and feet.

- Monitor intake and output closely. Include all oral and parenteral intake; amount of emesis; and number, volume, and presence of blood in stool. Urinary catheters increase the potential for urinary tract infection. When required, catheter care is extremely important.
- Maintain nutrition. Closely monitor for sodium and potassium restrictions. Provide high caloric and low protein diet. Total parenteral nutrition (TPN) may be used.
- Monitor laboratory tests for changes in electrolyte studies. Changes can occur with all phases of treatment.
- Maintain vascular access.
  1. A central line is common.
  2. Aseptic technique and dressing management are important to minimize infection.
  3. Proper flushing of the vascular access device is important to prevent thrombosis.

TAKE HOME POINTS

- Assessment for potential risk of ARF can prevent its occurrence.
- Early identification of ARF is easier to correct, and permanent damage to the kidney can be prevented.
- It is important to identify conditions when insufficient blood reaches the kidney, when the kidney may be damaged, or when there may be a potential obstruction below the kidney.
- Early changes in serum laboratory BUN and creatinine tests can signal the onset of ARF.

Do You UNDERSTAND?

DIRECTIONS: **Fill in the blanks.**

1. Renal failure caused by decreased flow to the kidney is called ______________________.
2. Renal failure caused by damage to the kidney itself is called ______________________.
3. Renal failure caused by obstruction of the urinary tract below the kidney is called ______________________.
4. Sufficient ______________________ is necessary for maintaining normal fluid and electrolyte balance.
5. ______________________ is the electrolyte imbalance that is the main cause of death in ARF.
6. Serum sodium lab values are ______________________, but the ______________________ are normal.
7. ______________________ occurs because of the lack of nitrogenous waste products being excreted in the urine.

Answers: 1. prerenal; 2. intrarenal; 3. postrenal; 4. urine; 5. Hyperkalemia; 6. low, total body stores; 7. Metabolic acidosis.

DIRECTIONS: **Fill in the squares to form the words that provide the missing links to connect the given words.**

8.

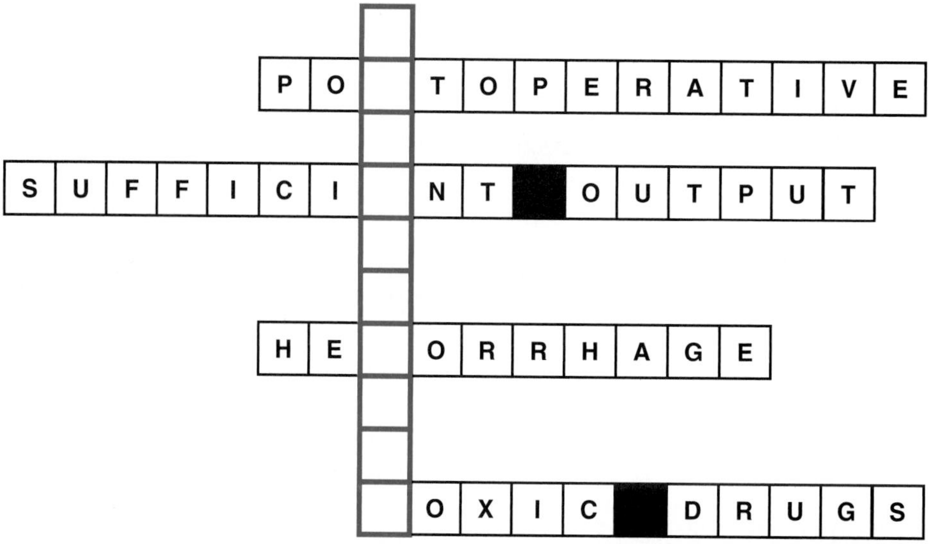

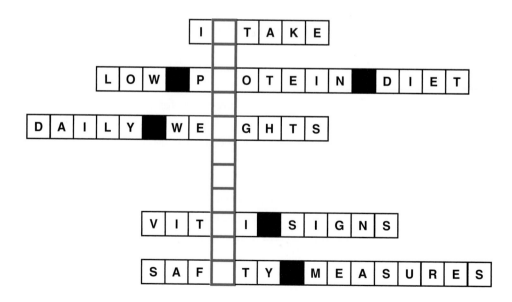

DIRECTIONS: **Fill in the squares to form the words that provide the missing links to connect the given words.**

9.

Answers: **8. assessment; 9. nursing care.**

What IS Crohn's Disease?

Crohn's disease is a chronic inflammation of the gastrointestinal (GI) tract. Although it can affect any part of the GI tract, it commonly affects the lower portion of the small intestine (ileum) and the right colon. Although it has some similarities with ulcerative colitis (another major inflammatory bowel disease), there are important differences. Ulcerative colitis is an inflammatory disease primarily of the left colon and rectum.

Crohn's and Colitis Foundation of America
www.ccfa.org

What You NEED TO KNOW

The small intestine plays an important role in digestion and the absorption of nutrients, fluid, and electrolytes. Potassium, zinc, magnesium, calcium, fats, vitamin B_{12}, iron, and fat-soluble vitamins are some of the nutrients that are not absorbed properly. Crohn's disease is a chronic disease with periods of no symptoms or mild symptoms interrupted by periods of acute illness. Many symptoms for Crohn's disease are related to malabsorption. Stress, anxiety, or depression can bring on acute symptoms.

Crohn's disease is characterized by the following:

- Abscesses, strictures, or perforation in affected bowel
- Diarrhea (3 to 20 semisoft to liquid stools per day)
- Foul-smelling bowel movements that float (**steatorrhea**)
- Urgency to pass stool at night
- Lower right abdominal pain (a classic symptom)
- Rectal and/or anal fissures
- Rectal bleeding (altered intestinal mucosa)
- Low-grade fever
- Chills
- Weight loss of 10% to 20%
- Anemia
- Kidney stones
- Malnutrition

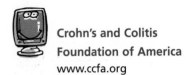

Fluid and electrolyte imbalances are related to diarrhea, malabsorption, poor nutrition, inflammation, and infection. Common electrolyte imbalances are hypokalemia, hypomagnesemia, and hypocalcemia (see Chapters 5, 7, and 8). Additionally, the patient will have a low serum albumin level, vitamin deficiencies (zinc, folic acid, and vitamin B_{12}), an elevated erythrocyte sedimentation rate, and fat in the feces (steatorrhea).

Common symptoms are edema, nervousness, numbness and tingling in hands and feet, fatigue, poor muscle coordination, decreased reflexes, anemia, mental depression and/or confusion, and foul-smelling stools.

TAKE HOME POINTS

- Crohn's disease is an inflammatory bowel disease characterized by lower right quadrant pain and foul-smelling stool.
- Fluid and electrolyte imbalances are related to diarrhea, malabsorption, poor nutrition, inflammation, and infection.

What You DO

Treatment involves relieving symptoms, controlling diarrhea, decreasing bowel inflammation, balancing fluids and electrolytes, replacing vitamins, and healing the intestinal wall. Drug therapy, nutrition and vitamin replacement, and correction of fluid and electrolyte losses are the cornerstones of treatment for patients with Crohn's disease.

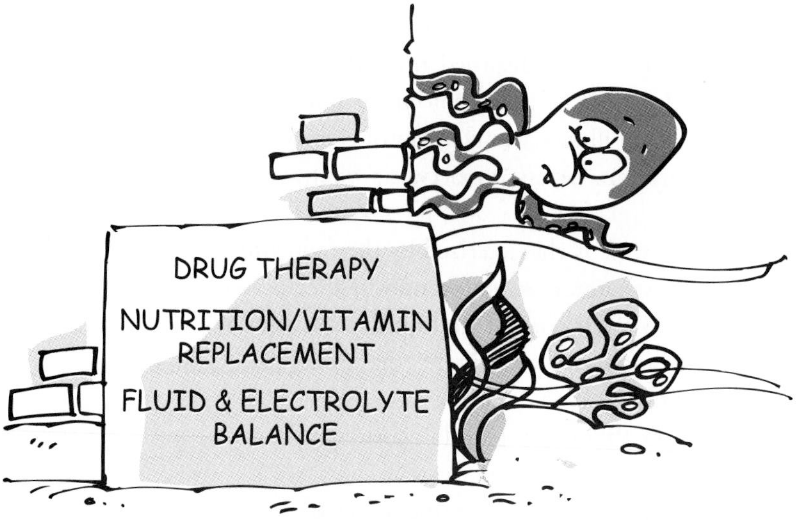

Drug therapy, nutrition and vitamin replacement, and correction of fluid and electrolyte losses are the cornerstones of treatment for patients with Crohn's disease.

The health care provider should do the following:

- Minimize the effects of malabsorption.
  1. Administer vitamins appropriately for maximum absorption. Vitamin B_{12} should be administered with meals.
  2. Begin a high-protein, low-fat, and low-fiber diet.
  3. Assess skin for breakdown. (Malabsorption of nutrients can lead to breakdown.)
- Assess fluid loss.

- Monitor routine vital signs.
- Monitor accurate intake and output.
  1. Record the number, consistency, odor, volume, and character of all bowel movements. (These factors are important indicators of disease progression.)
  2. Measure all emesis.
  3. Fluid intake should be sufficient to maintain urine output of at least 1200 to 1500 mL per day.
- During TPN administration, monitor daily serum electrolytes and compare to TPN formulation. Maintain aseptic technique when caring for an IV, especially the administration set and IV site to prevent sepsis.
- Monitor daily weight.
- Assess pain, and administer pain medications as prescribed.
- Administer steroids as prescribed. Remember, steroids can mask signs of inflammation and pain.

Do You UNDERSTAND?

DIRECTIONS: **Fill in the squares to form a word that is the missing link to connect the given words.**

1.

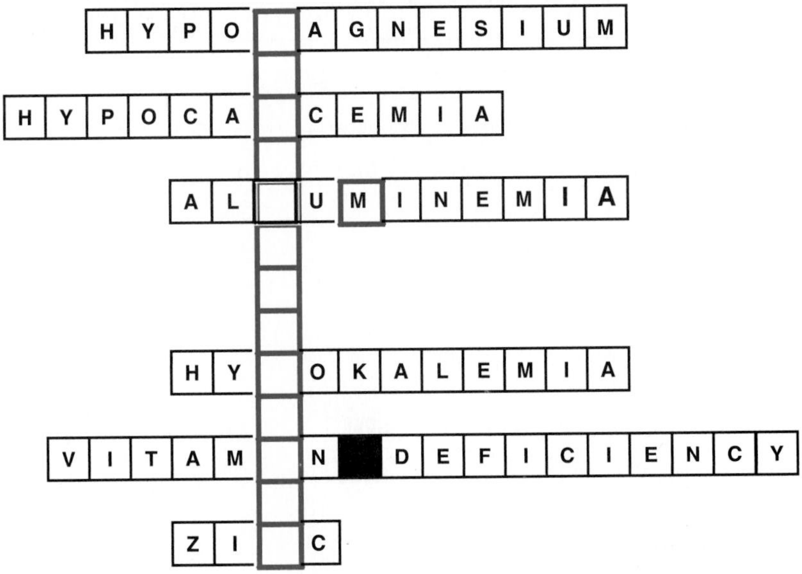

Answer: 1. malabsorption.

2.

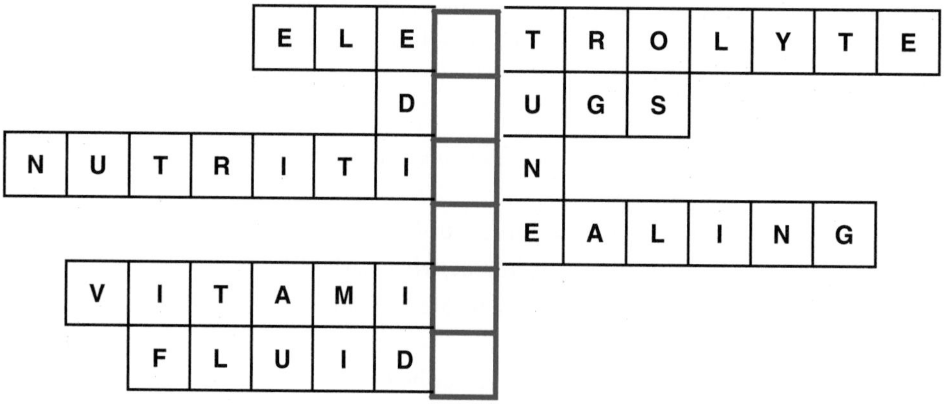

DIRECTIONS: **Unscramble the following characteristics associated with caregiving measures for patients with Crohn's disease.**

3. ______________________________ *(messessant)*
4. ______________________________ *(versaobniot)*
5. ______________________________ *(ruseamnemt)*
6. ______________________________ *(pricestodin)*
7. ______________________________ *(carcucay)*
8. ______________________________ *(woleb nevomsemt)*

Answers: **2. Crohn's; 3. assessment; 4. observation; 5. measurement; 6. description; 7. accuracy; 8. bowel movements.**

DIRECTIONS: Complete the crossword puzzle.

Across: Fluid and electrolyte

3. Polyuria leads to this
4. Lost buffering urine
5. Depleted with polyuria
7. Loss causes FVD
8. Most important electrolyte imbalance in DKA

Down: Outcome of fluid and electrolyte losses

1. Glucose in the urine
2. Increased serum glucose level causes serum _______________
6. Excessive breakdown of fats

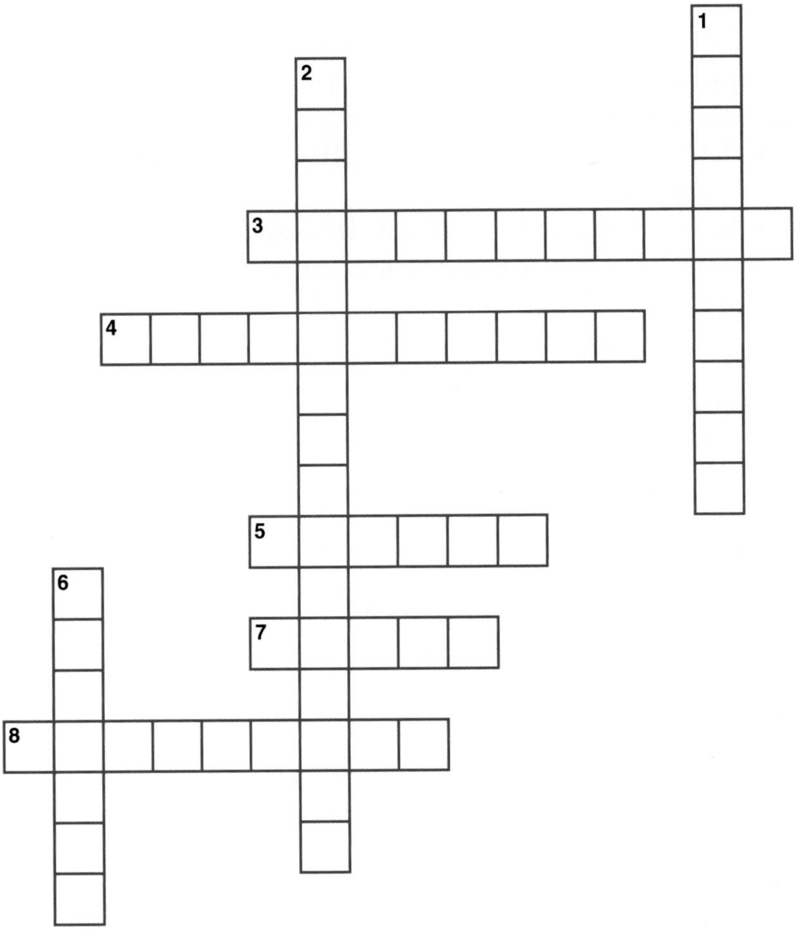

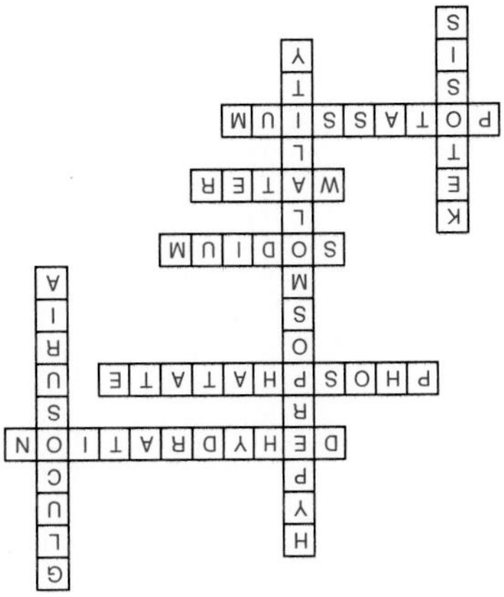

Answers:

References

Anderson KN, Anderson LE, Glanze WD: *Mosby's medical, nursing, and allied health dictionary,* ed 6, St Louis, 2002, Mosby.

Gahart BL, Nazareno AR: *Intravenous medications,* ed 21, St Louis, 2005, Mosby.

Glaser N, Barnett P, McCaslin I: Risk factors for cerebral edema in children with diabetic ketoacidosis. The Pediatric Emergency Medicine Collaborative Research Committee of the American Academy of Pediatrics, *N Engl J Med* 344(4):264-269, 2001.

Halperin ML: Fluid, electrolyte, and acid-base physiology: a problem-based approach, ed 3, Philadelphia, 1999, Saunders.

Ignatavicius DD, Workman ML: *Medical-surgical nursing critical thinking for collaborative care,* ed 4, Philadelphia, 2002, Saunders.

Macklin D, Chernecky C: *IV therapy,* St Louis, 2004, Saunders.

Macklin D, Chernecky C, Infortuna H: *Math for clinical practice,* St Louis, 2005, Mosby.

Umpierrez GE, Cuervo R, Karabell A: Treatment of diabetic ketoacidosis with subcutaneous insulin aspart, *Diabetes Care* 27(8):1873-1878, 2004.

NCLEX® Review

1. A 25-year-old white woman was admitted to the hospital with findings of extreme thirst, disorientation, warm and dry skin, and fruity-smelling breath. The initial nursing measure would be which of the following:
   1 Give orange juice with sugar.
   2 Obtain a serum glucose level.
   3 Encourage fluids.
   4 Withhold fluids.

2. The imbalance in diabetic ketoacidosis (DKA) is related to which of the following:
   1 Insulin's inability to enter the cell because of excess glucose
   2 Glucose's inability to enter the cell because of insufficient insulin
   3 Fat-metabolizing protein
   4 Protein-metabolizing fat

3. In response to metabolic acidosis, which of the following electrolyte imbalances occurs?
   1 Hyperkalemia
   2 Hypokalemia
   3 Hypernatremia
   4 Hyperphosphatemia

4. You have been assigned to take care of a patient who has been suffering from acute renal failure (ARF) for 3 days. Which of the following observations do you expect to find during a physical assessment?
   1 Hypotension, decreased central venous pressure (CVP), tachycardia, distended neck veins
   2 Flat neck veins, bradycardia, hypertension
   3 Hypertension, pitting edema, weight gain
   4 Shortness of breath, tachycardia, weight loss

5. When reviewing the physical assessment of a patient with Crohn's disease, you notice that the patient has numerous electrolyte imbalances and progressive weight loss. The primary reason for this condition is:
   1 Fluid volume overload
   2 Malabsorption
   3 Increased urine output
   4 Decreased urine output

6. Which of the following electrolyte imbalances is the main cause of death associated with acute renal failure?
   1 Hyperkalemia
   2 Hypokalemia
   3 Hypernatremia
   4 Hyponatremia

7. Which of the following serum chemistries are early indications of ARF?
   1 Decreased BUN and decreased creatinine
   2 Decreased BUN and increased creatinine
   3 Increased BUN and decreased creatinine
   4 Increased BUN and increased creatinine

8. Which of the following is the key indicator of fluid volume assessment?
   1 Blood pressure and urinary output
   2 Intake and output measurements
   3 Daily weights and blood pressure
   4 Daily weights and intake and output measurements

9. Which of the following insulin preparations may be administered IV?
   1 Lente
   2 NPH
   3 Regular
   4 Semilente

10. What are the two signs and symptoms characteristic of Crohn's disease?

11. Symptoms for HHNKS consist of __________, __________, __________, and __________.

12. True or False: With hyperglycemia, you can expect the skin to feel cold and clammy.

13. Define acute renal failure.

14. What is the cause of renal failure in patients with CHF?

15. Why do DKA and HHNKS lead to altered brain function and possibly coma?

NCLEX® Review Answers

1. 2 When you suspect DKA, obtaining a serum glucose level and arterial blood gases will provide confirmation. Giving orange juice with sugar is contraindicated in hyperglycemia because the serum glucose is already high in the patient. You would not encourage or withhold fluids if DKA is suspected. Treatment of the underlying insulin deficiency is most important.

2. 2 Insulin is required for glucose to enter the cells, where it is used for energy. With DKA, there is an abundance of glucose and low insulin. Fat-metabolizing protein and protein-metabolizing fat do not exist.

3. 1 With metabolic acidosis, potassium moves from the intracellular fluid (ICF) to the extracellular fluid (ECF), causing increased serum levels (hyperkalemia). With metabolic acidosis, potassium moves from the ICF to the ECF, causing increased serum levels. Sodium shifts from the ECF into the ICF, secondary to the loss of potassium. Phosphorous is lost in the urine with attempts to buffer acid.

4. 3 Patients with ARF and kidney damage suffer from fluid volume excess, which leads to hypertension, distended neck veins, pitting edema, and weight gain. Patients with ARF and kidney damage suffer from fluid volume excess. Decreased CVP and bradycardia are signs of fluid volume deficit. Distended neck veins are signs of fluid volume excess. Patients with ARF and kidney damage suffer from fluid volume excess. Flat neck veins and bradycardia are signs of hypotension. Hypertension is a sign of fluid volume excess. Shortness of breath and tachycardia are signs of fluid volume excess, but weight loss is not.

5. 2 The result of the inflammatory process of Crohn's disease is malabsorption. Fluids, electrolytes, and vitamins normally absorbed through the bowel wall cannot be absorbed and are thus excreted, leading to imbalances. Fluid volume deficit can occur with severe diarrhea. The primary system affected by Crohn's disease involves the small intestine and the right colon, not the kidneys.

6. 1 The inability to excrete potassium through the urine creates an increase in serum potassium. Cellular activity is sensitive to increased potassium with a rapid onset, which may lead to cardiac arrhythmias and cardiac arrest. Hypokalemia may occur with the return of urinary output and the inability of the kidney to concentrate urine; however, it may be treated. Hypernatremia may occur in patients with ARF; however, this is a gradual onset and is not associated with the primary cause of death. Hyponatremia is most commonly caused by a solute-induced diuresis and is observed in the late stages of ARF.

7. 4 BUN and creatinine are the best measures of renal function. Increased values represent an inability with the excretion process of the kidney. Decreased BUN and creatinine reflect adequate kidney function. Increased BUN is reflective of renal dysfunction, especially associated with an increased creatinine.

8. 1 Blood pressure reflects vascular fluid overload, and urinary output reflects renal function. Although these measures are necessary for the patient with fluid volume impairment, they are an indirect indicator of function. Weights may be influenced by other factors. Urinary output is a direct reflection of renal function. Weights and intake measurements are influenced by other factors and are not a direct reflection of renal function.

9. 3 Regular insulin is the only preparation that may be administered IV. Lente, NPH, and Semilente may not be administered IV.

10. Lower right quadrant pain and foul-smelling stool.

11. Severe hyperglycemia, absence of ketosis, profound dehydration, and neurologic changes. With HHNKs, there is enough insulin produced to prevent ketosis but not enough to prevent hyperglycemia.

12. False. With hyperglycemia the skin will be hot and dry.

13. Acute renal failure is a generic term to define the abrupt onset of decreased renal function and the retention of nitrogen waste products in the body.

14. Decreased blood flow to the kidneys. The heart is unable to pump sufficient volume to perfuse the kidneys.

15. Dehydration of brain cells. The elevated glucose levels in the blood causes water to shift from the ICF into the ECF causing cell dehydration.

Notes

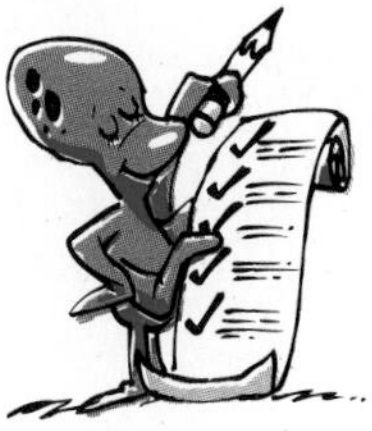

Chapter 15

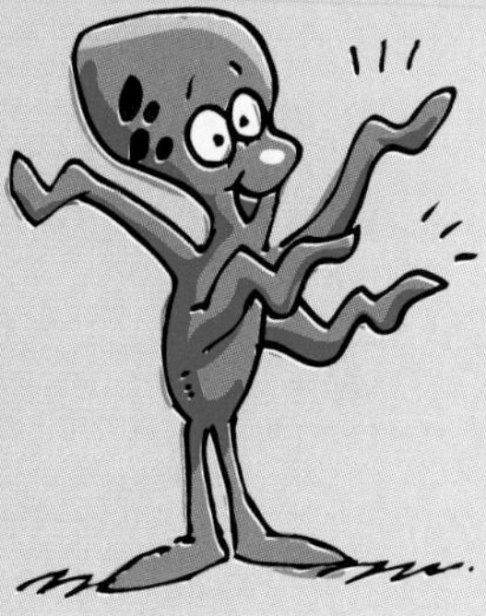

Health Care Problems of the Older Adult

What You WILL LEARN

After reading this chapter, you will know how to do the following:

- ✔ Define chronic obstructive pulmonary disease (COPD).
- ✔ Identify five treatments of COPD that will maintain functional independence, avoid repeated hospitalizations, and prevent infections and complications.
- ✔ Define four types of shock.
- ✔ Identify three major causes for each type of shock.
- ✔ Define heart failure.
- ✔ Identify four symptoms for left- and right-sided heart failure.

This chapter examines three representative disorders affecting fluid and electrolyte balance in the older adult:

- Chronic obstructive pulmonary disease
- Heart failure
- Shock

Although these conditions can occur in all age groups, they are common in the older adult (older than 65 years of age).

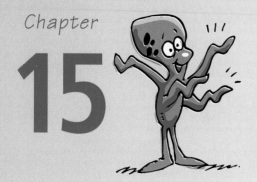

What IS Chronic Obstructive Pulmonary Disease?

Chronic obstructive pulmonary disease (**COPD**) is a prolonged, persistent disease process that affects the lower respiratory tract by increasing the resistance of airflow in the airways of the lung. The limited inspiratory and expiratory capacity of the lungs causes the body to have chronically reduced oxygen levels and/or chronically elevated amounts of carbon dioxide. The body has lower oxygen levels and higher carbon dioxide levels, with the loss of lung elasticity. Elastic lungs are able to force out carbon dioxide when exhaling. Lungs in the patient with COPD are less able to force air out during exhalation, similar to a paper bag filled with air.

This disorder is also called *chronic restrictive lung disease* (CRLD) or chronic airflow limitation (CAL).

The primary cause of COPD is smoking (80%). Pollution (including secondhand smoke and environmental pollutants), heredity, and infectious agents are less important contributors.

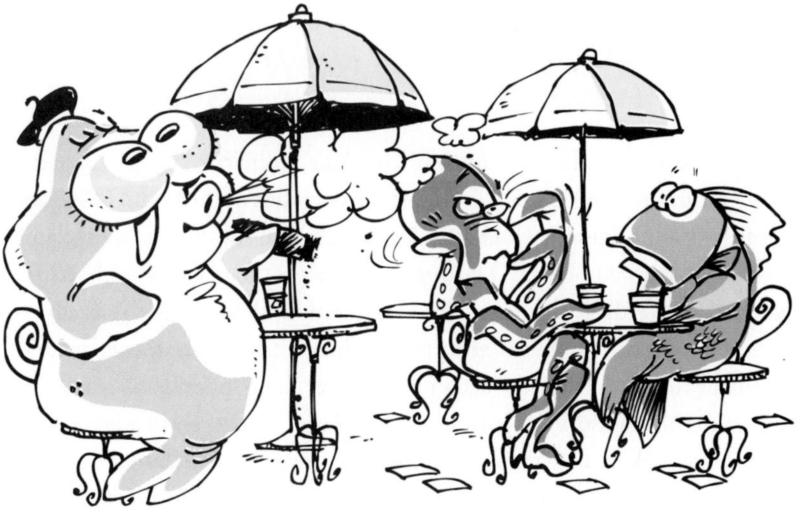

The primary cause of COPD is smoking.

Other risk factors for COPD include being male, living in a low socioeconomic status, and having had a childhood respiratory illness. COPD usually refers to some combination of chronic bronchitis, emphysema, and small-airway disease. Chronic bronchitis is a disorder affecting primarily the small and large airways. Emphysema is a disorder primarily affecting the alveoli.

The following are important facts about COPD as related to the older adult:

- COPD tends to worsen over time.
- A 70-year-old individual must work twice as hard to compensate for age-related compliance changes than he or she did at age 20.
- Evidence shows that older adults may not develop breathlessness (**dyspnea**) until they are at a substantially later stage of COPD than younger persons are when they develop it.
- The well-documented immune system decline with aging may mask commonly observed signs and symptoms of infections often associated with COPD.
- Decreased renal function is commonly associated with the older adult. This decrease impairs the renal compensatory mechanism.
- Older persons have the highest prevalence for heavy cigarette smoking in history, have had the longest potential exposure to air pollution and other environmental pollutants, and have experienced childhood illnesses before antibiotic use became common.

TAKE HOME POINTS

Chronic: persisting for a long time
Obstructive: clogging
Pulmonary: pertaining to the lungs
Disease: sickness

What You NEED TO KNOW

With COPD, the lung is unable to inhale sufficient oxygen or exhale enough carbon dioxide (CO_2) to meet the demands of the body. This occurs because of lung elasticity loss, lung hyperinflation, trapped air by collapsed alveoli, and mucus plugs. The process develops as patients with COPD gradually have difficulty with active respiration. The patient is unable to force air out of the lungs adequately; thus, carbon dioxide is retained. Gradually, carbon dioxide accumulates over long periods. Shortness of breath (**dyspnea**) during exertion (in early stages, but at rest in advanced disease) persists for years with a respiratory rate greater than 20 (**hypercapnia**). Chronic respiratory acidosis occurs. The renal system compensates for the respiratory acidosis by excreting hydrogen ions and conserving bicarbonate ($HCO_{3}-$) ions. Airway obstruction progresses, and hypoxemia may slowly develop. Hypercapnia (elevated carbon dioxide in blood) may develop.

The acid–base balance is the most common disturbance with COPD. Chronic respiratory acidosis that is completely or partially compensated for by the kidneys is commonly present.

Typical Arterial Blood Gases with COPD

pH < 7.35 or within lower limit of normal with complete renal compensation
pH < 7.35 without renal compensation as COPD progresses
$PaCO_2$ > 42 mm Hg (frequently 50–60 mm Hg or higher)
HCO_{3-} > 26 mEq/L (renal or metabolic compensation)
Base excess > +2 (renal or metabolic compensation)

Chest Medicine On-Line
www.priory.com/chest.htm

With carbon dioxide concentration ($PaCO_2$) chronically above 50 mm Hg, the respiratory center becomes relatively insensitive to carbon dioxide (CO_2) as the respiratory stimulant.

Typical Arterial Blood Gases with Acute Respiratory Acidosis

pH < 7.35
$PaCO_2$ can reach 120 mm Hg or higher (not compensated) metabolic alkalosis
HCO_{3-} > 26 mEq/L but not sufficient to compensate for sudden increase in $PaCO_2$
O_2 saturation below normal

TAKE HOME POINTS

1. For patients with COPD, the lungs are unable to inhale sufficient oxygen or exhale sufficient carbon dioxide to meet the demands of the body.
2. The causes of alteration in gas exchange are loss of lung elasticity, lung hyperinflation, collapsed alveoli that trap air, and mucus plugs.
3. Hypoxemia becomes the respiratory stimulus.

With acute hypoxemia, such as what might occur with pneumonia, the acidosis changes from chronic to acute respiratory acidosis (uncompensated).

Combined metabolic and respiratory acidosis occurs when the patient has severe diarrhea.

A complication of lung disease includes enlargement of the right ventricle of the heart (cor pulmonale). This can lead to right-sided heart failure.

Signs and Symptoms of COPD

With COPD, symptoms of emphysema, chronic bronchitis, or both (with one of them being predominant) are rare. Emphysema is more common with the older adult. Most of the symptoms are related to lung obstruction and respiratory acidosis: pursed lips breathing, tachypnea (respirations above 20/min), dyspnea, pink skin, orthopnea (must sit or stand to breathe), barrel-shaped chest, breathing with extrathoracic muscles, and abdominal bloating. Refer to your medical-surgical textbook for more in-depth information.

In addition to these symptoms, chronic respiratory acidosis symptoms include weakness and dull headache. It is important to identify symptoms that may indicate a negative change in the disease process. A reduction in short-term memory, restlessness, and confusion may be

TAKE HOME POINTS

- Clubbing of the fingertips occurs with chronic hypoxemia.
- Be certain not to dismiss the following symptoms as senility:
- Mental confusion and restlessness: symptoms of hypoxia.
- Malnutrition: common in patients with COPD because they are unable to eat and breathe at the same time, and they suffer a loss of appetite.
- Dehydration: increases the viscosity of mucous secretions.

misinterpreted as senility in older patients. However, these are symptoms that accompany increased hypoxemia and indicate a change in status. Infections are always a possibility with the older adult because of decreased immune function, compromised lung function, and secretion stasis. Infections can increase hypoxemia and change the chronic respiratory acidosis into acute respiratory acidosis.

Protein calorie malnutrition is common. The increased effort for breathing, coughing, and sputum production leads to a loss of appetite and an inability to eat and breathe at the same time. Poor nutrition is an identified problem with the older adult, which is complicated by COPD. Adults tend to become dehydrated because of altered renal function. Dehydration increases the thickness and stickiness (**viscosity**) of secretions, making coughing and expelling (**expectorating**) secretions difficult.

What You DO

- Patients with chronic hypoxemia and hypercarbia require lower levels of oxygen because hypoxia is the primary respiratory stimulant.
- Hydration may be restricted in some patients with renal failure or heart failure. Implement dietary education.

Treatment of COPD involves maintaining functional independence, avoiding repeated hospitalizations, and preventing infections and complications. Low-flow oxygen at least 15 hours a day, drug therapy, proper nutrition, and ensuring adequate fluid intake are common interventions.

- Thorough respiratory assessment is critical in the care of patients with COPD. Ongoing and careful evaluations lead to early recognition and intervention that may prevent complications.
- Administer pharmacologic agents as prescribed. Avoid sedatives and hypnotics because they can depress the ventilatory drive.
- Monitor and evaluate arterial blood gases (ABGs) as prescribed. A rapid rise in carbon dioxide concentration ($PaCO_2$) with a drop in pH suggests that the patient has fatigued respiratory muscles and may need mechanical ventilation. Administer oxygen therapy, usually at 2 to 3 L/min by nasal cannula.
- Promote adequate hydration, both oral and parenteral (1 to 2 L/day). Offer warm liquids to facilitate expectoration of secretions. Cold fluids may increase bronchospasms.
- Promote a diet high in calories and fats (decreases carbon dioxide production). Avoid caffeine (increases diuresis and promotes dehydration) and gas-producing foods (increases gas, pressure on diaphragm, and respiratory effort). Limit salt intake and include fiber to prevent

constipation. Nutrition is vital for maintaining energy, for muscle growth needed for respiratory function, and for improved resistance against infections.

TAKE HOME POINTS

- Thorough respiratory assessment is critical in the care of patients with COPD.
- Avoid sedatives and hypnotics (depresses ventilatory drive).
- A rapid rise in carbon dioxide concentration with a drop in pH suggests that the patient has fatigued respiratory muscles and may need mechanical ventilation.
- Patients with chronic hypoxemia and hypercarbia require lower levels of oxygen because hypoxia is the primary drive respiratory stimulus.
- Nutrition is vital for maintaining energy, for muscle growth needed for respiratory function, and for improved resistance against infections.

Do You UNDERSTAND?

DIRECTIONS: **Match the values most typically seen in patients with COPD.**

Column A	Column B
1. _____ $PaCO_2$	a. Low normal
2. _____ pH	b. +2 or greater
3. _____ HCO_{3-}	c. High normal
4. _____ Base excess	d. Greater than 42 mm Hg

DIRECTIONS: **Unscramble the following terms frequently associated with the treatment of patients with COPD.**

5. ______________________ *(taeioonxgny)*
6. ______________________ *(pseiioanrtr)*
7. ______________________ *(ximopahey)*
8. ______________________ *(geeyrn vtcaeioosnrn)*
9. ______________________ *(ndhaoyirt)*
10. ______________________ *(stessemans)*
11. ______________________ *(chemnaical taveinliton)*
12. ______________________ *(ttnniiour)*

What IS Shock?

The cardiovascular system is a closed, continuous system. There are three vital areas of the cardiovascular system that distribute oxygenated blood to the tissues: the heart as the cardiac pump, the vessels of the vascular system, and the circulating blood volume. The heart forces blood into the blood vessels of the body. The supply of blood is necessary for the delivery of oxygen and nutrients to the cells, which supports cell metabolism.

Answers: **1. d; 2. a; 3. c; 4. b; 5. oxygenation; 6. respiration; 7. hypoxemia; 8. energy conservation; 9. hydration; 10. assessment; 11. mechanical ventilation; 12. nutrition.**

Successful perfusion depends on cardiac output, circulating blood volume, and vascular tone. When any one of these elements becomes dysfunctional, *shock* may develop.

Shock is not one specific illness but a clinical syndrome (a combination of signs, symptoms, and effects). During shock, the body attempts to maintain cellular function until the cause of the poor tissue perfusion can be alleviated; otherwise, death will occur.

The following are important facts about shock as related to the older adult:

- The older adult has less reserve to control shock.
- The older adult is more susceptible to pH disturbances because of the reduced compensatory capability of the renal and respiratory systems.
- Older adults have less tolerance for hypovolemia.
- Patients on beta blockers or calcium channel blockers or patients with pacemakers may not become tachycardic or hypovolemic, which delays the diagnosis of shock.
- Heart failure is most common in older adults, with 75% occurring in adults older than 60 years of age.
- Because of neurologic or physical disability, older adults do not respond to thirst by increasing fluid intake.
- Older adults are more likely to have conditions that predispose them to bacterial infection.

There are four main classifications of shock: cardiogenic, hypovolemic, distributive, and obstructive.

Cardiogenic Shock

Cardiogenic shock relates to problems with the heart itself. A poorly functioning heart causes poor tissue perfusion. Fluid volume is not affected. With decreased contractility of the heart muscle the amount of blood pumped with each contraction is decreased, leading to increased ventricle filling and then to increased chamber size. Eventually, with low cardiac output comes systemic hypotension and/or pulmonary edema. Cardiogenic shock occurs in 5% to 10% of patients with an acute myocardial infarction (MI). Approximately 70% of cases are fatal despite treatment.

Cardiogenic shock can result from the following:

- Heart attack (MI)
- Previous MI
- Heart failure

- Arrhythmias
- Rupture of the wall between the heart's ventricles (main pumping chambers)
- Aneurysm (bulging) in a ventricle wall
- Prolonged open heart surgery involving heart/lung bypass
- Dysfunction or inflammation of the heart muscle (cardiomyopathy or myocarditis, respectively)
- Irregular heartbeat (too rapid or too slow)
- Defective heart valves, either real or artificial, including narrowing of the aortic valve, leading to decreased blood flow from the heart
- Increased thickness of the wall of one of the ventricles, blocking blood flow out of the heart

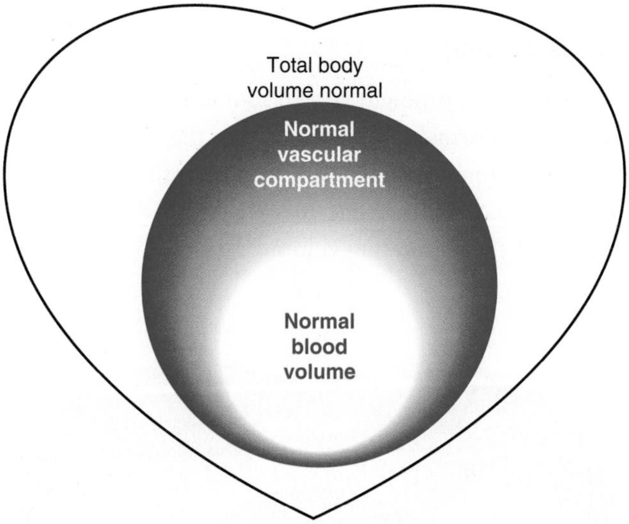

Hypovolemic Shock

Hypovolemic shock relates to a problem with the circulating blood volume. Rapid fluid loss characterizes hypovolemic shock.

Hypovolemic shock can result from the following:

- Hemorrhage (e.g., trauma, surgical procedures, ruptured aortic aneurysm)
- Fluid volume deficit (e.g., burns, severe vomiting, diarrhea, diabetes insipidus, diabetic ketoacidosis, sweating, third spacing)

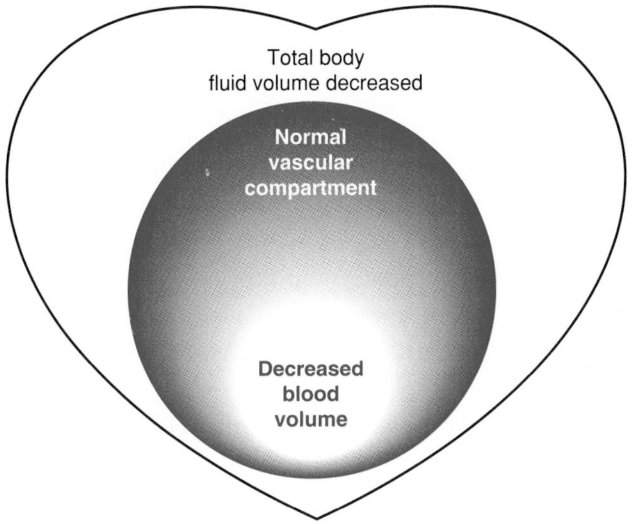

Distributive Shock

Distributive shock is a problem related to a loss of vascular tone (blood vessels dilate) or abnormal flow of fluids into the tissues, despite normal or increased heart function. The fluid volume is the same, but the veins are larger or the fluid volume is decreased because it has moved into the tissues and out of the circulating volume.

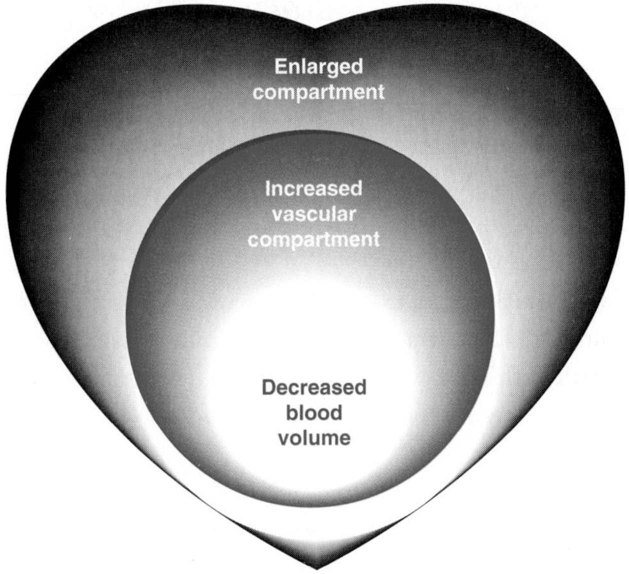

Distributive shock can result from the following:

- Drug overdose
- Bacterial infection in the blood (septic shock; release of bacterial toxins most often caused by gram-negative bacteria). The genitourinary or respiratory system is the most frequent source of infections; the older adult is more susceptible to septic shock.
- Anaphylaxis (severe, body-wide allergic reaction)
- Abnormal opening of blood vessels due to neurologic dysfunction (neurogenic shock), high spinal anesthesia, head trauma, vasovagal response
- Addisonian crisis (a severe adrenal gland insufficiency)

Obstructive Shock

Obstructive shock relates to the inability of blood to enter the heart because of an extracardiac obstruction. This obstruction prevents the heart muscle from functioning effectively, causing inadequate heart filling.

Obstructive shock can result from the following:

- Pericardial tamponade (build-up of fluid that puts pressure on the heart, preventing it from filling with enough blood)
- Massive pulmonary embolism (blockage of blood flow to the lungs by a blood clot, gas bubble, bit of tissue, or other object)
- Tension pneumothorax (collapse of the lungs caused by air that collects outside them due to a rupture in the lungs or chest wall)
- Severe high blood pressure in the vessels coursing through the lungs

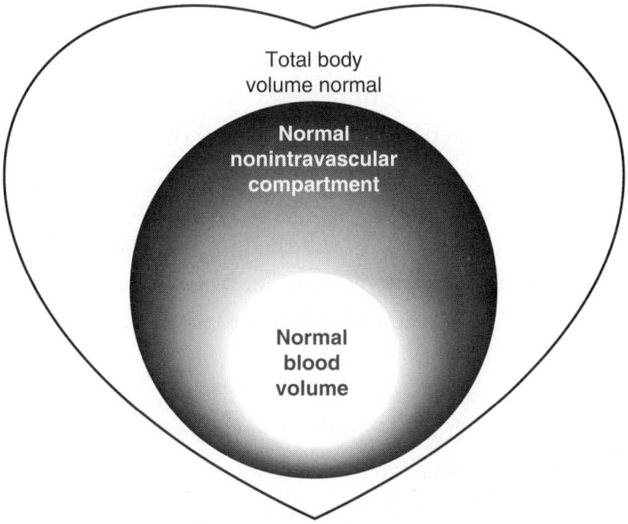

Inability of blood to enter heart.

A poorly functioning heart causes poor tissue perfusion. Approximately 70% of cases are fatal, despite treatment. Fluid volume is not affected. Risk factors for this type of shock are MI, previous infarction, HF, and arrhythmias.

What You NEED TO KNOW

Inadequate tissue perfusion leads to anaerobic metabolism (without oxygen). The four stages of shock are initial (early), nonprogressive (compensatory), progressive (compensatory mechanisms unable to maintain oxygen supply), and refractory (irreversible).

TAKE HOME POINTS

1. The heart, blood vessels, and circulating blood volume are responsible for maintaining hemodynamic tissue perfusion.
2. Shock results from a lack of perfusion.
3. Cardiogenic shock results from the poor pumping action of the heart.
4. Hypovolemic shock results from the decrease in circulating blood volume.
5. Distributive shock results from a loss of vascular tone.
6. Obstructive shock results from an extracardiac obstruction of cardiac output.

Fluid and Electrolyte Imbalances in Shock

Imbalance	Rationale
Increased ADH	Chemical compensation
Metabolic acidosis	Hypoperfusion and increased lactic acid because of anaerobic metabolism
Hyperkalemia	Decreased renal function, metabolic acidosis, release from injured cells
Respiratory alkalosis	Compensation for metabolic acidosis (compensated)
Respiratory acidosis	Respiratory failure, decreased respiratory rate, and decreased tidal volume (decompensated)
Decreased $PaCO_2$	Hypoxia
Increased anion gap	Excessive fixed acid accumulation
Decreased pH	Hypoperfusion and lactic acid production

ADH, Antidiuretic hormone.

Specific risk factors for shock with the older adult are as follows:

- **Cardiogenic:** Heart failure or diabetes
- **Hypovolemic:** Diuretic therapy, immobility, and decreased thirst response
- **Distributive:** Urinary tract infections, trauma, or cancer, as well as cerebrovascular accidents or diminished immune response
- **Obstructive:** Pulmonary hypertension, tension pneumothorax, pulmonary emboli, cardiac tamponade (post–open heart surgery), or thoracic tumors.

Although the cause of shock may be different, the major signs and symptoms are the result of the body's compensatory systems working to supply oxygen to the vital organs and, as shock progresses, are related to the body's inability to compensate. Symptoms common with all categories include the following:

- **Altered level of consciousness:** Early: apprehension and restlessness. Late: lethargy and coma (lack of oxygen to the brain)
- **Oliguria (compensatory):** Attempt to maintain sufficient circulating volume
- **Deep, rapid respirations (compensatory):** In an attempt to increase oxygen
- **Arterial blood gas (ABG) alterations:** Respiratory acidosis (decreased PaO_2, increased carbon dioxide concentration, and decreased pH)
- **Blood pressure (BP) changes:** Systolic BP under 90 mm Hg, diastolic pressure 30 mm Hg below normal reading
- **Pulse pressure:** Difference between the systolic and diastolic pressures; less than 20 mm Hg
- **Early sign:** BP between lying and sitting positions is 10 mm Hg or more
- **Pulse rate increases:** An attempt to increase perfusion
- **Weak or absent peripheral pulses:** When the systolic pressure falls below 80 mm Hg
- **Pale, moist, and cool skin**
- **Extreme thirst:** Compensatory response for altered volume
- **Nausea and vomiting:** Result of decreased gastrointestinal function (decreased central nervous system [CNS] stimulation because of hypoxia)
- **ECG changes:** May be evidence of myocardial ischemia or decreased pump function

Septic shock symptoms initially include fever, shaking chills, pounding pulse, flushed skin, and hyperventilation. Temperature will eventually become subnormal, pulse will become weak and "thready," and skin will become pale and cool as shock worsens.

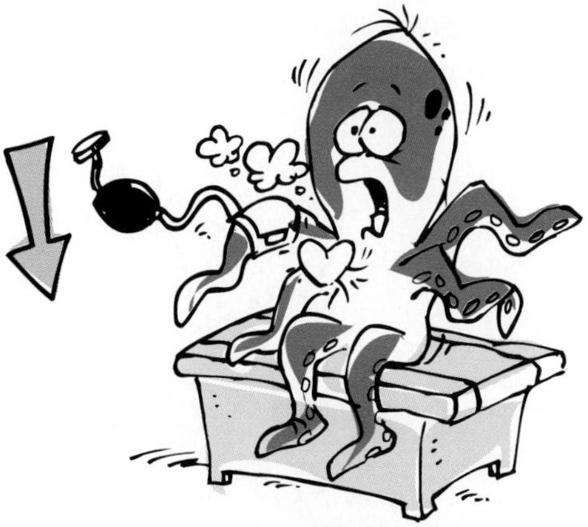

Septic shock symptoms include fever, shaking chills, bounding pulse, flushed skin, and tachypnea.

TAKE HOME POINTS

1. Identifying patients at risk for shock may aid in early identification of shock.
2. Changes in sensorium such as anxiety, irritation, or confusion may be an early indicator of impending shock.
3. Clinical manifestations of shock relate to the body's attempt to maintain function of the vital organs necessary for sustaining life.
4. Classic signs and symptoms of shock are increased pulse rate, decreased blood pressure, and increased respiratory rate.
5. With septic shock, fever, shaking chills, pounding pulse, and flushed skin occur initially.

What You DO

The primary treatment for shock is to sustain life support until the cause leading to shock is identified. Treatment involves correcting the underlying source of the problem. Treatment for the four types of shock focuses on the following:

Cardiogenic: Restoring coronary blood flow, reducing oxygen demand, and promoting fluid shift into intravascular compartment

Hypovolemic: Expanding circulating volume and preventing further loss

Distributive: Identifying the cause

Obstructive: Reducing the obstruction to improve cardiac output

Nursing measures involve early recognition, compensation support, and deterioration prevention. The rule of thumb is to give the patient what is lost!

- Maintain patent, large-gauge (20-gauge or larger) IV access so that IV fluids (see Chapter 16) can be successfully administered for volume expansion.
- Provide oxygen as prescribed.
- Monitor blood pressure, intake and output, central venous pressure (CVP), laboratory values, and ABGs to measure the effectiveness of treatment.
- Administer pharmacologic agents as prescribed. The use of pressor drugs (dopamine, norepinephrine, epinephrine, or vasopressin) enhances both coronary and cerebral blood flow. Other drugs aimed at correcting the underlying cause and preventing potential complications may also be given. Review your medical-surgical text for a complete description of nursing care.

TAKE HOME POINTS

Remember VIP
Ventilation: Increases oxygen and decreases carbon dioxide (always administer supplemental oxygen)
Infusion: IV fluids maintain an adequate intravascular volume
Pump function: Is supported to maximize cardiac output

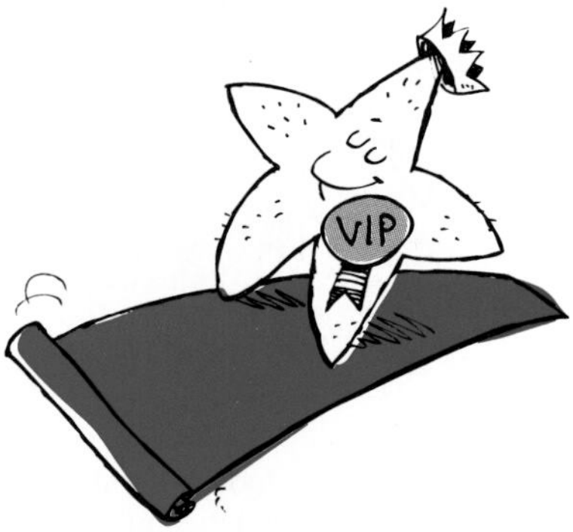

Sedatives, tranquilizers, and narcotics should not be given to the patient in shock.

Do You UNDERSTAND?

DIRECTIONS: **Match the imbalance in column A with the related cause in column B.**

Column A	Column B
1. _____ Metabolic acidosis	a. Decreased renal function
2. _____ Hyperkalemia	b. Increased lactic acid
3. _____ Hyperventilation	c. Inadequate tissue perfusion
4. _____ Hypoxia	d. Respiratory compensation

DIRECTIONS: **Place the answers to the clues in the puzzle, and fill in the squares to form the missing word that connects them.**

Down

5. Missing word

Across

6. Cardiac pump
7. Loss of tone
8. Loss with hemorrhage

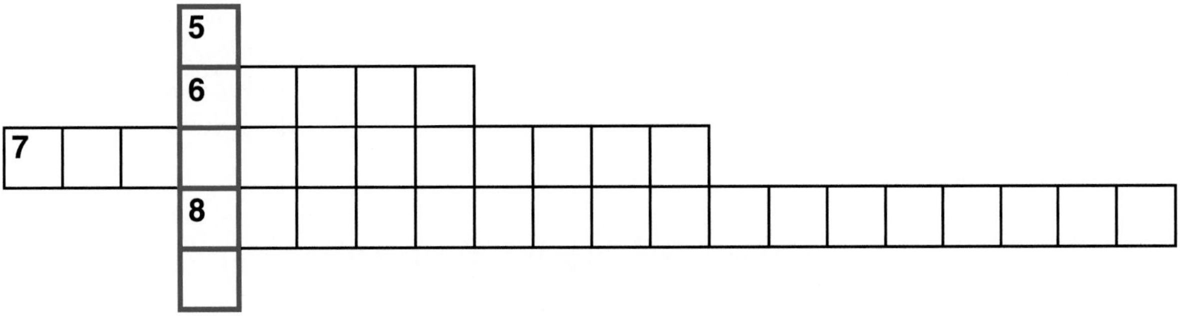

Answers: 1. b; 2. a; 3. d; 4. c; 5. shock; 6. heart; 7. blood vessels; 8. circulating volume.

DIRECTIONS: Place the answers to the clues in the puzzle.

9. Adequate oxygen to the cells is known as tissue ________________.
10. Metabolism without oxygen
11. Substance released when metabolism occurs without oxygen
12. The acid-base balance that occurs with 10 and 11.

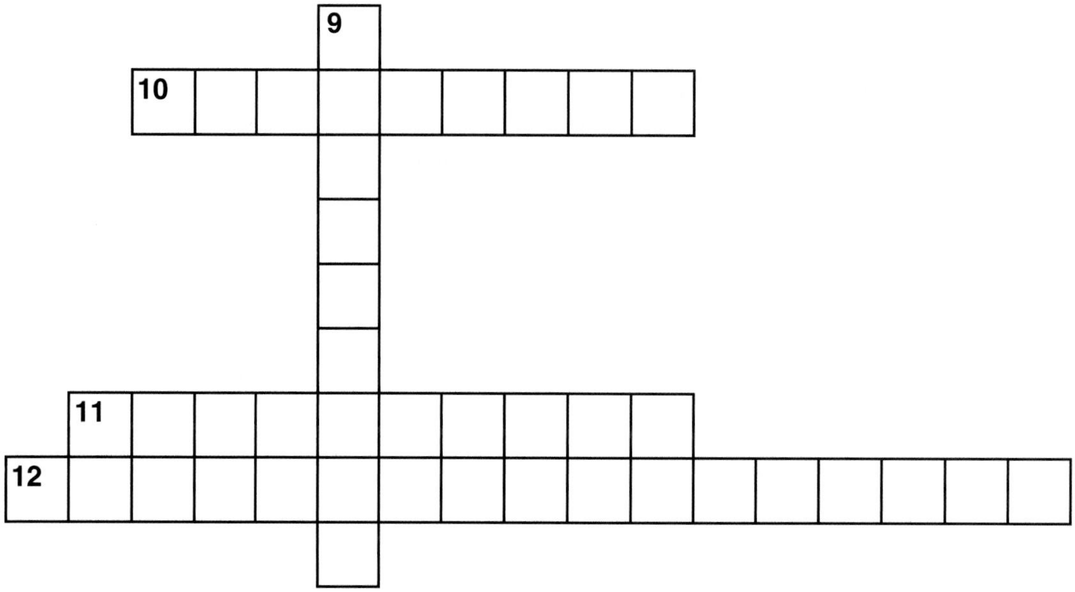

TAKE HOME POINTS

- Adequate perfusion of life-sustaining organs is imperative in clinical management.
- Adequate perfusion is the maintenance of vascular flow, pressure, and volume to meet the metabolic demands of the tissue.
- Early recognition of and intervention for shock can prevent further deterioration and death.

DIRECTIONS: Unscramble the following parameters that the health care provider monitors.

13. ______________________________ *(velel fo snessciontcous)*
14. ______________________________ *(ketain nad toutup)*
15. ______________________________ *(bal selauv)*
16. ______________________________ *(trialear dolob sages)*
17. ______________________________ *(tlaiv gsins)*

What IS Heart Failure?

Heart failure (HF) results when the heart muscle is unable to pump sufficient blood to meet the body's requirements. The heart can be affected on the right side, the left side, or both. Failure of one side eventually leads to failure of the other side.

Answers: **9. perfusion; 10. anaerobic; 11. lactic acid; 12. metabolic acidosis; 13. level of consciousness; 14. intake and output; 15. lab values; 16. arterial blood gases; 17. vital signs.**

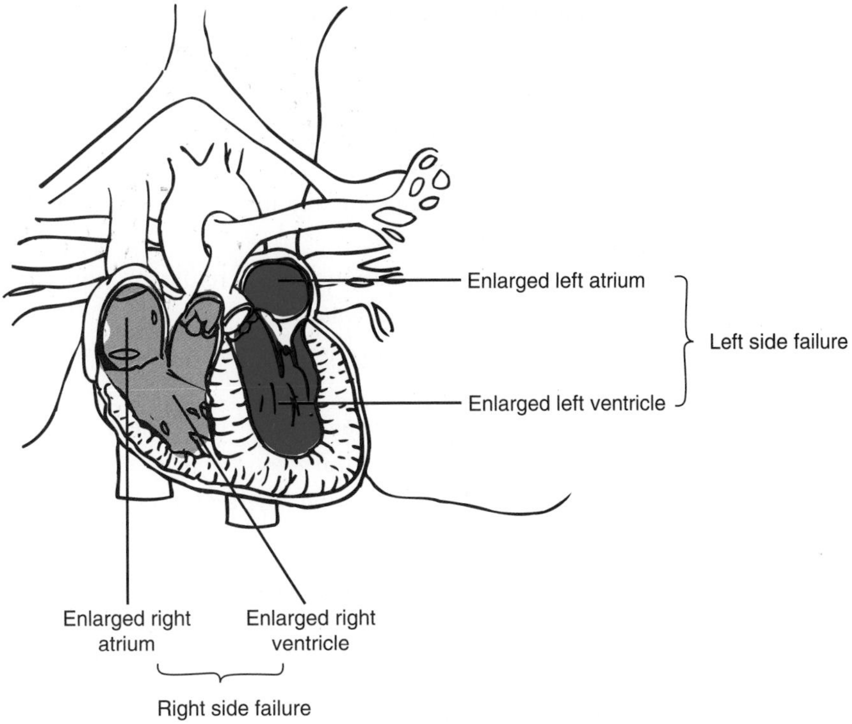

Heart failure.

The following are important facts about HF as related to the older adult:

- HF is most common in older adults, with 75% occurring in adults older than 60 years of age.
- HF is the most frequent cause of hospitalization in older adults.
- HF occurs more often in men than in women.

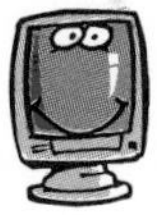

American Heart Association
www.amhrt.org
HeartINFO
www.heartinfo.org

What You NEED TO KNOW

Causes of HF are MI, coronary heart disease, cardiomyopathy, valvular disease, hypertension, and pulmonary hypertension. Left-sided HF occurs when the blood coming from the lungs cannot be pumped into circulation. This causes blood to back up in the lungs (hypertension, coronary artery disease, and valve disease). HF usually begins with left-sided failure. Right-sided failure is usually the result of left-sided failure. Right-sided HF occurs when the right ventricle does not completely empty (left-sided HF, right ventricular MI, and pulmonary hypertension).

When the blood is not pumped into the lungs from the systemic circulation, blood backs up in the veins. The body is able to compensate for the HF for an extended period. Eventually, compensatory mechanisms lead to a further decrease in pump function. Compensatory mechanisms include the following:

- Increased heart rate initially improves cardiac output, but as the rate increases, output falls.
- Sympathetic stimulation volume results in more forceful contraction and improved stroke volume.
- Arterial constriction caused by sympathetic stimulation increases tissue perfusion.
- Sodium and water retention by the kidneys increases the blood volume returning to the heart.
- Myocardial wall thickening (**hypertrophy**) improves the force of contractions.

Mechanisms that Cause Fluid and Electrolyte Imbalances in Patients with Heart Failure

Imbalance	Cause
Hyponatremia	Dilutional effect of increased water retention Decreased blood volume to the kidney causes increase in aldosterone and ADH secretion
Increase in extra-cellular water	Sodium is retained; there is high total sodium Water is retained in larger amounts than sodium
Increased hydrostatic pressure	Increased venous blood volume leads to movement of fluid into the interstitial tissues (edema) and lungs (pulmonary edema)
Hypokalemia	Aldosterone promotes potassium secretion Some diuretics are used to reduce edema and, in the process, further potassium loss
Mild metabolic acidosis	Decreased circulation Elimination of acids Hypoxia leads to increased lactic acid from anaerobic metabolism Decreased ability to excrete hydrogen with low urine output Hypokalemia
Respiratory alkalosis	Compensate for metabolic acidosis
Respiratory acidosis (pulmonary edema)	Increased pulmonary congestion Increased carbon dioxide retention

Signs and Symptoms of Heart Failure

The symptoms of HF are related to the side of the heart that is impaired. Symptoms related to left-side failure are related to decreased cardiac output, pulmonary congestion, and hypoxia. These symptoms are tachypnea, dyspnea (during exertion), orthopnea, paroxysmal nocturnal dyspnea, pulmonary edema, tachycardia, fatigue, dizziness, confusion, and oliguria.

Symptoms of right-side failure are related to systemic venous congestion. These symptoms include edema, weight gain, distended neck veins, enlarged liver (**hepatomegaly**), ascites, enlarged spleen, anorexia, nausea and vomiting, and increased BP.

Usually a patient presents with a combination of these symptoms because both sides of the heart are commonly performing improperly.

TAKE HOME POINTS

- HF occurs when the heart cannot pump sufficient blood to meet the metabolic requirements of the body.
- Left-sided HF causes pulmonary congestion and decreased systemic circulation. Symptoms are related mainly to the compromised lung function and hypoxia.
- Right-sided HF causes systemic venous congestion. Symptoms are related mainly to increased hydrostatic pressure and increased blood volume.

What You DO

Treatment for HF involves reducing the workload of the heart, improving cardiac contractility, and identifying and correcting the underlying cause.

Because the older adult may have impaired renal and liver function and diseases such as COPD, the treatment of HF requires continual monitoring. (Review your medical-surgical textbook for a complete review of nursing interventions.)

- Monitor and evaluate the functioning of the heart. (Assess response to activity and a low-sodium diet.)
- Determine the effectiveness of prescribed medications, and recognize early toxicities. (Measure intake and output, daily weights, and vital signs.)
- Observe for symptoms signaling disease progression (vital signs, heart sounds, ABGs, and lab values).
- Institute interventions to lessen the workload of the heart, decrease venous return (low-salt diet and diuretics as prescribed), and increase cardiac contractility and cardiac output (administer drugs as prescribed, such as digitalis and/or vasodilators).

TAKE HOME POINTS

- Treatment for HF involves reducing the workload of the heart, improving cardiac contractility, and identifying and correcting the underlying cause.
- Preexisting conditions make assessment of the patient with HF extremely complex.

Do You UNDERSTAND?

DIRECTIONS: Select the appropriate cause for each symptom.

Symptom

1. _____ Abdominal distention
2. _____ Cyanosis
3. _____ Edema
4. _____ Jugular venous distention
5. _____ Orthopnea
6. _____ Rapid, shallow breathing

Cause

a. Right-sided heart failure
b. Left-sided heart failure

DIRECTIONS: Fill in the blanks.

7. HF occurs when the ______________ cannot ______________ sufficient blood to meet the body's requirements.
8. Laboratory values for sodium indicate ______________, although the total body store is ______________, because of the ______________ of increased water retention.
9. Aldosterone promotes the excretion of ______________.
10. Left-sided HF symptoms are related to ______________ ______________ ______________, ______________ ______________, and ______________.
11. Right-sided HF symptoms are related to ______________ ______________ ______________.

Answers: 1. a; 2. b; 3. a; 4. a; 5. b; 6. b; 7. heart, pump; 8. hyponatremia, high, dilutional effect; 9. potassium; 10. decreased cardiac output, pulmonary congestion, hypoxia; 11. systemic venous congestion.

DIRECTIONS: **Find the nine hidden signs, symptoms, and imbalances that need to be assessed.**

DYSPNEA
ORTHOPNEA
SECRETIONS
PURSED-LIP BREATHING
HYPOXEMIA
MALNUTRITION
TACHYPNEA
RESPIRATORY ACIDOSIS
DEHYDRATION

I	R	H	J	W	Q	A	E	N	P	Y	H	C	A	T	Y	H	U	O	R
Y	O	E	S	D	F	R	T	W	J	U	H	L	O	P	M	N	V	C	L
D	X	Z	S	V	G	S	E	Z	E	E	H	W	K	T	L	Y	G	R	E
E	D	F	F	P	K	E	B	V	C	C	X	Z	Z	A	L	N	O	U	Y
H	M	I	O	B	I	C	B	W	Q	R	E	T	Y	C	I	U	P	P	I
Y	C	C	V	S	S	R	H	J	K	L	L	G	T	H	E	E	V	A	Z
D	R	A	T	T	U	E	A	M	M	N	B	V	T	Y	C	C	X	E	Z
R	E	I	N	Y	Y	T	S	T	U	I	O	A	P	P	L	S	S	N	W
A	V	M	Z	Z	Q	I	R	E	O	T	E	Y	O	N	P	L	L	P	J
T	J	E	O	P	M	O	N	B	B	R	V	J	J	E	P	L	F	O	F
I	W	X	X	S	S	N	H	J	B	K	Y	L	O	A	Y	G	I	H	J
O	M	O	V	V	X	S	W	P	Q	R	R	A	I	O	U	C	S	T	B
N	L	P	N	N	L	L	I	H	G	F	D	S	C	A	A	W	E	R	T
U	I	Y	I	U	Y	L	R	E	A	W	Q	A	S	I	T	Y	U	O	P
T	Y	H	F	F	D	H	H	J	E	F	D	S	A	A	D	Z	X	C	C
V	V	B	G	E	A	M	A	L	N	U	T	R	I	T	I	O	N	L	O
O	Y	F	S	U	K	L	N	M	P	O	U	I	Y	Y	T	O	S	B	B
T	T	R	E	W	D	C	B	N	S	O	P	L	M	I	H	N	V	I	C
G	U	H	Y	P	O	M	A	C	Y	R	H	C	R	A	C	K	L	E	S
P	N	E	U	L	M	U	E	C	D	Y	Y	U	K	J	J	C	X	W	Q

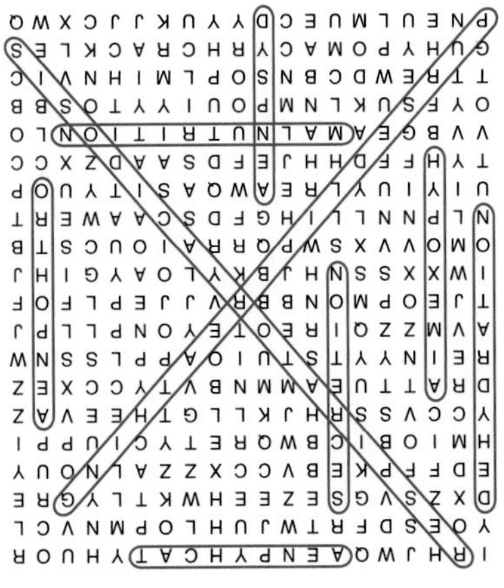

Answers

References

Anderson KN, Anderson LE, Glanze WD: *Mosby's medical, nursing, and allied health dictionary,* ed 5, St Louis, 1998, Mosby.

Duthie EH, *Practice of geriatrics,* ed 3, Philadelphia, 1998, Saunders.

Graber MA: *University of Iowa family practice handbook,* ed 3, St Louis, 1999, Mosby.

Hodgson GB: *Saunders nursing drug handbook 2000,* Philadelphia, 2000, Saunders.

Hostetler MA: *Shock, cardiogenic,* 2004. Available online at www.emedicine.com.

Ignatavicius DD, Workman ML, Mishler MA: *Medical-surgical nursing across the health care continuum,* ed 3, Philadelphia, 1999, Saunders.

Josephson DL: *Intravenous infusion therapy for nurses: principles and practices,* Albany, NY, 2000, Delmar.

Kolecki P: *Shock, hypovolemic,* 2004. Available online at www.emedicine.com.

Valdes E: *University of Iowa family practice handbook,* ed 3, St Louis, 1999, Mosby.

Welk TA: Clinical and ethical considerations of fluid and electrolyte management in the terminally ill patient, *J Intraven Nurs* 22(1):43, 1999.

NCLEX® Review

1. A postoperative patient who has been alert and oriented becomes anxious and confused and is hyperventilating. The most appropriate nursing action is to:
   1 Institute safety precautions.
   2 Orient the patient to surroundings, time, place, and person.
   3 Assess the patient's vital signs.
   4 Calm and reassure the patient.

2. A 57-year-old man presents in the emergency room with a blood pressure of 50/30 mm Hg, pulse of 142 beats per minute, and capillary refill of 4 seconds. The most appropriate fluid replacement is:
   1 D_5W at 125 mL/hr
   2 D½W at 500 mL/hr
   3 5% albumin at open rate
   4 0.9% normal saline or lactated Ringer's solution at open rate

3. Which of the following nursing measures demonstrates that the nurse understands the goal of oxygen therapy for patients with chronic obstructive pulmonary disease (COPD)?
   1 Encourage the patient to take deep breaths.
   2 Administer oxygen at a low (2 L) rate.
   3 Notify the health care provider that the patient is hypoxemic.
   4 Titrate the oxygen rate to maintain carbon dioxide concentration ($PaCO_2$) at 90% or above.

4. Which of the following instructions should the health care practitioner include in his or her dietary instructions to patients with COPD?
   1 Drink a glass of water before eating to help clear secretions.
   2 Restrict fluid intake.
   3 Exercise before eating to increase appetite.
   4 Puree foods and add supplements rich in calories.

5. Mr. Garcia has been diagnosed with heart failure (HF). The health care provider has prescribed diuretics. Which of the following is the most appropriate measure the nurse should include in the patient's instructions?
   1 Notify the health care provider if weight decreases more than 2 pounds in 1 day.
   2 Take a diuretic only when dependent edema is present.
   3 Drink at least eight glasses of water a day.
   4 Hold the diuretic medication if pulse is less than 60 or greater than 120 beats per minute.

6. The therapeutic regimen for a patient with HF includes rest, analgesics, and oxygen therapy. The health care practitioner understands that the purpose of these measures is to:
   1 Increase blood pressure.
   2 Decrease contractility of the heart.
   3 Increase venous return.
   4 Decrease workload on the heart.

NCLEX® Review Answers

1. 3 Altered vital signs will help determine whether the patient is in early shock. Instituting safety precautions is an appropriate action, but the potential for shock is life threatening and requires immediate attention. Confusion is not related to neurologic deficit but is the first sign of hypoxia; thus, there is no need to orient to time, place, surroundings, or person. Shock is a life-threatening event. Immediate intervention is necessary to ensure a positive outcome. Calming and reassuring the patient must be secondary to shock treatment.

2. 4 The patient requires volume expansion; thus you would administer 0.9% normal saline or lactated Ringer's at open rate. D_5W at 125 mL/hr and D1/2W at 500 mL/hr are contraindicated with shock. Although 5% albumin at open rate is hyperosmotic, it contains neither electrolytes nor enough fluid volume to expand the circulatory compartment.

3. 2 Administering oxygen at a low (2 L) rate will promote optimal oxygenation. Encouraging the patient to take deep breaths is contraindicated. Deep breathing tires the patient; the patient does not have the lung function for this action to improve oxygenation. There is no need to notify the health care provider that the patient is hypoxemic because hypoxemia is normal with COPD. Hypoxemia is the primary respiratory stimulus. Titration of the $PaCO_2$ saturation to 90% could disrupt ventilation.

4. 4 Pureeing foods and adding supplements rich in calories to the diet maximizes calorie intake and minimizes effort. Drinking a glass of water before eating promotes a feeling of fullness and decreases the amount of food the patient will eat. Limiting fluids will cause dehydration, which increases the viscosity of secretions, making expectorating difficult. Activities need to be planned throughout the day so the patient with COPD does not become exhausted. Rest is needed before mealtimes to conserve energy for the activity of eating and to promote more consumption.

5. 1 The purpose of diuretics is to promote the excretion of sodium and water and to reduce intravascular volume. Loss of more than 2 pounds in 24 hours can lead to fluid and electrolyte imbalances such as hypokalemia. Diuretics should be taken as prescribed. Blood tests are required to determine the need for a change in prescription. Patients with HF are predisposed to fluid volume overload and may need to restrict fluid intake; thus they would not be encouraged to drink eight glasses of water per day. Diuretics have no direct action on the heart rate and should not be held if pulse is less than 60 or greater than 120 beats per minute; this measure is appropriate for digitalis therapy.

6. 4 Rest reduces metabolic needs and tissue oxygen need. Analgesics relieve pain and promote relaxation. Oxygen therapy increases oxygen saturation. All of these measures effectively reduce the workload of the heart. The higher the blood pressure, the greater the resistance, making the heart work harder to force blood into the vascular system. Increased blood pressure increases the workload on the heart and is not desirable with COPD. The more forceful the contractions of the heart, the more volume of blood is ejected into the circulatory system, increasing tissue perfusion. Decreased contractility requires tissue perfusion. Decreased contractility increases the workload on the heart. Increased venous return increases the workload of the heart with the increased blood volume and can lead to pulmonary congestion.

Notes

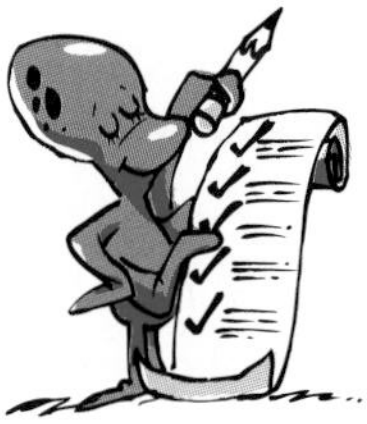

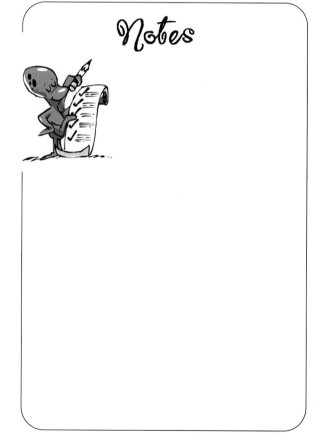

Interventions for Maintaining Fluid and Electrolyte Balance

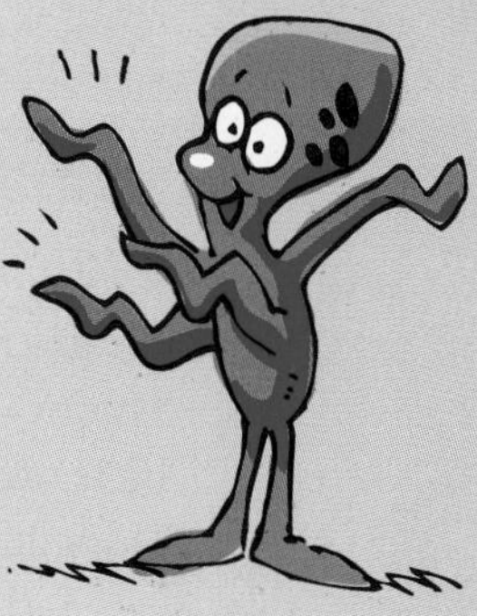

Chapter 16

What You WILL LEARN

After reading this chapter, you will know how to do the following:

- ✔ Identify four patient populations that are candidates for enteral feeding.
- ✔ Identify seven nursing interventions for the patient receiving enteral feedings.
- ✔ Identify four factors that affect the choice of IV solution.
- ✔ Identify four nursing interventions for the patient receiving IV therapy.
- ✔ Identify 11 factors that influence patient selection for dialysis.

Patients who are unable to follow regular diets require interventions to maintain fluid and electrolyte balance. Enteral and parenteral therapy are alternatives to oral intake. Patients with renal failure (see Chapter 14) who are unable to excrete fluid and metabolic wastes need dialysis to maintain proper fluid and electrolyte balance. This chapter examines enteral feeding, intravenous solutions, partial and total parenteral nutrition, and dialysis.

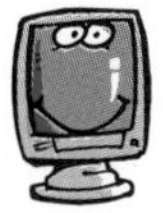

American Society for Parenteral and Enteral Nutrition
www.nutritioncare.org

What IS Enteral Feeding?

Enteral nutrition (**tube feeding**) is the delivery of nutrients directly into the gastrointestinal (GI) tract. Enteral nutrition is used when the patient cannot meet nutritional requirements by normal oral intake, has increased nutritional needs, or is unable to eat. Enteral feeding is more physiologic, easier, cheaper, and safer than parenteral therapy.

What You NEED TO KNOW

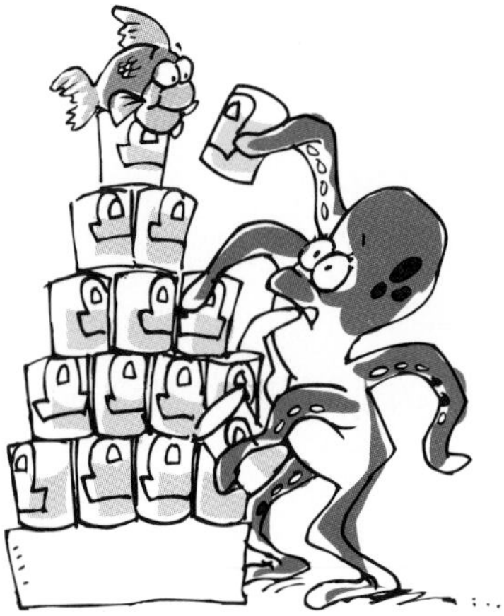

Patients who are candidates for enteral feeding must have a functioning GI tract, cannot maintain adequate oral intake, cannot swallow because of neuromuscular damage, or cannot eat because of the severity of the illness.

Indications for enteral feedings include:

- Inadequate calorie intake
- Severe malnutrition
- Preoperative and postoperative nutrition
- Inability to eat (e.g., cancer of the face, jaw, mouth, throat, esophagus, stomach, and surgery of head and neck).

Contraindications for enteral feedings include disorders in which the GI tract is not intact or needs to be rested (e.g., intestinal obstruction, paralytic ileus, peritonitis, upper-GI bleeding, severe malabsorption diseases, intractable vomiting, diarrhea, increased potential for aspiration of stomach contents).

There are six different categories of enteral feedings available. The choice is based on the nutritional needs of the patient.

1. Standard formulas that require normal digestion (Isocal and Osmolite)
2. Chemically defined formulas that require little or no digestion (Vital High Nitrogen [HN])
3. Special formulas designed for limited function of kidney, liver, and lung (Hepatic Aid II Instant Drink [liver], Pulmocare [lung], and Travasorb Hepatic Diet [kidney])
4. Formulas with increased calories or protein to meet metabolic needs (Ensure HN, Criticare HN, and Megace)

5. Modular formulas that meet single or combined nutrient requirements (MCT oil [fat] and Casec [nitrogen])
6. Blender-processed foods that require complete digestion

Enteral feedings are administered through tubes that are inserted either through the nose and passed into the stomach (nasogastric [NG] tubes) or into the duodenum (NDT) or jejunum (NJT). Nasogastric tubes are used for short-term treatment. Gastrostomy or jejunostomy tubes are used for patients requiring long term feedings. These tubes are percutaneously placed into the stomach or jejunum through the abdomen. This type of placement has a higher risk for infection than the NG placement.

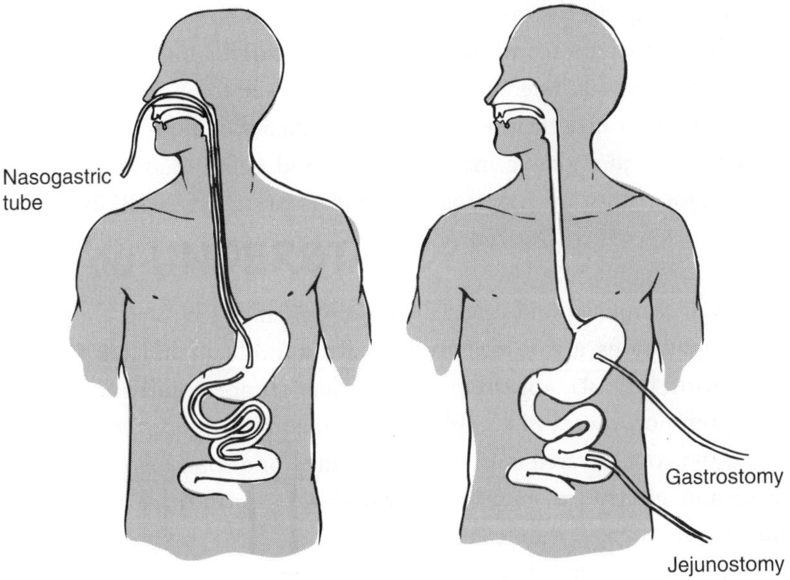

Tube feedings can be administered once by bolusing a small amount through a syringe; intermittently, by infusing a larger amount over a specified interval by gravity or electronic infusion device; or continuously at a low rate by an electronic infusion device.

What You DO

Nursing interventions include the following:

- Assess the GI system. Check for residuals, abdominal distention, pain, and nausea and vomiting.

LIFE SPAN

Older adults, especially women, are at risk for malnutrition because of chronic diseases, decreased intake (food and fluid), medications, poverty, and social isolation.

TAKE HOME POINTS

Raw eggs should not be used in blender-processed food because they may contain salmonella.

TAKE HOME POINTS

Enteral feedings require a functioning GI tract.

There are three enteral feeding delivery methods: bolus, intermittent, and continuous.

Nasogastric tubes are used for short-term therapies.

Gastrostomy tubes are used for long-term therapies.

- Minimize the potential for aspiration. Identify patients at risk for aspiration. Check tube placement and elevate the head of the bed at least 30 degrees during continuous infusion and 30 minutes after each intermittent or bolus infusions.
- Maintain the equipment to minimize formula contamination and loss of feeding tube patency. Allow refrigerated feedings to reach room temperature before administration, flush tube as prescribed, change feeding bag every 24 hours, and fill bag with no more than a 4-hour supply (with continuous infusions). It has been determined that diarrhea is related to bacterial contamination.
- Administer the prescribed flow rate. This action allows physiologic functioning and absorption.
- Maintain hydration with the administration of enteral nutrition.
- Monitor formula tolerance. Every 4 hours, check and record bowel-movement consistency, volume, and frequency. Verify therapy effectiveness by monitoring intake, output, and daily weights, as well as laboratory tests by monitoring blood urea nitrogen (BUN), electrolytes for hyperkalemia and hypernatremia imbalances, and glucose levels.
- Prevent complications, especially aspiration and electrolyte problems.

Complications are related to four areas: problems related to tube placement, formula, digestion, and patient's underlying disease. The most common causes of complications are administration of a formula that is too concentrated or at too rapid a rate, or a combination of both. Fluid and electrolyte imbalance through vomiting, diarrhea, osmotic diuresis, and dehydration can occur.

Hyperkalemia and hypernatremia are common electrolyte imbalances. These conditions are related to hyperglycemia and the resulting increased serum osmolarity and osmotic diuresis. Hypomagnesemia can occur with prolonged diarrhea. With the respiratory-compromised patient, carbon dioxide (CO_2) retention can occur with overfeeding of excessive carbohydrates (excessive carbon dioxide is produced). Check your medical-surgical textbook for a complete review.

- Aspiration of tube contents is a constant threat and can lead to death.
- Do not use microwave ovens to warm feedings.

TAKE HOME POINTS

- Nursing responsibilities are related to equipment maintenance, administration of feeding, and monitoring the patient for tolerance, effectiveness, and potential complications.
- Assessment of gastric motility is essential with enteral feedings.
- Hydration must be maintained with addition to the administration of enteral nutrition. Administer supplemental water.
- Complications occur secondary to tube placement, feeding formulation, digestion, and the underlying disease.

Do You UNDERSTAND?

DIRECTIONS: **Fill in the squares to form a word that is the missing link that connects the given words.**

1.

D	U	O	D		N	U	M										
					A	S	O	G	A	S	T	R	I	C			
					U	B	E										
			J		J	U	N	E	M								
			G		A	V	I	I	Y								
			G		S	T	R	I	C								
			E		E	C	T	R	O	N	I	C	■	P	U	M	P

DIRECTIONS: **Unscramble the following methods for administering enteral feedings.**

2. ______________________ *(sonciutoun)*
3. ______________________ *(retientmittn)*
4. ______________________ *(sobul)*

DIRECTIONS: **Match the complications in column A with the nursing interventions in column B.**

Column A	**Column B**
5. _____ Hyperglycemia and hypoglycemia	a. Large amounts of diarrhea, vomiting, profuse sweating
6. _____ Hyponatremia	b. Dilute formula and increase concentration slowly
7. _____ Hyperosmolar nonketotic syndrome	c. Extra water is needed with elevated temperature, extensive tissue breakdown
8. _____ Hypernatremia	d. Monitor serum glucose levels

Answers: **1. enteral; 2. continuous; 3. intermittent; 4. bolus; 5. d; 6. a; 7. b; 8. c.**

DIRECTIONS: **Complete the nursing measure crossword puzzle on the following page.**

Across

11. For 30 minutes, after completing bolus feeding *(4 words)*
13. Minimize potential for aspiration.
14. To prevent fluid and electrolyte imbalances, administer ________.
17. Off-white, mucus-laden aspirate comes from which body organs?
18. Flush tube to maintain ________.

Down

9. ________ intake and output
10. Measure ________ before administering intermittent feedings.
12. Abbreviation for blood urea nitrogen
13. Infection control measure associated with continuous infusions
15. ________________ flow rate to maintain prescribed flow rate.
16. Measuring ________ is an intervention to monitor excess water loss or gain.

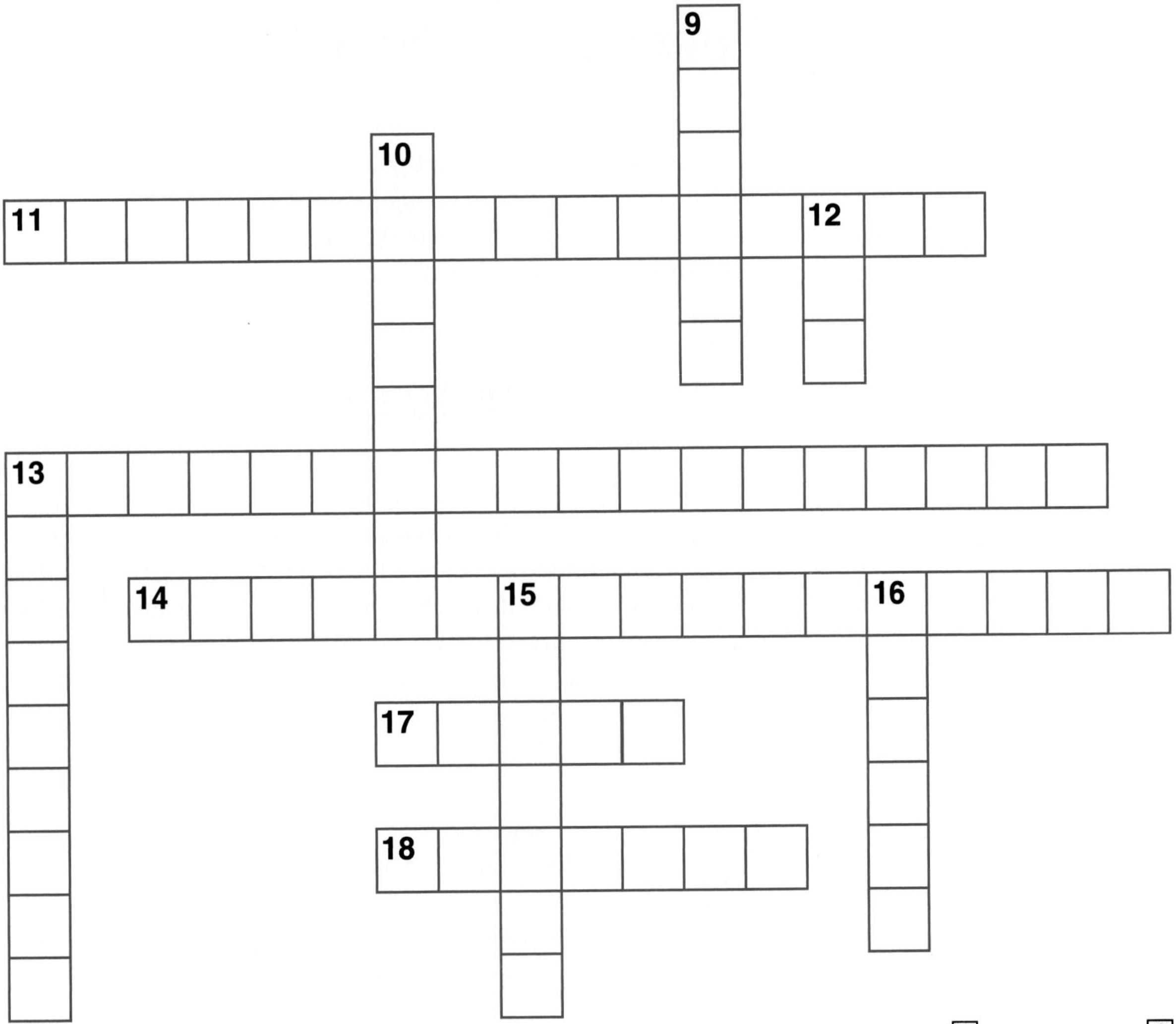
9
10
11
12
13
14
15
16
17
18

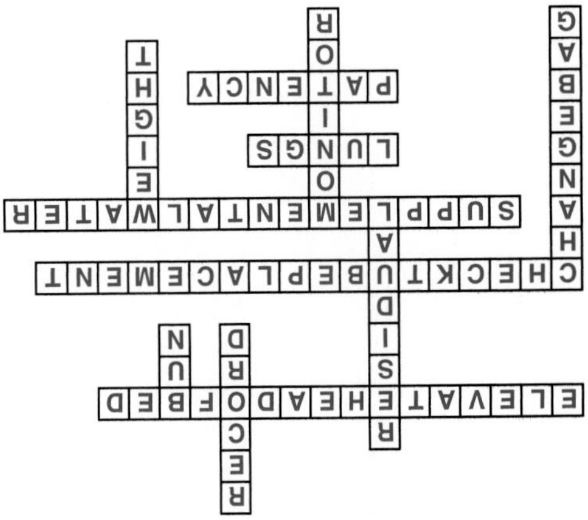
CHANGE BAG
MONITOR
PATENCY
WEIGHT
LUNGS
SUPPLEMENTAL WATER
CHECK TUBE PLACEMENT
RESIDUAL
BUN
RECORD
ELEVATE HEAD OF BED

Answers:

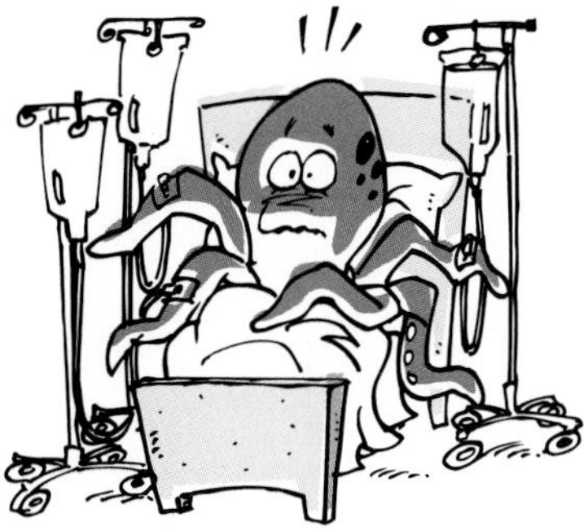

What IS Intravenous Therapy?

Intravenous (IV) *therapy* is the administration of fluids and electrolytes directly into the circulating blood system through a vein.

An IV catheter placed in either a peripheral vein or a central vein is used. The type of therapy, length of therapy, and quality of venous access determines which route is chosen.

What You NEED TO KNOW

The purpose of IV therapy is to maintain daily fluid or electrolyte requirements or replace lost fluids or electrolytes. When patients are unable to meet daily requirements through oral intake, IV fluids are given. Standard IV solutions do not meet daily caloric, protein, or fat requirements. Only solutions containing dextrose have calories. Solutions containing 5% dextrose have 170 calories per 1000 mL. Higher dextrose solutions have more calories (10% dextrose contains 340 calories per 1000 mL). Patient factors that affect the choice of solution include:

- Renal function
- Daily maintenance requirements
- Existing fluid and electrolyte imbalances
- Clinical status

Normal blood osmolarity is approximately 270 to 300 mOsm/L. Osmolarity describes the amount of osmotic pressure exerted by the particles in the solution. Parenteral solutions are classified as hypotonic, isotonic, or hypertonic.

Hypotonic: Osmolarity less than 270 mOsm/L. These solutions cause fluid to shift from the extracellular fluid (ECF) into the intracellular fluid (ICF) and interstitial spaces. Hypotonic solutions decrease the intravascular volume. An example is 0.45% NaCl.

Isotonic: Osmolarity between 270 and 340 mOsm/L. These solutions expand the ECF. Examples are 0.9% NaCl, lactated Ringer's (LR).

Hypertonic: Osmolarity less than 340 mOsm/L. These solutions are used to replace electrolytes and shift fluid from the interstitial spaces into the ECF (3% NaCl).

Dextrose solutions: Dextrose solutions do not contain electrolytes unless combined with an electrolyte solution. After the dextrose is rapidly metabolized, these solutions become less tonic, and the osmolarity effect is changed into an effect similar to nondextrose solutions. Once the dextrose is metabolized, only water remains. Continual administration of dextrose solutions can lead to electrolyte imbalances and water intoxication.

Osmolarity at the time of administration is:

D_5W and D_5 0.225% NaCl—isotonic
D_{10}, D_5 0.9% NaCl, D_5 0.45% NaCl, D_5 RL—hypertonic

Parenteral solutions can be either crystalloid or colloid.

Crystalloid solutions form a true solution and can pass through a semipermeable membrane. Crystalloids must be given in three to four times the volume to expand the vascular space. Examples include dextrose solutions, saline solutions, lactated Ringer's, Ringer's, and sodium bicarbonate.

Colloid solutions do not dissolve completely and do not pass through a semipermeable membrane. Examples include dextran, albumin, and artificial blood substitutes (hetastarch).

IV solutions can be administered continuously using large-volume solutions (250 to 1000 mL); over 2 to 24 hours; intermittently, using small volume solutions (50 to 100 mL); by piggyback or secondary infusions; with an as needed (PRN) adapter administered over 30 minutes to 2 hours; or using a direct IV push of an extremely small volume.

LIFE SPAN

Older patients have decreased adipose tissue and decreased skin elasticity, making veins difficult to stabilize for venipuncture. The veins are fragile and require changes in technique, such as using a blood pressure cuff rather than a tourniquet to puncture and cannulate the vein successfully.

Common Intravenous Solutions

Solution	Indications	Precautions	Incompatibilities
D_5W	Replace water and low-calorie needs Dehydration Hyperkalemia Spares body protein; provides nutrition	Do not use in head trauma (increases cerebral edema) Can cause water intoxication if used with early postoperative patient or continuously Do not use with fluid overload (CHF) Contraindicated with diabetes	Whole blood Ampicillin Erythromycin Warfarin Fat emulsions Sodium bicarbonate Dilantin (phenytoin) B_{12}

Continued

Common Intravenous Solutions—cont'd

Solution	Indications	Precautions	Incompatibilities
0.9% saline	Replace ECF Hyponatremia Hypochloremia Water overload Mild metabolic acidosis Medication diluent IV irrigant Compatible with blood	Does not contain any free water or calories Can cause fluid overload Can cause hypokalemia Can cause hypernatremia Can cause hyperchloremic acidosis Administered cautiously to those with renal or circulatory impairment, to older adults, and to those with sodium retention (CHF) or glucocorticoids (causes sodium retention)	Amphotericin B Mannitol Diazepam Fat emulsion Chlordiazepoxide Methylprednisolone Warfarin Whole blood Ampicillin Erythromycin
D_5 0.45% NaCl	Rehydrate; has free water, salt, and calories	Use caution with CHF, pulmonary edema, urinary obstruction, steroid therapy May falsely elevate BUN level Contraindicated with diabetic coma	Amphotericin B Mannitol Diazepam
Ringer's	Replacement of fluid and electrolytes (dehydration, vomiting, diarrhea, burns) Volume expander Contains no calories	Do not use with CHF, renal insufficiency, or sodium retention Does not contain enough potassium or calcium to be used as a maintenance fluid	Ampicillin Cefamandole Diazepam Erythromycin Methicillin Potassium Phosphate Sodium bicarbonate Whole blood
Lactated Ringer's	Resembles blood serum No free water Rehydration Burns, dehydration, DKA, salicylate overdose	Can cause hypernatremia, hyperkalemia Can exacerbate CHF, edema, and sodium retention Contraindicated with liver disease, Addison's disease, severe metabolic acidosis and alkalosis, profound hypovolemia and hyperkalemia	Ampicillin Cefamandole Diazepam Erythromycin Phosphate Sodium bicarbonate

BUN, Blood urea nitrogen; *CHF*, cardiac heart failure; *IV*, intravenous; *DKA*, diabetic ketoacidosis; *ECF*, extracellular fluid.

Comparison of Intravenous Delivery Methods

Advantages	Disadvantages
CONTINUOUS	
Constant serum levels can be maintained	Drug incompatibility Accidental bolus infusion (fluid overload) Flow rate can be erratic if not infused with an electronic flow device
INTERMITTENT	
Risk for incompatibilities reduced Large drug doses can be administered at a lower concentration per milliliter Decreased risk of fluid overload	Potential for speed shock when accidentally infused at a rapid rate Loss of venous access because of catheter dislodging or occlusion from improper flushing Phlebitis
BOLUS	
Rapid results Ability to monitor response	Speed shock Phlebitis

TAKE HOME POINTS

- Standard IV solutions replace fluids and electrolytes.
- Solutions containing dextrose provide some calories.
- Standard IV solutions do not meet nutritional requirements.
- Renal function, daily maintenance requirements, existence of fluid and electrolyte imbalances, and clinical status influence solution selection.

- Do not administer hypotonic solutions to patients with low blood pressure, as this will worsen hypotension.
- Hypertonic osmolarity solutions are extremely irritating to veins. Administer slowly to prevent hypervolemia.

What You DO

The health care provider should understand all aspects of parenteral therapy. These aspects include indications, expected outcomes, complications, and appropriate interventions required to achieve positive outcomes. Specific actions include the following:

- Administer IV fluids at the prescribed rate.
- Monitor vital signs, intake and output, daily weight, and blood chemistry.
- Monitor the IV site and administration set at least every 2 hours and more frequently with patients who are at risk for potential complications (the best intervention for preventing complications).

  Phlebitis: Inflammation of the lining of the vein. Irritation is caused by chemical (solution or drug), mechanical (catheter size or placement, restraints, or tape over tip of catheter), or bacterial (lack of aseptic techniques) causes. The site will be tender with red streaks, swelling,

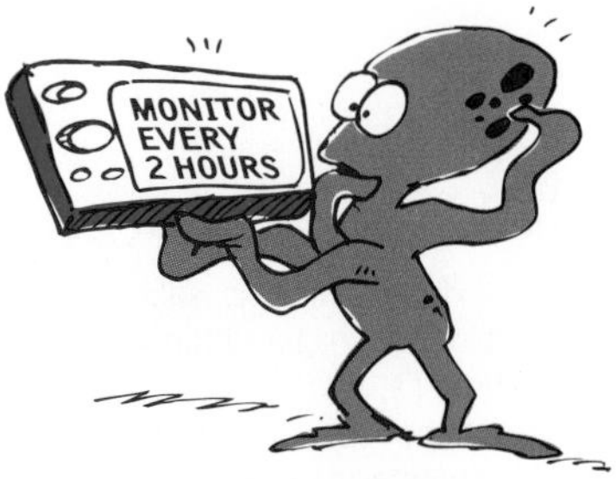

Remember to monitor the IV site, rate, and check type of solution at least every 2 hours for standard IV fluids. More frequent monitoring is required when solutions are mixed with medications.

TAKE HOME POINTS

- Solutions are categorized by how their osmolality compares with normal blood osmolarity. The same is known as isotonic; higher is known as hypertonic; or lower is known as hypotonic.
- The osmolarity of parenteral solutions determines whether the blood volume is expanded, remains constant, or is decreased.
- Dextrose solutions contain some calories but no electrolytes.
- Continuous administration of dextrose solutions can lead to electrolyte imbalances and water intoxication.

and/or cord (feels hard to touch like a piece of cord). Routine site rotation for 96 hours is performed to limit the occurrence of phlebitis. Always use the smallest catheter in the largest vein.

Infiltration: Fluid escaping the vein into surrounding tissue. If the fluid is a vesicant, the common term is extravasation. To identify infiltration, apply pressure 3 inches above the insertion site. If the IV flow continues to run, infiltration has occurred. The presence of blood return is not a sign of vein integrity. Preventive actions include routinely checking the site, avoiding bony prominences for the insertion site, and never placing any restraints or tight clothing over or above an infusion site.

Fluid overload: Caused by too rapid an infusion rate for the body's compensatory mechanisms.

Sepsis: Systemic blood infection. Factors that increase the risk for sepsis are the lack of aseptic technique, an immunocompromised patient, the number of manipulations of the central venous catheter, the jugular placement, poor dressing management, and a contaminated fluid or administration set. Preventive measures that minimize sepsis risk are routine dressing changes and the use of strict aseptic techniques in all aspects of IV care.

Do You UNDERSTAND?

DIRECTIONS: **Match the solutions in column A with the appropriate corresponding descriptions in column B.**

Column A	Column B
1. _____ D_5W	a. Does not contain free water
2. _____ Normal saline	b. True solution
3. _____ D_5 1/2NS	c. 230 to 350 mOsm/L
4. _____ Lactated Ringer's	d. Do not use with head trauma
5. _____ Ringer's	e. Resembles blood serum
6. _____ Crystalloid	f. Less than 375 mOsm/L
7. _____ Colloid	g. Do not use with cardiac heart failure
8. _____ Isotonic	h. May falsely elevate BUN
9. _____ Hypertonic	i. Less than 250 mOsm/L
10. _____ Hypotonic	j. Dextran

TAKE HOME POINTS

- Dextrose solutions, saline solutions, lactated Ringer's, Ringer's, and sodium bicarbonate can pass through a semipermeable membrane.
- Dextran and albumin increase intravascular osmotic pressure because they cannot pass through a semipermeable membrane.

Answers: 1. d; 2. a; 3. h; 4. e; 5. g; 6. b; 7. j; 8. c; 9. f; 10. i.

DIRECTIONS: Unscramble the following jumbled nursing measures necessary with patients receiving IV therapy.

11. ______________________ *(sternimiad dliufs ta pcreisbred tera)*
12. ______________________ *(troimon vi tise)*
13. ______________________ *(crerod kineat nad tupout)*
14. ______________________ *(laidy thewisg)*

Never play catch-up with IV fluids.

DIRECTIONS: Match the following complications in column A to the appropriate associated nursing measure in column B.

Column A	Column B
15. _____ Phlebitis	a. Monitor venous distention
16. _____ Infiltration	b. Monitor vital signs
17. _____ Fluid overload	c. Restart IV
18. _____ Sepsis	d. Cold compress

TAKE HOME POINTS

- Monitor IV insertion site at least every 2 hours and more frequently if patient is at risk for infiltration or phlebitis.
- Administer fluids at the prescribed rate. Never play catch-up.
- Monitor vital signs, intake and output, daily weights, and blood chemistry to determine therapy effectiveness and potential complications.
- Common complications associated with IV therapy are infiltration, phlebitis, fluid overload, and sepsis.

What IS Parenteral Nutrition?

Parenteral nutrition is a complex mixture of dextrose (carbohydrate), amino acids (protein), lipids (fats), electrolytes, vitamins, and trace elements that promotes tissue synthesis, repair, and growth. This specialized formulation is used as a source of nutrition for patients who are unable to ingest or use enough food to maintain metabolic function. Parenteral nutrition is administered intravenously either through peripheral or central veins. There are two major types of parenteral nutrition: peripheral parenteral nutrition and total parenteral nutrition.

What You NEED TO KNOW

The goals of parenteral nutrition are to sustain nutritional balance when oral or enteral routes are not acceptable, to preserve or restore positive nitrogen balance, to prevent malnutrition, and to promote wound healing and correct nutritional deficits.

Answers: **11. administer fluids at prescribed rate; 12. monitor IV site; 13. record intake and output; 14. daily weights; 15. c; 16. d; 17. a; 18. b.**

Peripheral parenteral nutrition (PPN) is for short-term use, with the patient being able to eat again in 7 to 10 days. PPN is supplemental nutrition to prevent malnourishment. The dextrose content of PPN is 5% to 10%, allowing it to be infused through a peripheral vein. Examples are Procal and Amine. PPN is not nutritionally complete. The low dextrose content does not provide sufficient calories to increase body mass. PPN should not be used with volume-restricted patients.

Patient criteria include the following:

- Maintained on less than 2400 calories/day
- Good nutritional status and no required weight gain
- NPO but no fluid restriction
- No option of central venous access
- PPN is used before *total parenteral nutrition* is started or after it is discontinued

Total parenteral nutrition (TPN) is for long-term nutrition support (more than 14 days). TPN is a high-caloric formulation (dextrose content of 20% to 70%) that is nutritionally complete, reverses starvation, and promotes tissue synthesis. A central vein is required for administration because of the high dextrose content. Patients on TPN are more prone to fluid and electrolyte imbalances than patients on PPN.

Patient criteria include the following:

- Requires more calories than can be obtained with PPN
- Has long-term poor nutritional status
- Has weight loss greater than 10%
- Has increased metabolic needs (for burns and trauma)
- Requires bowel rest (for pancreatitis, inflammatory bowel disease, and bowel obstruction)
- Is unable to eat (as with cancer or coma)
- Will not eat (as with anorexia nervosa)

Comparison of Peripheral and Total Parenteral Nutrition

PPN	TPN
Short-term	Long-term
Dextrose content 5%-10%	Dextrose content 20%-70%
Administered through peripheral vein	Administered through central vein
Not nutritionally complete	Nutritionally complete

Nitrogen balance is the cornerstone of monitoring the therapy effectiveness of parenteral nutrition. Nitrogen balance is the relationship between the intake of nitrogen and its excretion in urine and feces. Positive nitrogen balance occurs when there is a greater intake of nitrogen than is excreted. Tissue synthesis can occur with positive nitrogen balance. Negative nitrogen balance occurs when more nitrogen is excreted than is taken in. Tissue destruction and muscle wasting occurs with negative nitrogen balance.

Individuals on TPN are prone to fluid and electrolyte imbalances.

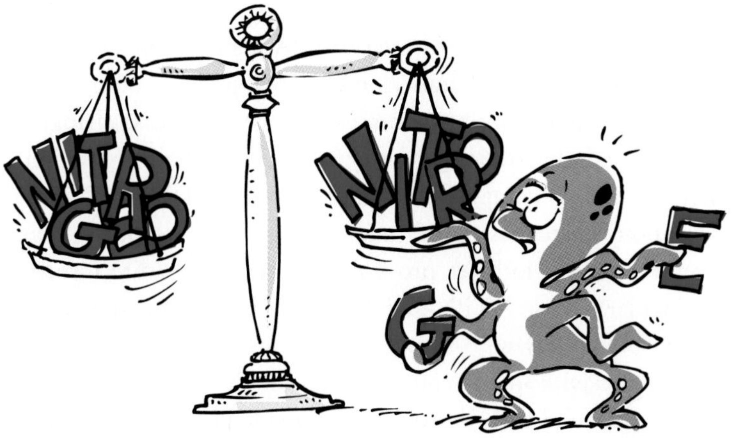

It is important to monitor the nitrogen balance of those receiving parenteral nutrition.

TAKE HOME POINTS

- PPN should not be used with a volume-restricted patient.
- PPN is prescribed for short-term use with patients who need some support to prevent malnourishment.
- TPN is prescribed for long-term use to promote tissue synthesis and overcome malnourishment.

What You DO

Because the goal of parenteral therapy is nutritional support, establishing baseline data of the patient's condition before beginning the therapy is important. The health care provider should:

- **Gather baseline data.** These data should include weight, height, white blood count with percent of lymphocytes, BUN level, hemoglobin and hematocrit, and blood chemistry. These baseline findings will be compared with the patient's ongoing condition to determine response to therapy, nitrogen balance, fluid and electrolyte balance, and the presence of infection.
- **Obtain daily weights.** Weight gain may be a result of fluid retention or tissue growth. Weight loss may be a result of hypovolemia or insufficient calories. Acceptable weight gain for a patient on TPN is 1 pound per day.
- **Monitor vital signs, intake and output, serum glucose, and blood chemistry to determine the state of nitrogen balance.** Changes in

any of these parameters may be an early indicator of complications, as well as fluid and electrolyte imbalances.

- **Maintain prescribed infusion rate.** Too rapid or too slow a rate may result in complications such as hyperglycemia or hypoglycemia, circulatory overload, and other fluid and electrolyte imbalances. TPN solutions should be initiated and discontinued at a gradual rate. An electronic infusion pump is required for the administration of TPN.
- **Maintain infection control measures.** A high glucose concentration of TPN provides a medium for bacterial growth. Some measures include changing solution containers every 24 hours, changing the routine IV administration set every 72 hours (24 hours with lipids) or when integrity is compromised (the Centers for Disease Control and Prevention guidelines), and maintaining strict aseptic technique. A central venous catheter provides bacteria with a direct entry into the vascular system. A TPN line should not be used for any other infusions or blood draws.

Patients receiving parenteral nutrition are at risk for complications associated with fluid and electrolyte imbalances. Identification of patients at risk for developing complications is important. Some examples include:

- Very young patients
- Older adults
- Patients with glucose intolerance
- Patients with impaired renal function
- Patients with fistulas
- Intubated patients
- Patients receiving diuretics or steroids

Complications associated with parenteral nutrition are grouped into three categories:

Metabolic: Because a patient's condition is neither stagnant nor totally predictable, imbalances can occur at any time. Some common imbalances are overhydration or underhydration, hyperkalemia or hypokalemia, hypernatremia or hyponatremia, hyperglycemia or hypoglycemia (glucose metabolism), mineral imbalances (especially related to elevated or below normal phosphorous, magnesium, and calcium), and nutritional imbalances related to overfeeding or underfeeding of proteins, carbohydrates, and fats.

Common Fluid and Electrolyte Imbalances with TPN

Imbalance	Cause	Intervention	Tip
Altered hydration	Overhydration or underhydration Osmolarity of formula	Accurate intake and output Daily weights Skin assessment Monitor BUN, Na+, H & H.	Weigh with same scale and with comparable clothing weight.
Hypokalemia	Metabolic acidosis Osmotic diuresis Increased need for tissue repair	Increase K+ in formulation.	Insulin should not be administered unless serum potassium level is within normal range.
Hypophosphatemia	Respiratory alkalosis Excessive glucose in formula Inadequate replacement	Increase amount in formulation.	Phosphorus is necessary for production of cell energy.
Hypoglycemia	Abrupt disruption of infusion	Gradually initiate and discontinue infusion. Maintain steady rate of infusion once maintenance flow rate is obtained.	Monitor Accucheck. Ensure connections within system. Danger: If disruption of TPN occurs for any reason, start infusion of $D_{10}W$ until TPN infusion is restarted. Do not rely on infusion pump. Compare amount left in container with amount infused.
Hyperglycemia (common)	Carbohydrate intolerance Rapid TPN infusion Sepsis Stress Hypokalemia	Decrease dextrose content. Increase calories from fat. Decrease rate of administration. Administer sliding-scale insulin. Monitor blood glucose.	Danger: Potential for hyperglycemic hyperosmolar nonketotic coma
Acid base imbalances	Improper formulation for metabolic needs	Change formulation.	Lead to fluid and electrolyte imbalances.
Hypercalcemia	Excessive replacement	Alter formulation.	Nausea and vomiting can cause additional fluid and electrolyte imbalances.

TAKE HOME POINTS

- Tissue synthesis can occur with positive nitrogen balance.
- Monitoring daily weight, BUN, and blood chemistry is necessary to determine whether positive nitrogen balance is being maintained.
- Ongoing assessment and monitoring of patients receiving parenteral nutrition are required to prevent metabolic complications.
- Proper care of the solution, administration set and central venous catheter can help prevent technical and septic complications.

Technical: Related to the central venous catheter (e.g., air embolism, occlusion, pneumothorax).

Septic: Related to the care and maintenance of the administration system (solution, administration set, and central venous catheter) that can cause bacterial, fungal, or viral contamination.

Do You UNDERSTAND?

DIRECTIONS: **Place either PPN or TPN next to the appropriate statement.**

1. _____ Short-term use
2. _____ Supports tissue synthesis
3. _____ Requires a central line
4. _____ Dextrose content 5% to 10%
5. _____ Long-term use
6. _____ Can be given through a peripheral IV
7. _____ Nutritionally complete
8. _____ NPO but no fluid restriction
9. _____ Bowel rest
10. _____ Nutritionally incomplete

Answers: 1. PPN; 2. TPN; 3. TPN; 4. PPN; 5. TPN; 6. PPN; 7. TPN; 8. PPN; 9. TPN; 10. PPN.

DIRECTIONS: Find the words related to parenteral nutrition.

DAILY WEIGHTS	**GLUCOSE TESTING**
BLOOD CHEMISTRIES	**NITROGEN BALANCE**
ASEPTIC TECHNIQUE	**CONCENTRATION TOLERANCE**
BACTERIAL MEDIUM	

A	A	S	E	P	T	I	C	T	E	C	H	N	I	Q	U	E	S	R	T
D	U	A	I	O	N	T	I	C	V	E	C	H	G	U	L	E	M	E	A
A	M	N	U	I	E	E	U	Q	I	N	U	Y	N	T	I	R	E	D	R
I	C	H	J	K	C	I	O	P	P	O	K	J	I	R	H	Y	G	T	F
L	M	H	J	K	L	O	I	H	F	D	S	E	T	S	X	C	V	B	N
Y	O	P	M	B	C	X	N	Z	C	V	B	S	N	M	M	L	K	J	H
W	G	F	D	S	E	R	T	C	Y	U	I	E	U	U	I	O	L	P	O
E	L	K	K	J	M	J	H	B	E	M	F	T	Y	T	O	A	S	D	Z
I	O	O	N	I	T	R	O	G	E	N	B	A	L	A	N	C	E	R	G
G	E	W	R	T	E	A	S	H	P	U	T	I	O	N	I	M	G	E	I
H	K	L	Z	X	C	V	C	U	O	Q	M	R	P	U	I	O	N	C	T
T	U	M	O	P	C	D	Z	X	V	O	M	O	A	P	L	L	F	N	D
S	Q	I	I	B	O	V	B	O	P	K	I	U	N	T	V	C	C	A	X
G	L	U	C	O	S	E	T	E	S	T	I	N	G	O	I	M	V	R	B
Q	W	S	L	E	D	R	F	T	G	H	Y	H	U	J	I	O	K	E	P
Z	A	B	S	X	D	C	F	V	G	D	B	H	N	J	M	K	N	L	M
L	P	K	O	J	I	H	U	G	Y	F	T	D	R	S	E	A	W	O	Z
B	A	C	T	E	R	I	A	L	M	E	D	I	U	M	I	O	N	T	S

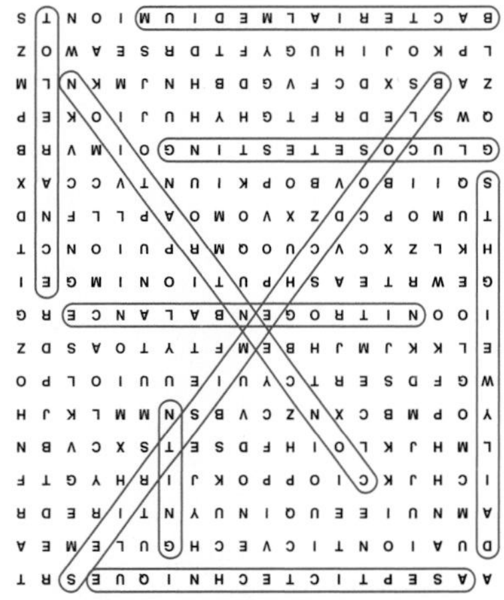

Answers:

DIRECTIONS: Complete the following equation:

11. Nitrogen intake that is ____________________ *(greater or less)* than nitrogen excretion = positive nitrogen balance.

DIRECTIONS: Fill in the blanks.

12. Monitoring ______________ ___________, ________, and ______________ ______________ is necessary to determine whether positive nitrogen balance is being maintained.
13. Proper care of the solution, administration set, and central venous catheter can help prevent ____________________________ and ____________________________ complications.

What IS Dialysis?

Kidney Dialysis Foundation
kdf.org.sg

Dialysis is a therapeutic process to replace the waste-excretion function of the renal system. Dialysis removes excess fluid and waste products while restoring fluid and electrolyte balance.

What You NEED TO KNOW

There are two methods of dialysis: hemodialysis and peritoneal dialysis. Each method replicates the physiologic diffusion and osmosis processes of the renal system by using an alternate filtration system. Hemodialysis removes wastes at a faster rate than peritoneal dialysis.

Patient selection includes the following:

- Creatinine greater than 0.9 mg/dL (severe renal failure)
- Poison removal
- Excessive drug removal
- Correction of serious electrolyte and/or acid-base imbalances
- End-stage renal failure

Dialysis is initiated when:

- Diuretics do not affect fluid overload.
- Severe hyperkalemia is present.
- Pericarditis is present.

Answers: 11. greater; 12. daily weights, BUN, blood chemistry. 13. technical, septic.

- Uncontrolled hypertension is present.
- Neurologic symptoms are present and progressive (confusion).
- General renal failure symptom progression (vomiting, anemia, or pruritus) is present.

Short-term risks for dialysis include electrolyte imbalance, shock, infection, and emotional distress. Longer-term risks include anemia, hypotension, neurologic complications, pericarditis, osteodystrophy, and peritonitis.

The most common complications of hemodialysis are hypotension and leg cramps, which are caused by the rapid changes in fluid and electrolyte imbalances. Other complications include infection, cardiac dysrhythmias, hemolysis, and hypoxemia.

The most common complications of peritoneal dialysis are peritonitis, hyperglycemia, and respiratory distress. Complications related to the catheter include sluggish fill and emptying times, dialysate leakage, and bowel perforation.

TAKE HOME POINTS

- Dialysis is a process whereby fluids and waste excretion are removed from the blood, restoring chemical and electrolyte balance.
- Dialysis is used when the renal system is ineffective.
- Both hemodialysis and peritoneal dialysis use diffusion and osmosis through a semipermeable membrane to remove metabolic wastes and fluid from the body.

What You DO

Nursing responsibilities involve assessing the effectiveness of the dialysis process and monitoring for potential complications. Maintaining optimal fluid volume balance and minimizing symptoms are primary goals of nursing interventions. Complications are possible but preventable with careful nursing care.

Specific interventions include the following:

- Weigh before and after dialysis.
- Monitor vital signs before and after dialysis. Changes may be the initial sign of complications.
- Evaluate electrolyte and glucose values before and after dialysis.
- With hemodialysis, observe the patient for bleeding during dialysis and for 1 hour after dialysis. Heparin is given prophylactically to avoid the formation of blood clots within the dialyzer membrane and tubing.
- Assess the dialysis catheter site for redness, swelling, and discharge. These are early signs of catheter site infection that can be a precursor to sepsis.
- With peritoneal dialysis, observe the color and consistency of drainage. Normal drainage is clear. Initial returns may be bloody until

the peritoneum adjusts to the process. Color denotes the type of drainage. Cloudy or opaque drainage is the most common change, which is a sign of peritonitis. Brown drainage is a sign of bowel perforation. Clear yellow drainage is a sign of bladder perforation.

TAKE HOME POINTS

- Nursing responsibilities involve assessing the effectiveness of dialysis and monitoring for potential complications.
- The most common complications with hemodialysis are hypotension and leg cramps.
- The most common complications with peritoneal dialysis are peritonitis, hyperglycemia, and respiratory distress.
- There is a potential for hemorrhage with hemodialysis.
- It is important to observe the color and consistency of peritoneal dialysis drainage. Cloudy or opaque peritoneal dialysis drainage is the most common sign of peritonitis.

Do You UNDERSTAND?

DIRECTIONS: **Unscramble these words related to dialysis.**

1. ______________________________ *(triflaiont)*
2. ______________________________ *(dialhemsosey)*
3. ______________________________ *(retioplean ticavy)*
4. ______________________________ *(merpmiesbeale neambrem)*
5. ______________________________ *(ssmoois)*
6. ______________________________ *(sifufidon)*

DIRECTIONS: **Fill in the blank.**

7. Dialysis is initiated when ____________ ____________ does not respond to diuretics, severe ____________ or ____________ or pericarditis is present, hypertension is ____________, or with ____________ ____________ in symptom progression.
8. A creatinine greater than 0.9 mg/dL denotes ____________ renal failure.
9. The most common complications of hemodialysis are ____________ and ____________ ____________.
10. The most common complications of peritoneal dialysis are ____________, ____________, and ____________ ____________.
11. Nursing responsibilities involve ____________ the effectiveness of the dialysis process and ____________ for potential complications.

Answers: **1. filtration; 2. hemodialysis; 3. peritoneal cavity; 4. semipermeable membrane; 5. osmosis; 6. diffusion; 7. severe overload, hyperkalemia, hypercalcemia, uncontrolled, renal failure; 8. severe; 9. hypotension, leg cramps; 10. peritonitis, hyperglycemia, respiratory distress; 11. assessing, monitoring.**

References

Hanchett M: Infusion outcome analysis in the new millennium: what advanced practitioners need to know, *J Vascul Access Devices* 6(1):18, 2001.

Hand H: Continuing professional development: fluid management: the use of intravenous therapy, *Geriatr Nurs Home Care* 11(9):43, 2001.

Hankins J et al: *Infusion therapy in clinical practice*, ed 2, Philadelphia, 2001, Saunders.

Ignatavicius DD, Workman ML: *Medical-surgical nursing critical thinking for collaborative care,* ed 4, St Louis, 2002, Saunders.

Josephson DL: *Intravenous infusion therapy for nurses: principles and practices,* ed 2, Albany, NY, 2004, Delmar.

Klotz RS: The effects of intravenous solutions on fluid and electrolyte balance, *J Intraven Nursing* 21(1):20, 1998.

Macklin D: Phlebitis, *Am J Nurs* 103(2):55, 2003.

Macklin D, Chernecky C: *IV therapy,* St Louis, 2004, Saunders.

Notes

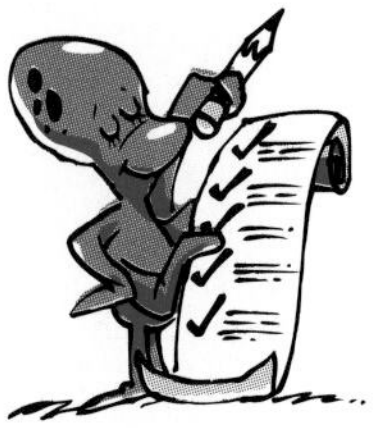

NCLEX® Review

1. A patient is receiving an IV solution of $D_5$1/2 normal saline at 125 mL/hr continuously. The urinary output for the past 2 hours equals 23 mL. The most appropriate action for the staff is to:
   1 Check the IV site for infiltration.
   2 Decrease the rate of the IV fluid.
   3 Increase the rate of IV fluid.
   4 Notify the physician.

2. Which of the following is the most likely cause of a patient developing diarrhea when being fed enterally?
   1 Concentration of the formula is too high.
   2 Feedings are too cold.
   3 The patient is overhydrated with too much water.
   4 Rate of infusion is too fast.

3. Which of the following patients is the most appropriate candidate for TPN?
   1 A 54-year-old man with chronic renal failure
   2 A 26-year-old woman with an acute exacerbation of inflammatory bowel disease
   3 A 58-year-old woman who has been held NPO (nothing by mouth) for 3 days postoperatively.
   4 A 35-year-old man with uncontrolled diabetes

4. Immediately after completion of hemodialysis, the patient attempts to get out of bed and becomes weak and unsteady. The most likely cause is:
   1 Hepatitis
   2 Hyperglycemia
   3 Hypovolemia
   4 Infection

5. Which of the following nursing measures is most appropriate for patients receiving peritoneal dialysis?
   1 Administer anticoagulant before initiation of dialysis exchange.
   2 Aspirate contents to confirm catheter placement.
   3 Monitor serum glucose.
   4 Palpate access site for a thrill or bruit.

6. The best nursing measure to prevent aspiration as a result of tube feedings is to:
   1 Elevate the head of the bed at least 30 degrees.
   2 Offer fluids every 2 hours.
   3 Turn, cough, and breathe deeply every 3 hours.
   4 Warm the feedings to room temperature.

7. What is the cornerstone of monitoring the therapy effectiveness of parenteral nutrition?

8. The health care practitioner observes that the peritoneal dialysis drainage is cloudy. This is a sign of which of the following:
   1 Bladder perforation
   2 Bowel perforation
   3 Normal drainage
   4 Peritonitis

9. Which of the following parenteral solutions increases intravascular osmotic pressure?
   1 0.45% NaCl
   2 Dextran
   3 D_5W
   4 Ringer's

10. Which of the following statements is true?
    1 Both hemodialysis and peritoneal dialysis use diffusion and osmosis through a semipermeable membrane to remove metabolic wastes and fluid from the body.
    2 Dialysis is a process whereby fluids and waste excretion are replaced in the blood, which maintains chemical and electrolyte balance.
    3 Dialysis is used only when the renal system is effective.
    4 Peritoneal dialysis removes wastes and fluids at a faster rate than hemodialysis.

11. What are the two most common electrolyte imbalances related to enteral feeding?

12. Which type of IV fluid decreases the intravascular volume?

13. True or False: It is important to keep IV fluids infusing as prescribed. When fluids are running behind, you should increase the rate until the infusion is caught up.

14. True or False: PPN is nutritionally complete.

15. True or False: TPN Patients on TPN are more prone to fluid and electrolyte imbalances.

NCLEX® Review Answers

1. **4** The patient presents with decreased output, and immediate medical intervention is required. Although monitoring the IV site is important, the patient is in acute distress. Although it is true that the patient does not need additional fluid, the low output requires immediate medical intervention. The patient demonstrates a fluid imbalance. Increasing the rate of the IV increases the fluid intake and contributes to the potential for fluid volume overload.

2. **1** Concentrated formulas pull fluid into the intestine, causing diarrhea. Temperature of the feedings contributes to discomfort and hypothermia. Hydration with water increases urinary output. Although the infusion rate may affect absorption, diarrhea does not always occur.

3. **2** Acute bowel disease is an indication for bowel rest and requires replacement of calories to maintain positive nitrogen balance. Chronic renal failure does not impair a person's ability to eat or require excess caloric intake. Short-term nutritional support is not an indication for TPN, but rather an indication for PPN. Diabetes does not impair a patient's ability to eat or require excess caloric intake.

4. **3** Excess fluid loss from dialysis is a common complication and is reflected with hypotension. The signs and symptoms of hepatitis are not related to dialysis. Hyperglycemia is not a complication of hemodialysis. Although generalized weakness is a symptom of infection, currently, there are no other findings to support this option. Because the weakness occurred immediately after completion of dialysis, it is probably a sign of hypovolemia as a result of dialysis.

5. **3** Glucose may be absorbed from the dialysate during exchanges. Anticoagulants are given with hemodialysis to prevent clot formation as the blood passes through the dialyzer and tubing. Aspiration of contents confirms nasogastric tube placement. Palpation of the access site for a thrill or bruit indicates an arteriovenous shunt or graft for hemodialysis, not peritoneal dialysis.

6. **1** Elevating the head of the bed prevents the backflow of fluids into the respiratory system. Fluid management does not prevent risk for aspiration. The patient is at the greatest risk for aspiration during the feeding process. Temperature of the feedings does not prevent the risk for aspiration.

7. Nitrogen balance.

8. **4** Cloudy drainage is a sign of infection from the peritoneal cavity. Clear, yellow drainage is a sign of bladder perforation. Brown drainage is a sign of bowel perforation. Clear drainage is a sign of normal drainage.

9. **2** Dextran is a colloid solution that does not dissolve completely and does not pass through a semipermeable membrane. 0.45% NaCl is

a hypotonic, crystalloid solution that causes fluid to shift from the ECF into the ICF and interstitial spaces and decreases the intravascular volume. D_5W is a crystalloid, isotonic solution that expands into the ECF. Ringer's is a crystalloid solution that passes through a semipermeable membrane.

10. 1 Each method replicates the physiologic diffusion and osmosis processes of the renal system by using an alternate filtration system. Dialysis removes fluids and waste excretion, restoring chemical and electrolyte balance. Dialysis is used when the renal system is ineffective. Hemodialysis removes wastes and fluids at a faster rate than peritoneal dialysis.

11. Hyperkalemia and hypernatremia. These conditions are related to hyperglycemia and the resulting increased serum osmolarity and osmotic diuresis.

12. Hypotonic such as 0.45% NaCl. These solutions cause fluid to shift from the extracellular fluid into the intracellular fluid and the interstitial spaces. Hypotonic solutions decrease the intravascular volume.

13. False. IV fluids should be administered at the prescribed rate. Never play catch-up.

14. False. PPN is not nutritionally complete. The low dextrose content does not provide sufficient calories to increase body mass.

15. True. Because a patient's condition is neither stagnant nor totally predictable, imbalances can occur at any time. Identification of patients at risk, such as very young or older patients; patients with glucose intolerance; and patients with impaired renal function.

Notes

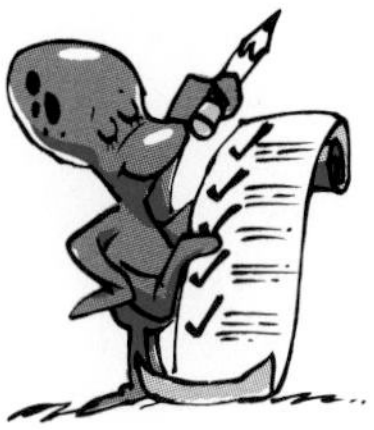

Notes

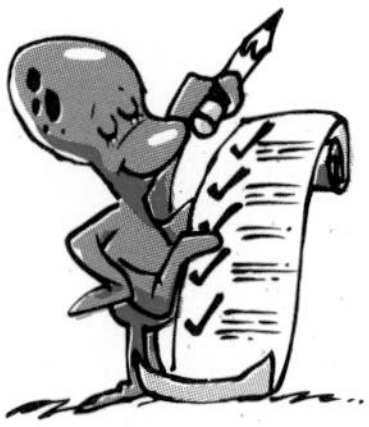

Index

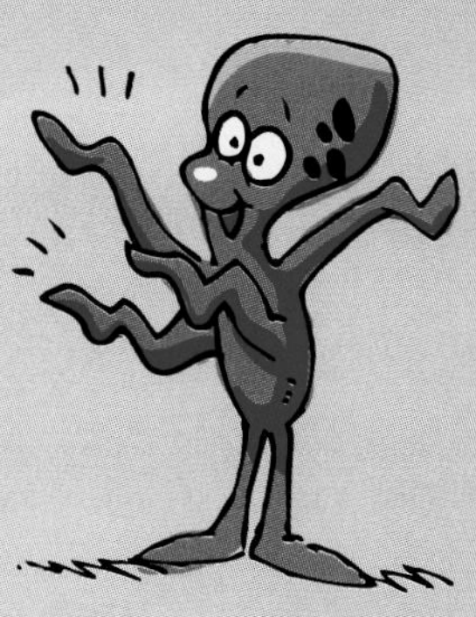

Page numbers followed by *t* indicate tables.